Biomechanics
of Musculoskeletal
INJURY

Biomechanics of Musculoskeletal INJURY

William C. Whiting, PhD
California State University, Northridge

Ronald F. Zernicke, PhD
University of Calgary

UNIVERSITY OF WOLVERHAMPTON
LIBRARY

Acc No. 2206042	CLASS 535
CONTROL 0873227794	617.
	470
DATE -4 MAY 2000 SITE WV	44. WHi

Human Kinetics

Library of Congress Cataloging-in-Publication Data

Whiting, William Charles.
 Biomechanics of musculoskeletal injury / William C. Whiting,
Ronald F. Zernicke.
  p. cm.
 Includes bibliographical references and index.
 ISBN 0-87322-779-4
  1. Musculoskeletal system--Wounds and injuries.
 2. Musculoskeletal system--Mechanical properties. I. Zernicke,
Ronald F. II. Title.
 RD680.W47 1998
 617.4'7044--dc21   97-41020
                   CIP

ISBN: 0-87322-779-4

Acquisitions Editor: Loarn Robertson; **Developmental Editor:** Kristine Enderle; **Assistant Editor:** Laura Hambly; **Copyeditor** Karen Bojda; **Proofreader:** Kathy Bennett; **Indexer:** Gerry Lynn Messner; **Graphic Designer:** Nancy Rasmus; **Graphic Artist:** Denise Lowry; **Photo Editor:** Boyd LaFoon; **Cover Designer:** Jack Davis; **Photographer (interior):** Tom Roberts (pp. 146, 151, 171, 172); **Mac Illustrator:** Craig Ronto; **Medical Illustrator:** Beth Young; **Line Artist:** Dianna Porter; **Printer:** Braun-Brumfield

Printed in the United States of America 10 9 8 7 6 5 4 3 2

Human Kinetics
Web site: http://www.humankinetics.com/

United States: Human Kinetics, P.O. Box 5076, Champaign, IL 61825-5076
1-800-747-4457
e-mail: humank@hkusa.com

Canada: Human Kinetics, 475 Devonshire Road, Unit 100, Windsor, ON N8Y 2L5
1-800-465-7301 (in Canada only)
e-mail: humank@hkcanada.com

Europe: Human Kinetics, P.O. Box IW14, Leeds LS16 6TR, United Kingdom
(44) 1132 781708
e-mail: humank@hkeurope.com

Australia: Human Kinetics, 57A Price Avenue, Lower Mitcham, South Australia 5062
(088) 277 1555
e-mail: humank@hkaustralia.com

New Zealand: Human Kinetics, P.O. Box 105-231, Auckland 1
(09) 523 3462
e-mail: humank@hknewz.com

To my mother Charlotte,
and in loving memory of my father Richard.
William C. Whiting

To Kathy, Kristin, and Eric.
Ronald F. Zernicke

Contents

Foreword

I am excited and pleased about this new volume, *Biomechanics of Musculoskeletal Injury*, because it is definitely not a standard description of biomechanical concepts and their relevance to applied topics. The authors, Bill Whiting and Ron Zernicke, have created an exciting story that goes far beyond a simple collection of topics related to injury. The book is a strong tool for comprehending injury mechanisms; it reflects the authors' excellent understanding of the function of the human body in general and of the different biological tissues in particular. The book is a result of extensive scientific work of the authors themselves, but it does not overemphasize their own contributions to the field. On the contrary, a great deal of material is incorporated from other sources and researchers of the highest international standard.

Production of this volume is both welcome and necessary. The first chapter, "Introduction to Injury," poses the question of why there was a need to write a specific biomechanics book on injury mechanisms. The reasons are presented in a very pragmatic and comprehensive way. The book challenges, not only the readers, but many scientific disciplines to explore injury mechanisms from different perspectives.

The importance and relevance of the material presented in this book can be seen, clearly, from the standpoint of public health policies. The authors state this very well in their conclusion to chapter 1: "Can we eliminate injury? The answer is no. Can we reduce the incidence and severity of injury? The answer is assuredly yes. Thus we embark on our exploration of the biomechanical aspects of injury, with the goals of increasing awareness of its importance to individuals and to society as a whole, and identifying ways in which biomechanics can contribute to the problem's solution."

The chapters after the "Introduction" follow a very basic format—from structure to function, and mechanisms are emphasized throughout. For example, chapter 2 "Biological Tissue: Classification, Structure, and Function" was written with the following question in mind: "How do the principles presented have relevance to injury mechanism or injury prevention?" This strategy is characteristic of all remaining chapters: "Biomechanical Concepts" (chapter 3), "Tissue Biomechanics and Adaptation" (chapter 4), "Mechanisms of Injury" (chapter 5), "Lower-Extremity Injuries" (chapter 6), "Upper-Extremity Injuries" (chapter 7), and "Head, Neck, and Trunk Injuries" (chapter 8).

Biomechanics of Musculoskeletal Injury is comprehensive and includes requisite details throughout the text. This is a scholarly production where considerable depth is necessary. Nevertheless, the material is easy to read and comprehend. Thus, the book will be accessible to readers with a basic background in anatomical, mechanical, and biological aspects of the human body. Because of the wide coverage of the basic mechanisms of musculoskeletal injuries, this book will likely become required reading for many students and researchers in biomechanics, orthopedics, physiotherapy, and rehabilitation.

Paavo V. Komi
Professor of Biomechanics
University of Jyväskylä
Jyväskylä, Finland

Preface

Ben Franklin, in a letter to a colleague, noted that ". . . in this world nothing is certain but death and taxes." We suggest adding a third inevitability from which there seems no escape: physical injury. Most injuries are a mere annoyance, some result in temporary disability, while the most dreaded are those few which cause permanent impairment or even death. Whatever the severity of the injury, however, most have a mechanically related etiology. The purpose of this book is to explore the mechanical bases of musculoskeletal injury in order to better understand the mechanisms involved in causing the injury, the effect of injury on musculoskeletal tissues, and ultimately, based on our current knowledge of biomechanics, how injury might be prevented.

Biomechanics of Musculoskeletal Injury was written primarily for undergraduate students in the fields of exercise science, kinesiology, human movement studies, physical education, biomechanics, physical therapy, and athletic training. Nonetheless, the book may serve as a supplemental reference for practitioners in the fields of orthopedics, rheumatology, physical medicine and rehabilitation, physical therapy, chiropractic medicine, ergonomics, and health and safety science.

In developing and teaching courses on the biomechanics of injury over the past 20 years, we have relied on a piecemeal collection of research and review articles, as well as book chapters, to provide our students with the requisite background to understand the broad spectrum of injury mechanics. Some good reference texts are available which address injury from a clinical perspective, but we have found none that contain the complete range of coverage that we provide here.

We begin in chapter 1 with an introduction to biomechanics as an interdiscipline and explore the mechanical aspects of injury, briefly assessing the prevalence of injury in our society and the physical, monetary, and emotional costs which result.

Chapter 2 establishes the structural foundation necessary to appreciate both the normal function of the human musculoskeletal system and how injury may affect this function. Included is a brief discussion of embryology and tissue development and how these processes play a role in determining the morphology and mechanical behavior of the mature human structure. We highlight the details of particular connective tissues (bone, cartilage, tendon, and ligament) which are most often involved in injuries of the musculoskeletal system. Chapter 2 concludes with an examination of arthrology, or joint mechanics; we emphasize this, because many of the most functionally disabling injuries afflict various joints.

Chapter 3 presents the basic biomechanical concepts essential for a greater understanding of injury mechanics. These mechanical parameters, such as force, stress and strain, stiffness, and elasticity, are examined in the context of connective tissue injuries. Although mathematics is inextricably intertwined with biomechanics, we have kept mathematical calculations to a minimum, emphasizing instead the concepts on which the mechanics of the phenomena are based.

Chapter 4 integrates the topics presented in earlier chapters and elucidates how connective tissues respond to mechanical loading, in both normal and abnormal environments, and how these tissues are tested experimentally to quantify their mechanical behavior. A multitude of factors affect the musculoskeletal system's responses when forces are applied to tissues. A collection of these factors, such as age, gender, nutrition, and exercise are discussed with emphasis on how an individual might, with an understanding of the responses involved, intervene to lessen the chance or severity of injury.

With a foundation in the scientific bases of tissue structure and function in place, we progress, in chapter 5, to the exploration of injury mechanisms. Beginning with a general discussion of injury concepts (such as acute versus chronic loading, and modes of tissue failure), we continue with a regionally based sample of common injuries, emphasizing for each the mechanical aspects of the injury. We begin with the lower extremity (chapter 6), looking in detail at injuries such as inversion ankle sprains, stress fractures, compartment syndromes, and meniscal tears. Subsequent chapters examine injuries of the upper extremity (chapter 7) (e.g., rotator cuff tears, impingement syndrome, epicondylar stress syndromes, carpal tunnel syndrome), and head, neck, and trunk (chapter 8) (e.g., concussion, intervertebral disc injury).

Understanding the mechanical responses of biological tissues and the associated injury mechanisms will assist our efforts in reducing the chances that we may fall victim to that third inevitability in life: physical injury.

Acknowledgments

A project of this scope involves the outstanding contributions of many more people than the two listed on the book's cover. We extend our grateful appreciation to these friends and colleagues. We thank Rainer Martens and the staff at Human Kinetics for sharing our belief in the importance of this project, in particular the initial encouragement of Rick Frey and Rick Washburn, and in recent months the devoted efforts of Kristine Enderle, Laura Hambly, and Loarn Robertson. We acknowledge the hundreds of professional colleagues and thousands of students who have shaped our philosophies, guided our progress, and provided inspiration for our professional work over the past two decades. Lastly, and most importantly, we thank our families for their support, patience, and love while we worked to complete this project. Without them, our work and lives would have little meaning.

Credits

Figure 1.1   From *The History of Orthopaedics* (Figs. 6 & 13, p. 9) by D. LeVay, 1990, Lancashire, England: Parthenon Publishing Group. Copyright 1990 by Parthenon Publishing Group. Reprinted by permission.

Figure 1.2   From *Andreas Vesalius of Brussels: 1514-1564.* (Plate 31) by C.D. O'Malley, 1964, Berkeley: University of California Press. Copyright 1964 by The Regents of the University of California. Reprinted by permission.

Figure 1.3   From *Leonardo Da Vinci's Elements of the Science of Man* (Fig 1.1, p. 10, & Fig. 10.7, p. 236) by K.D. Keele, 1983, New York: Academic Press. Copyright 1983 by Academic Press. Reprinted by permission.

Figure 1B.1   From *The History of Orthopaedics* (Fig. 18, p. 26) by D. LeVay, 1990, Lancashire, England: Parthenon Publishing Group. Copyright 1990 by Parthenon Publishing Group. Reprinted by permission.

Figure 2.1   From *Medical Embryology* (2nd ed.) (Fig. 3.3, p. 41) by J. Langman, 1969, Baltimore: Williams & Wilkins. Copyright 1969 by Williams & Wilkins. Reprinted by permission.

Figure 2.2   From *Medical Embryology* (2nd ed.) (Fig. 5.1, p. 55) by J. Langman, 1969, Baltimore: Williams & Wilkins. Copyright 1969 by Williams & Wilkins. Reprinted by permission.

Figure 2.3   From *Bloom and Fawcett: A Textbook of Histology* (12th ed.) (Fig. 2.1, p. 58) by D.W. Fawcett, 1994, New York: Chapman & Hall. Copyright 1994 by Chapman & Hall. Adapted by permission.

Figure 2.5   From *Medical Embryology* (2nd ed.) (Fig. 2.9, p. 132) by J. Langman, 1969, Baltimore: Williams & Wilkins. Copyright 1969 by Williams & Wilkins. Reprinted by permission.

Figure 2.6   From "Anterior angulation deformity of the radial head" by H. Ellman, 1975, *Journal of Bone and Joint Surgery, 57A,* (Fig. 1, p. 777). Copyright 1975 by the Journal of Bone and Joint Surgery, Inc. Reprinted by permission.

Figure 2.8a From *Bloom and Fawcett: A Textbook of Histology* (12th ed.) (Fig. 7.4, p. 185) by D.W. Fawcett, 1994, New York: Chapman & Hall. Copyright 1994 by Chapman & Hall. Reprinted by permission.

Figure 2.8b From *Basic Biomechanics of the Musculoskeletal System* (2nd ed.) (Fig. 2.3, p. 34) by M. Nordin & V.H. Frankel, 1989, Philadelphia: Lea & Febiger. Copyright 1989 by Lea & Febiger. Reprinted by permission.

Figure 2.10 From "Form and function of articular cartilage" (Fig. 18, p. 21) by H.M. Mankin, V.C. Mow, J.A. Buckwalter, J.P. Iannotti, & A. Ratcliffe, 1994. In: S.R. Simon (Ed.), *Orthopaedic Basic Science*, Park Ridge, IL: American Academy of Orthopaedic Surgeons. Copyright 1994 by American Academy of Orthopaedic Surgeons. Reprinted by permission.

Figure 2.12 From "Metabolic and circulatory limitations to $\dot{V}O_2$max at the whole animal level" (p. 319-331) by P.E. di Prampero, 1985. In: *The Journal of Experimental Biology*, 115, Cambridge: The Company of Biologists Ltd. Copyright 1985 by The Company of Biologists Ltd.

Figure 2.13 From *Molecular Biology of the Cell* (2nd ed.) (Fig. 11-4, p. 615) by B. Alberts, D. Bray, J. Lewis, M. Raff, K. Roberts, & J. Watson, 1989. New York: Garland Publishing. Copyright 1989 by Garland Publishing Inc. Reprinted by permission.

Figure 2.14 From *Molecular Biology of the Cell* (2nd ed.) (Fig. 11-16, p. 617) by B. Alberts, D. Bray, J. Lewis, M. Raff, K. Roberts, & J. Watson, 1989. New York: Garland Publishing. Copyright 1989 by Garland Publishing Inc. Reprinted by permission.

Figure 3.47a Reprinted from *Journal of Biomechanics*, 1, A. Viidik, "A rheological model for uncalcified parallel-fibered collagenous tissue," 9, Copyright 1968, with kind permission from Elsevier Science Ltd, The Boulevard, Langford Lane, Kidlington OX5 1GB, UK.

Figures 3B.2 and 3B.3 Photos courtesy of Insurance Institute for Highway Safety.

Figure 3B.4 Reprinted from *Journal of Biomechanics*, 24(6), T. Nambu, B. Gasser, E. Schneider, W. Bandi, & S.M. Perren, "Deformation of the distal femur: A contribution towards the pathogenesis of osteochondrosis dissecans in the knee joint," 426, Copyright 1991, with kind permission from Elsevier Science Ltd, The Boulevard, Langford Lane, Kidlington OX5 1GB, UK.

Figure 4.3 From "Form and function of bone" (Fig. 48, p. 167) by F.S. Kaplan, W.C. Hayes, T.M. Keaveny, A. Boskey, T.A. Einhorn, & J.P. Iannotti, 1994. In: S.R. Simon (Ed.), *Orthopaedic Basic Science*, Park Ridge, IL: American Academy of Orthopaedic Surgeons. Copyright 1994 by American Academy of Orthopaedic Surgeons. Adapted by permission.

Figure 4.4 From "Growth, physical activity, and bone mineral acquisition" (Fig. 8.2, p. 240) by D.A. Bailey, R.A. Faulkner, & H.A. McKay, 1996. In: *Exercise and Sport Sciences Reviews*, 24, Baltimore: Williams & Wilkins. Copyright 1996 by the American College of Sports Medicine. Reprinted by permission.

Figure 4.6 From "Joint loading-induced alterations in articular cartilage" (p. 82) by M. Tammi, K. Paukkonen, I. Kiviranta, J. Jurvelin, A.-M. Säämänen, & H.J. Helminen, 1987. In: H.J. Helminen, I. Kiviranta, M. Tammi, & A.-M. Säämänen. (Eds.), *Joint Loading*, Bristol: Wright. Adapted by permission.

Figure 4.7 From "Biomechanics of ligaments and tendons" (Fig. 12, p. 145) by D.L. Butler, E.S. Grood, F.R. Noyes, & R.F. Zernicke, 1978. In: *Exercise and Sport Sciences Reviews*, 6, Baltimore: Williams & Wilkins. Copyright 1978 by the American College of Sports Medicine. Reprinted by permission.

Figure 4.8 (a, b) From "Biomechanics of ligaments and tendons" (Figs. 10 & 11, p. 144) by D.L. Butler, E.S. Grood, F.R. Noyes, & R.F. Zernicke, 1978. In: *Exercise and Sport Sciences Reviews*, 6, Baltimore: Williams & Wilkins. Copyright 1978 by the American College of Sports Medicine. Reprinted by permission.

Figure 4.9 From "The biomechanical and morphological changes in the medial collateral ligament of the rabbit after immobilization and remobilization" by S.L.-Y. Woo, M.A. Gomez, T.J. Sites, P.O. Newton, C.A. Orlando, & W.H. Akeson, 1987, *Journal of Bone and Joint Surgery, 69A* (Fig. 11, p. 1210). Copyright 1987 by the Journal of Bone and Joint Surgery, Inc. Adapted by permission.

Figure 4.10   From "Site and mechanical conditions for failure of skeletal muscle in experimental strain injuries" by J.G. Tidball, G. Salem, & R.F. Zernicke, 1993, *Journal of Applied Physiology, 74* (Figs. 4 & 5, p. 1283). Copyright 1993 by the American Physiological Society. Reprinted by permission.

Figure 4.11   From "Site and mechanical conditions for failure of skeletal muscle in experimental strain injuries" by J.G. Tidball, G. Salem, & R.F. Zernicke, 1993, *Journal of Applied Physiology, 74* (Figs. 6 & 7, p. 1284). Copyright 1993 by the American Physiological Society. Reprinted by permission.

Figure 4.12   From "Site and mechanical conditions for failure of skeletal muscle in experimental strain injuries" by J.G. Tidball, G. Salem, & R.F. Zernicke, 1993, *Journal of Applied Physiology, 74* (Fig. 8, p. 1285). Copyright 1993 by the American Physiological Society. Reprinted by permission.

Figure 5.4   From "Myotendinous junction injury in relation to junction structure and molecular composition" (Fig. 12.3, p. 426) by J.G. Tidball, 1991. In: *Exercise and Sport Sciences Reviews,* Baltimore: Williams & Wilkins. Copyright 1991 by American College of Sports Medicine. Reprinted by permission.

Figure 5.5b   From "Tendon and ligament insertion. A light and electron microscopic study" by R.R. Cooper & S. Misol, 1970, *Journal of Bone and Joint Surgery, 52A* (Fig. 1-A, p. 3). Copyright 1970 by the Journal of Bone and Joint Surgery, Inc. Reprinted by permission.

Figure 5.6a   From "Shoulder injuries" (Fig. 8, p. 320) by M.J. Julin & M. Mathews, 1990. *The Team Physicians Handbook* (1st ed.), by Mellion, Philadelphia: Hanley and Belfus, Inc. Copyright 1990 by Hanley and Belfus. Reprinted by permission.

Figure 5.6b   From "Imaging of shoulder instability" by P.B. Gusmer & H.G. Potter, 1995, *Clinics in Sports Medicine, 14(4)* (Fig. 5, p. 780). Copyright 1995 by W.B. Saunders Company. Reprinted by permission.

Figure 5B.1a   From "Implant selection for total hip arthroplasty" (Fig. 6.20, p. 86) by W.T. Stillwell, 1987. In: *The Art of Total Hip Arthroplasty,* New York: Harcourt Brace Jovanovich. Copyright 1987 by Harcourt Brace Jovanovich Publishers. Reprinted by permission.

Figure 5B.1b   From "Implant selection for total hip arthroplasty" (Fig. 6.19, p. 86) by W.T. Stillwell, 1987. In: *The Art of Total Hip Arthroplasty,* New York: Harcourt Brace Jovanovich. Copyright 1987 by Harcourt Brace Jovanovich Publishers. Reprinted by permission.

Figure 6.8   From "Special concerns of the pediatric athlete" (Fig. 10.7, p. 139) by M.S. Moreland, 1994. In: *Sports Injuries: Mechanisms, Prevention, Treatment,* Philadelphia: Williams & Wilkins. Copyright 1994 by Williams & Wilkins. Reprinted by permission.

Figure 6.10   From "Myotendinous junction injury in relation to junction structure and molecular composition" (Fig. 12.2, p. 425) by J.G. Tidball, 1991. In: *Exercise and Sport Sciences Reviews,* Baltimore: Williams & Wilkins. Copyright 1991 by American College of Sports Medicine. Reprinted by permission.

Figure 6.13   From "Tibial meniscal dynamics using three-dimensional reconstruction of magnetic resonance images" by W.O. Thompson, F.L. Thaete, F.H. Fu, & S.F. Dye, 1991, *American Journal of Sports Medicine, 19(3)* (Fig. 7, p. 214). Copyright 1991 by American Orthopaedic Society for Sports Medicine. Adapted by permission.

Figure 6.20   From "Force ratios in the quadriceps tendon and ligamentum patellae" by H.H. Huberti, W.C. Hayes, J.L. Stone, & G.T. Shybut, 1984, *Journal of Orthopaedic Research, 2* (Fig. 3, p. 51). Copyright 1984 by Orthopaedic Research Society. Adapted by permission.

Figure 6.22 From "Patellofemoral contact pressures: The influence of q-angle and tendofemoral contact" by H.H. Huberti & W.C. Hayes, 1984, *Journal of Bone and Joint Surgery, 66A* (Fig. 2, p. 717). Copyright 1984 by the Journal of Bone and Joint Surgery, Inc. Adapted by permission.

Figure 6.25 From "Exertional compartment syndromes" (Fig. 14-9, p. 218) by S.J. Mubarak, 1981. In: *Compartment Syndromes and Volkmann's Contracture*, Philadelphia: W.B. Saunders. Copyright 1981 by W.B. Saunders Company. Reprinted by permission.

Figure 6.26 From "Tibial stress reaction in runners: Correlation of clinical symptoms and scintigraphy with a new magnetic resonance imaging grading system" by M. Fredericson, A.G. Bergman, K.L. Hoffman, & M.S. Dillingham, 1995, *American Journal of Sports Medicine, 23(4)* (Fig. 2, p. 472-481). Copyright 1995 by the American Orthopaedic Society for Sports Medicine. Reprinted by permission.

Figure 6.29b From "Subtalar joint: Morphology and functional anatomy" (Fig. 5.2, p. 34; Fig. 5.3, p. 35) by B.J. Sangeorzan, 1991. In: *Inman's Joints of the Ankle* (2nd ed.), by J.B. Stiehl, Baltimore: Williams & Wilkins. Copyright 1991 by Williams & Wilkins. Reprinted by permission.

Figure 6B.1 From "Human patellar-tendon rupture" by R.F. Zernicke, J. Garhammer, & F.W. Jobe, 1977, *Journal of Bone and Joint Surgery, 59A* (Fig. 1, p. 180; Fig. 3, p. 181). Copyright 1977 by the Journal of Bone and Joint Surgery, Inc. Adapted by permission.

Figure 6B.2 From "Biomechanical evaluation of bilateral tibial spiral fractures during skiing—a case study" (Fig. 1, p. 244) by R.F. Zernicke, 1981. In: *Medicine and Science in Sports and Exercise, 13(4)*, Baltimore: Williams & Wilkins. Copyright 1981 by the American College of Sports Medicine. Reprinted by permission.

Figure 7.9 From "Kinetics of baseball pitching with implications about injury mechanisms" by G.S. Fleisig, J.R. Andrews, C.J. Dillman, & R.F. Escamilla, 1995, *American Journal of Sports Medicine, 23(2)* (Figs. 4-6, p. 236, 238). Copyright 1995 by American Orthopaedic Society for Sports Medicine. Adapted by permission.

Figure 8.3 From "Head injury in motor vehicle crashes: Human factors, effects, and prevention" (Fig. 4-1, p. 58) by D.V. McGehee, 1996. In: *Head Injury and Postconcussive Syndrome*, New York: Churchill Livingstone. Copyright 1996 by W.B. Saunders Company. Adapted by permission.

Figure 8.6 From "Cerebral concussion and traumatic unconsciousness: Correlations and experimental and clinical observations" by A.K. Ommaya & T.A. Gennarelli, 1974, *Brain, 97,* (Fig. 1, p. 634). Copyright 1974 by permission of Oxford University Press.

Figure 8.8 From *Gunshot Wounds: Pathophysiology and Management* (2nd ed.) (Figs. 2-1 to 2-5, p. 8 and Figs. 2-11 to 2-12, p. 15) by K.G. Swan & R.C. Swan, 1989, St. Louis: Year Book Medical Publishers, Inc. Copyright 1989 by Year Book Medical Publishers, Inc. Adapted by permission.

Figure 8.10 Reprinted from *Journal of Biomechanics, 28,* A.K. Ommaya & T.A. Gennarelli, "Facial injury: A review of biomechanical studies and test procedures for facial injury assessment," 6, Copyright 1995, with kind permission from Elsevier Science Ltd, The Boulevard, Langford Lane, Kidlington OX5 1GB, UK.

Figure 8.17 From "The epidemiologic, pathologic, biomechanical, and cinematographic analysis of football-induced cervical spine trauma" by J.S. Torg, J.J. Vegso, M.J. O'Neill, & B. Sennett, 1990, *The American Journal of Sports 18(1),* (Fig. 2, p. 52; Fig. 3, p. 53). Copyright 1990 by the American Orthopaedic Society for Sports Medicine. Reprinted by permission.

Figure 8.20 Reprinted from *Pain, 58,* L. Barnsley, S. Lord, & N. Bogduk, "Whiplash injury," 284, Copyright 1994, with kind permission of Elsevier Science – NL, Sara Burgerhartstraat 25, 1055 KV Amsterdam, The Netherlands.

Figure 8.28   From "Biomechanics of the lumbar spine" (Fig. 10-13, p. 192) by M. Lindh, 1989. In: M. Nordin & V.H. Frankel (Eds.), *Basic Biomechanics of the Musculoskeletal System* (2nd ed.), Philadelphia: Lea & Febiger. Copyright 1989 by Lea & Febiger. Reprinted by permission.

Figure 8.30   From "Spondylolysis and spondylolisthesis in the athlete" (Fig. 3, p. 520) by J. T. Stinson, 1993. In: *Clinics in Sports Medicine, 12(3)*, Philadelphia: W.B. Saunders. Copyright 1993 by W.B. Saunders Company. Adapted by permission.

Figure 8.32   From "Towards a better understanding of low-back pain: A review of the mechanics of the lumbar disc" by A. Nachemson, 1975, *Rheumatology and Rehabilitation, 14(3)*, (Fig. 1, p. 131). Copyright 1975 by permission of Oxford University Press.

Figure 8B.1   From "Mechanism and dynamics of closed head injuries (preliminary report)" by K. Sano, N. Nakamura, K. Hirakawa, H. Masuzawa, K. Hashizume, & T. Hayashi, 1967, *Neurologia Medico-Chirurgica, 9* (Fig. 1, p. 22). Copyright 1967 by the Japan Neurosurgical Society. Adapted by permission.

Table 2.2   From "Anatomy, physiology, and mechanics of skeletal muscle" (Table 1, p. 100) by W.E. Garrett, Jr., & T.M. Best, 1994. In: S.R. Simon (Ed.), *Orthopaedic Basic Science*, Park Ridge, IL: American Academy of Orthopaedic Surgeons. Copyright 1994 by American Academy of Orthopaedic Surgeons. Adapted by permission.

Table 2.3   From *Kinesiology and Applied Anatomy* (Table 2.1, p. 24) by P.J. Rasch, 1989, Philadelphia: Lea & Febiger. Copyright 1989 by Lea & Febiger. Reprinted by permission.

Table 4.2   From *Musculoskeletal Conditions in the United States* (Table 2-2, p. 47) by A. Praemer, S. Furner, & D. Rice, 1992, Park Ridge, IL: American Academy of Orthopaedic Surgeons. Copyright 1992 by American Academy of Orthopaedic Surgeons. Adapted by permission.

Table 5.1   From "Soft tissue athletic injury" (Table 44.7, p. 761) by W.B. Leadbetter, 1994. In: F.H. Fu & D.A. Stone (Eds.), *Sports Injuries: Mechanisms, Prevention, Treatment* (p. 733-780), Baltimore: Williams & Wilkins. Copyright 1994 by Williams & Wilkins. Reprinted by permission.

Table 5.2   From "Head Injuries" (Table 47.3, p. 827) by D.W. Marion, 1994. In: F.H. Fu & D.A. Stone (Eds.), *Sports Injuries: Mechanisms, Prevention, Treatment* (p. 813-831), Baltimore: Williams & Wilkins. Copyright 1994 by Williams & Wilkins. Reprinted by permission.

Table 5.4   Adapted from "Soft tissue athletic injury" (Table 44.6, p. 761) by W.B. Leadbetter, 1994. In: F.H. Fu & D.A. Stone (Eds.), *Sports Injuries: Mechanisms, Prevention, Treatment* (p. 733-780), Baltimore: Williams & Wilkins. Copyright 1994 by Williams & Wilkins. Reprinted by permission.

Table 7.3   From "Arthroscopic debridement and decompression for selected rotator cuff tears. Clinical results, pathomechanics, and patient selection based on biomechanical parameters" by S.S. Burkhart, 1993, *Orthopedic Clinics of North America, 24(1)* (Table 3, p. 115). Copyright 1993 by W.B. Saunders Company. Adapted by permission.

Table 8.2   From "Assessment of coma and impaired consciousness. A practical scale" by G. Teasdale & B. Jennett, 1974, *Lancet, 2* (p. 81-83). Copyright 1974 by Lancet. Adapted by permission.

Table 8.3   From "Traumatic brain swelling and edema" (Table 14.1, p. 332) by J.D. Miller, 1993. In: P.R. Cooper (Ed.), *Head Injury* (3rd ed.), Baltimore: Williams & Wilkins. Copyright 1993 by Williams & Wilkins. Reprinted by permission.

Table 8.6   From "Evaluation and management of spondylolysis and spondylolisthesis" by C.B. Stillerman, J.H. Schneider, & J.P. Gruen, 1993, *Clinical Neurosurgery, 40* (Table 18.1, p. 385). Copyright 1993 by Williams & Wilkins. Reprinted by permission.

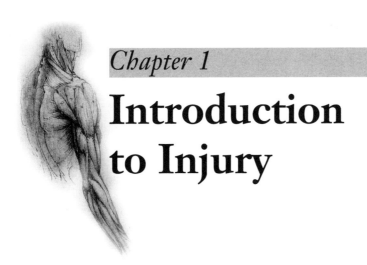

Chapter 1

Introduction to Injury

All injury leaves pain in the memory except the greatest injury,
that is death, which kills memory with life.
Leonardo da Vinci, 1452-1519

Injury is an unfortunate fact of everyday life. While some individuals sustain injuries of greater severity more frequently than others, no one is spared the pain, distraction, and incapacity caused by injury. Along with injury come the inevitable physical, emotional, and economic costs, as well as loss of time and normal function.

The impact of these costs and losses is staggering. More than eight million people in the United States can be expected to die from injuries. In 1996 the National Safety Council (U.S.) estimated that the annual cost of injury in the United States is nearly $435 billion and that about 40% of admissions to hospital emergency rooms or hospital clinics are for treatment of injury. The actual number of emergency room visits in the United States in 1993 represented by this proportion was estimated at more than 36 million (Stussman 1996).

Injury is justifiably considered one of the most serious public health problems in the developed countries. In the United States unintentional injury ranks immediately after heart disease, cancer, cerebrovascular disease (stroke), and chronic obstructive pulmonary disease as a leading cause of death. If homicides and suicides are added to the definition of injury, death due to injury vaults into third place, trailing only heart disease and cancer (National Safety Council 1996).

The impact of injury-related death is more significant than the impact of death from other causes when considered from the perspective of the potential life span remaining. Individuals fatally injured in 1985 had an average remaining life span of 36 years compared with the 12 and 16 years average remaining life span for those dying of cardiovascular disease and cancer, respectively (Rice et al. 1989). Estimates by the National Center for Health Statistics (1995) confirm these findings. Using years of potential life lost (YPLL) as a measure of impact, the NCHS identified unintentional injuries as the leading cause of death, outpacing both cancer and heart disease.

The foregoing injury fatality statistics paint only a portion of the picture of the impact of injury. Nonfatal accident statistics are even more astounding. Disabling injuries affect millions of individuals each year. National Safety Council estimates from the United States indicate that every 10 minutes, two people are killed and about 370 suffer a disabling injury, at a cost of $8.3 million. On average, there are 11 deaths from unintentional injury and about 2,200 disabling injuries every hour during the year. Despite successful efforts at injury reduction in some areas, such as automobile crashes, we should expect that a large proportion of us will be victims of injury.

A Definition of Injury

It will become clear in the following chapters that many injuries have a mechanical cause. Forces and force-related factors can lead to injury and may influence the severity of injury. Before delving into the multiple facets of injury, we start with a working definition of *injury:* Injury is the damage, caused by physical trauma, sustained by tissues of the body. This definition is narrower and less encompassing than generally accepted notions of injury, but it provides us with a working definition that is useful within the context of the biomechanics of musculoskeletal injury.

Biomechanics can be defined as the area of science that is interested in the application of mechanical principles to biological problems. A momentary reflection on this definition reveals that the number of potential areas of study in biomechanics is immense. Topics as diverse as blood-flow dynamics, human gait, prosthetic design, and biomaterials fall under the rubric of biomechanics. The mechanical causes and effects of forces applied to the human musculoskeletal system are the primary focal points of our text within the broader area of biomechanics.

As we explore injury biomechanics, a few key terms will recur, so let us define them at the outset.

What's in a Word: *Accident* or *Injury?*

Hear the word *accident* and most people envision an event which is unexpected, by chance, unintentional, or, as insurance companies like to say, an "act of God." The term *accident,* in the context of discussing injury, is an ambiguous and misleading descriptor. Accident implies a degree of human error or involvement, but that is not always the case. Accident is often used synonymously with injury in practical situations. This is unfortunate and inaccurate since not all accidents involve injuries and not all injuries are accidental in nature.

Suchman (1961) provided a list of indicators that increase the likelihood that an event is accidental. These indicators are the degree of expectedness, avoidability, and intention. If an event is unexpected, unavoidable, and unintentional, it likely is "accidental."

No single definition of *accident* will likely satisfy everyone. So what should be done? In some scientific circles the word *accident* is gradually being replaced with more specific terminology. What were formerly accidental injuries are now specified as being unintentional or intentional injuries. Car accidents are now commonly termed motor vehicle crashes. Some organizations, such as the National Safety Council, no longer officially include the word *accident* in their professional vocabularies, although other organizations (e.g., the Federal Highway Administration, the World Health Organization) still use *accident* in their official reporting.

Confusion will likely continue for some time as the following example suggests. The National Safety Council annually publishes a comprehensive and useful volume of safety statistics that documents the prevalence of injury and its costs. The foreword of the 1994 edition begins by noting that "many organizations, including the National Safety Council, have decided to eliminate the term 'accident' from their official vocabularies." And the title of this National Safety Council publication? *Accident Facts.*

The first, *mechanics*, is the branch of science that deals with the effects of forces and energy on bodies. Second, a *mechanism* is defined as the fundamental physical process responsible for a given action, reaction, or result. Chapters 6 through 8 will examine in detail the biomechanics of many musculoskeletal injuries.

Perspectives on Injury

A comprehensive consideration of musculoskeletal injury presents tremendous challenges, demanding a detailed examination of many areas of study. Exploration of the biomechanics of injury is an interdisciplinary endeavor. Among the disciplines involved are anatomy, physiology, mechanics, kinesiology, medicine, engineering, and psychology. The problem of musculoskeletal injuries cannot be addressed effectively by each discipline examining it in isolation. Rather, interdisciplinary approaches are required to ensure optimal progress in addressing the problem.

Individuals with an interest in the study of injury include physicians, occupational therapists, kinesiologists, prosthetists, orthotists, nurses, physical therapists, chiropractors, osteopaths, ergonomists, safety engineers, athletic trainers, coaches, and athletes. Each of these individuals has his or her own perspective on injury; injury can be viewed from many different general perspectives.

Historical Perspective

Musculoskeletal injuries have ancient origins. Evidence of lesions in vertebrate fossils and pathologies in dinosaur bones suggest that injury is as old as life itself. Skeletal remains of the earliest humans show evidence of arthritis and fractures, suggesting that at no time have we been exempt from the effects of injury. The nature of injuries can provide insight into the history of an era. Some ancient Egyptian skeletons, for example, show a fracture of the left ulna, perhaps a result of self-defense from a blow by a club. Today, these types of fractures are sometimes called nightstick fractures. Evidence of musculoskeletal disorders is commonly seen in the art of ancient civilizations, often in the statues and wall paintings of a given era (figure 1.1).

Attempts to treat the injured are nearly as old as injury itself. Archeologists have uncovered evidence of splints and primitive surgical implements

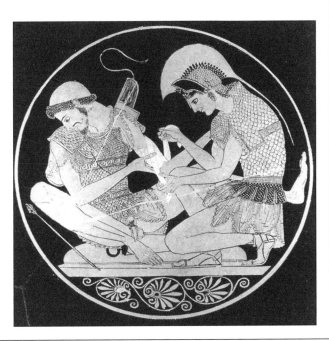
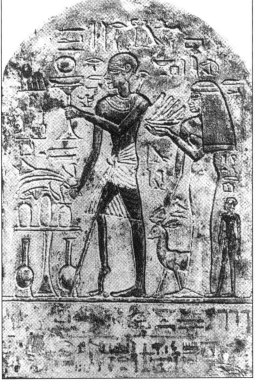

Figure 1.1   Historical artistic depictions of injury.
Reprinted from LeVay 1990.

Hippocrates and Injury

Hippocrates (460-377 B.C.), the "father of medicine," treated numerous injuries in his role as physician and described in detail many of the orthopedic conditions he encountered. Although some of his descriptions were flawed in light of our current understanding, he successfully treated injuries on a regular basis and related his techniques and results in documentary form. His descriptions of treating shoulder dislocations, for example, gave numerous artists the material to depict the procedures. Hippocrates, with biomechanical insight, noted that even an old dislocated shoulder could be reduced, "for what could not correct leverage move?" (LeVay 1990, 24).

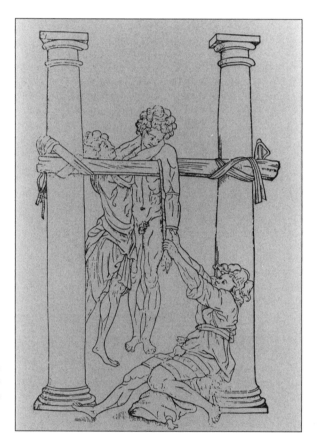

Figure 1B.1   Depiction of historical technique of reducing a shoulder dislocation using a large wooden beam.
Reprinted from LeVay 1990.

Among the many other injuries Hippocrates described were acromioclavicular dislocation ("I know many otherwise excellent practitioners who have done much damage in attempting to reduce shoulders of this kind"), spinal deformities (with vertebrae "drawn into a hump by diseases"), and leg fractures ("All bones unite more slowly if not placed in their natural position and immobilized in the same position, and the callus is weaker") (LeVay 1990, 26-37).

Hippocrates exhibited great insight in this summary observation:

All parts of the body which have a function, if used in moderation and exercised in labours to which each is accustomed, thereby become healthy and well-developed: but if unused and left idle, they become liable to disease, defective in growth, and age quickly. This is especially the case with joints and ligaments, if one does not use them (LeVay 1990, 30).

(obsidian knives). Surgical instruments such as forceps, scissors, and knives that were used by Indian surgeons about 1000 to 600 B.C. predate Hippocrates by several centuries.

The evolution of medical practice into a specialized profession with rational tenets of practice is generally acknowledged to have begun with Hippocrates. Though their knowledge of anatomy was scant and their procedures often crude by modern standards, Hippocrates and other Greek physicians established the foundations that are the basis for the study and treatment of injury today.

Besides the physicians of the day who studied and treated injury, some of history's great names, often heralded for other pursuits and accomplishments, noticed injury in some form and accorded it recognition in their work. The Greek poet Homer in his classic *Iliad* wrote often of both trauma and treatment, describing more than one hundred specific wounds and injuries.

With the decline of the Greek empire, much of the accumulated Greek knowledge shifted to Byzantium (Asia Minor), Alexandria, and then to Rome. Notable among practitioners of this era was Galen (A.D. 129-199). Galen's work is generally credited with defining, for better or worse, the direction of medical treatment for the next 1,500 years. Among his contributions were an appreciation for the nature of muscle contraction; a fundamental understanding of anatomy (though human dissection was still centuries away); the treatment of spinal deformities such as kyphosis, scoliosis, and lordosis; and the use of pressure bandages to control limb hemorrhage (LeVay 1990). Soon after Galen's death the Roman Empire declined, and with its abrupt fall in A.D. 476 western civilization entered the Dark Ages, and progress in medical science virtually ceased.

However, the entire world did not suffer the ravages of Europe's Dark Ages. In China during the Tang Dynasty (A.D. 619-901), for example, surgery (including orthopedic treatment of fractures and dislocations) was recognized as a special branch of medicine (LeVay 1990). Later, as Europe emerged from the Dark Ages, renewed creative energies were applied to medical problems of the time. Anatomical investigation flourished, most notably by Vesalius (1514-1564) whose anatomical drawings still inspire wonder today (figure 1.2). As knowledge of human anatomy advanced, so too did understanding of how the body functions.

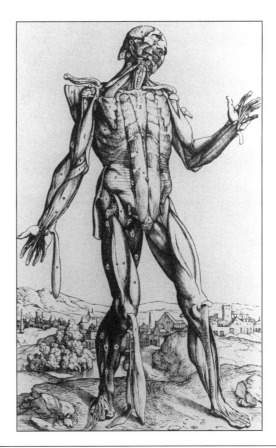

Figure 1.2   A "muscle man" from Vesalius's *Fabrica*. Reprinted from O'Malley 1964.

Leonardo da Vinci (1452-1519), perhaps the best-known figure of the Renaissance, was intrigued by the nature of pain and trauma. In his art we find exquisite depiction of painful expressions. In his scientific writing we also find many references to trauma, especially that caused by what he termed percussion (impact). From his deep interest in human anatomy, da Vinci was well aware that the joints in the body serve as shock absorbers. Noticing that the pain produced by landing from a jump on the heels is much greater than when landing on the toes, he deduced that "that which gives more resistance to a blow suffers most damage." Da Vinci had an abiding fascination with the body's senses, and in particular with the sense of pain (figure 1.3). Though he knew that pain served an important protective function, he also saw it as the "chief evil" in life, concluding that "the best thing is the wisdom of the soul; the worst thing is pain of the body" (Keele 1983). The insights of da Vinci and other great thinkers of the Renaissance era may seem elementary, even naive, in comparison to current levels of understanding, but compared to the knowledge that

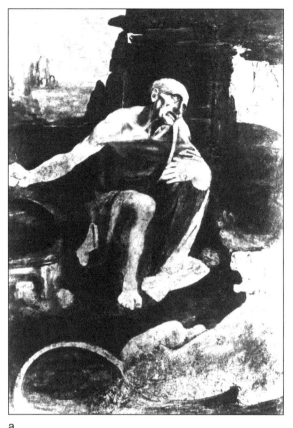
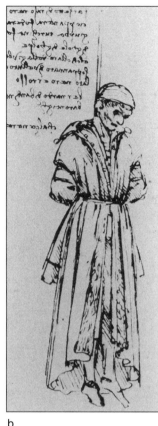

a   b

Figure 1.3   Leonardo da Vinci's visions of pain and trauma. (*a*) St. Jerome, a picture of pain. (*b*) The hanging of Bernado di Bandino Baroncelli.

Reprinted from Keele 1983.

had been available and accepted for many centuries, their breakthroughs were extraordinary.

With the advent of the Industrial Revolution in the 19th century, medical progress accelerated. Many of the problems that had previously been impossible to address were suddenly tractable. Admittedly, the industrial age created many new problems, notably injuries caused by machinery, but at the same time it brought a welcomed prospect for rapid developments in medicine. With the discovery of anesthesia and antiseptics, surgical success improved dramatically. Advances such as clinical arthroscopy, pioneered by Bircher in the early 1900s, showed early on the promise of rapidly developing technologies.

Progress continues today, and advancements in the diagnosis and treatment of injury show no sign of slowing. Just decades ago the suggestion of the practicality of joint replacement, laser surgery, advanced imaging techniques (e.g., magnetic resonance imaging), microsurgery, and computer- or robot-assisted surgery were dismissed as futuristic speculation. Continuing advancements in materials

science, computer technology, nanotechnology, robotics, and genetic engineering promise even more spectacular advances in the future. While technological progress extends great promise, we must not forget that it can be a two-edged sword. The technological saber swung in one direction has the potential to prevent or aid in the diagnosis and treatment of injury, but wielded in the opposite direction, it has potential for creating or exacerbating injury as well. As long as injury remains an unfortunate fact of everyday life, the challenges will undoubtedly change but not likely disappear.

Epidemiological Perspective

Questions about injuries such as How many? How often? What kind? and To whom? are endemic to epidemiology. *Epidemiology* is the study of the incidence, distribution, and control of disease and injury in a given population. In most cases the distinction between disease (e.g., measles) and injury (e.g., torn ligament) is clear. In other cases the picture is less clear, and deciding whether a malady is a disease or an injury may not be obvious. In our text we focus on musculoskeletal injuries, but you should keep in mind that diseases may enter the picture and that certain diseases can predispose an individual to injury (e.g., osteoporosis can lead to bone fractures).

Epidemiological studies are typically of two kinds: descriptive and analytical. The first of these, *descriptive epidemiology*, describes the frequency and distribution of a particular injury in a given population. This may appear at first glance to be a straightforward task, and in many cases it is. On the other hand, identification and classification of a particular injury can be a thorny problem either because the clinical manifestations are similar while the underlying pathology differs, or because there may be multiple injuries resulting from a single incident, which makes classification difficult. Descriptive studies rely on categorizing incidents according to the severity of the injury, the location where the injury took place (e.g., in a factory), the type of disability, the subset of a population affected, and the type of activity. Care must be taken in classifying injuries so that the resulting categories are mutually exclusive (Is an injury suffered in a truck crash a vehicular injury or a work-related injury?), exhaustive (Is there a category for every injury?), and useful (Does the classification system have practical and meaningful application?).

The second approach, *analytical epidemiology*, goes beyond description and attempts to pinpoint the causal relations involved in injury. Investigators must exercise care in assigning causal relations to injury by ruling out the possibility of either coincidence or mere correlation. Analytical studies typically are more difficult and time consuming than descriptive ones, and thus the latter predominate.

As in any discipline, terminology is essential for a productive discussion of the biomechanics of musculoskeletal injury. With respect to the epidemiology of injury, we briefly highlight a few central terms, including incidence, prevalence, risk factor, injury rate, and relative risk. Many people use the terms *incidence* and *prevalence* interchangeably, assuming that these terms are synonymous and give a sense of how many injuries are happening. In fact, incidence and prevalence are distinctly different terms and, when analyzing injuries, provide very different estimates. Injury *incidence* is defined as the number of new injuries in a fixed time period divided by the number of people at risk (Steiner, Norman, & Blum 1989). In contrast, injury *prevalence* is the number of people with an injury divided by the number of people at risk.

A *risk factor* is something that contributes to increasing the probability of an injury. Examples of injury risk factors include occupation, activity pattern, age, sex, history of previous injuries, recreational pursuits, and environmental conditions. Another widely used epidemiological term is *injury rate*, which is the number of injuries in a population divided by a reference measure. A reference measure can be the number of people in a population being studied, the number of hours of exposure, the number of miles run or innings played, or some other reference of interest. Examples of injury rates would include estimates such as metatarsal stress fractures per 1,000 runners or severe concussions per 100,000 hours of football participation.

The term *relative risk* can be used as a measure of the likelihood of an injury happening in one group versus another group. Relative risk is calculated as the injury incidence in group A divided by the injury incidence in group B. You could calculate the relative risk of shinsplints, for example, if you knew the respective incidence data of shinsplints in a group of female long-distance runners versus a group of age-matched sedentary females.

As with any statistical measure, care must be exercised to ensure that injury rates are calculated from data that are reliable and that conclusions based on rates are valid. We caution that care and clear thinking are warranted before using or accepting any statistical measures, including those for rates of injury.

Many organizations, including the National Safety Council, insurance companies, law enforcement agencies, the Occupational Safety and Health Administration (OSHA), and traffic safety boards, routinely collect and publish accident and injury data. For two primary reasons, much of the available injury data are for injury-related deaths. First, the catastrophic nature of fatalities makes them prominent, and second, death statistics are generally easy to compile. Less attention is paid to the documentation of nonfatal injuries, especially those of a minor nature that may never be reported at all. This raises the question, What percentage of all injuries is actually reported? The answer to that question is unknown. Certainly many injuries are never officially recorded, and therefore the published statistics must be considered underestimates of the true injury toll.

In the United States the 1995 unintentional-injury deaths totaled an estimated 90,000 (National

Safety Council 1996). The rate of unintentional-injury deaths in the United States is 37.0 per 100,000 population. Worldwide, the rates vary greatly from 10.7 in São Tomé e Príncipe, an island nation off the west coast of Africa, to 83.1 in Hungary. Variation in rates around the world is attributed to the influence of many economic, social, and cultural factors. For 61 nations reporting statistics to the World Health Organization over the years 1986 to 1992, annual deaths due to unintentional injury exceeded 500,000. Because the most populous countries of China, India, and Russia were not included, this number no doubt grossly underestimates the actual total (National Safety Council 1994).

Deaths due to injury are proportionately higher in the young. Overall, injury is the leading cause of death among individuals aged 1 to 44. In 1995 accidental injury was the number 2 cause of death in young adults (ages 25-44), according to U.S. Centers for Disease Control and Prevention (CDCP). Injury had been first, but in 1995 AIDS surpassed accidents as the top killer of young adults. In children, however, injury is still the leading cause of death.

Statistics for nonfatal injuries are just as daunting. In the United States in 1993, for example, the National Safety Council (1994) estimated that more than 18 million disabling injuries occurred. Virtually all nonfatal injury statistics are approximations based on hospital or commission records or extrapolations from interview surveys. Regarding the biomechanics of musculoskeletal injury, we find that much of the epidemiological information cannot be used easily because it is described according to circumstances (e.g., injury due to automobile collision) rather than by the specific causal agent or mechanism.

Health Professionals' Perspective

A health professional can be involved at any point in injury prevention or treatment. Many professionals are involved in preventive strategies to try to reduce the incidence and severity of injuries. At the organizational level, groups such as the National Safety Council, the Centers for Disease Control and Prevention, and the Consumer Product Safety Commission perform injury prevention analyses. At the individual level, safety engineers, ergonomists, safety consultants, job supervisors, parents, teachers, coaches, and many others are in positions to stress the tenets of safety and injury prevention.

Severe injuries often require immediate medical attention. Emergency medical personnel, such as paramedics, emergency room physicians, and support staff, provide this often life-saving emergency diagnosis and treatment. Less-severe injuries may require non-emergency treatment. Physicians, athletic trainers, and other allied health professionals perform these less-urgent diagnostic and treatment tasks. Many injuries, especially those requiring surgical treatment, require rehabilitation to ensure a return to preinjury performance levels. Rehabilitation personnel (e.g., physical therapists, occupational therapists) perform these essential services.

Economic Perspective

In addition to the physical and emotional costs associated with injury, the financial costs of injury are enormous. Since public policy decisions are often based on fiscal considerations, the economic perspective of injury requires comment.

In comparison to long-recognized public health hazards such as cardiovascular disease and cancer, only in the last two decades has injury been recognized as a true public health hazard. The publication of *Injury in America* (Committee on Trauma Research 1985) helped bring injury into the public health spotlight and prompted the U.S. Congress to commission a study on the economic and non-economic impact of injury. Results of that study showed that injury has a tremendous effect on both individuals and society as a whole (Rice et al. 1989). By including direct costs (medical and nonmedical), morbidity costs (value of goods and services not produced because of the injury), and mortality costs (the present value of remaining lifetime earnings adjusted for the person's life expectancy at the time of death), the estimated annual cost of injury is estimated at nearly $200 billion (Runge 1993). To further emphasize the magnitude of the problem in the United States alone, consider the following facts (Max, Rice, & MacKenzie 1990):

- Each year at least two million individuals are hospitalized as a result of an injury.
- Injuries account for 10% of hospital discharges and 16% of hospital days.
- Injuries sustained by those aged 15 to 44 result in 3.7 million years of life lost due to premature death and another 2.7 million years of lost productivity due to either temporary or permanent disability.

- For every person hospitalized for an injury, nearly 25 people sustain injuries that, while not necessitating hospitalization, require medical attention.

The National Safety Council (1996) estimated the total cost of unintentional injuries for 1995 at more than $430 billion. This total included estimates of economic costs of fatal and nonfatal unintentional injuries together with employer costs, vehicle damage costs, fire losses, wage and productivity losses, medical expenses, and administrative expenses. If to that $430 billion you add the more than $776 billion estimated cost for lost quality of life from those injuries, the resulting comprehensive cost of injury for 1995 alone was greater than $1.2 trillion.

In summarizing his discussion on the cost of injury, Runge (1993) issues a challenge to physicians to become more involved as advocates for injury prevention and control, thereby contributing to efforts at limiting the present cost of injury. This advice to physicians should be heeded by everyone, since we all pay the price that injury exacts.

Psychological Perspective

The most obvious consequence of injury is the direct, physical damage to bodily tissues. Often overlooked are the psychological factors that may be involved before, during, and after the actual injury. These factors can influence the likelihood and severity of injury and the course of healing and rehabilitation. Aspects of injury in which psychological factors may be integrally involved include risk behaviors and predisposition to injury, human error and accidents, theories of causation, risk evaluation, and emotional response to injury.

A person's likelihood of being injured depends largely on the particular task in which he or she is engaged, the environment in which the injury occurs, and the person's psychological state. Some activities such as playing football or occupations such as oil drilling are inherently riskier than others. Certain environments, such as rugged outdoor terrain or construction sites, are more risk laden than others. In addition, certain psychological states, such as inattention, distraction, fatigue, or stress, may predispose one to injury. Regarding stress, Andersen and Williams (1988) proposed a theory of stress responsivity that suggests a strong relation between the likelihood of injury and stress factors such as stress history, personality factors, and coping resources.

Key points from a discussion of the role of human error, accident causation, and risk evaluation in injury prevention and control by Sanders and McCormick (1993) highlight the importance of including psychological factors in the overall context of injury analysis:

- Human error (defined as an inappropriate or undesirable human decision or behavior that reduces, or has the potential for reducing, effectiveness, safety, or system performance) is responsible for most, if not all, events leading to injury. Human error leading to injury most often occurs from the direct action of the injured person, but also may be an indirect human error, such as a poor decision made by an engineer in designing a particular product or device.

- Human error may be reduced by (1) selecting people with appropriate skills and capabilities to perform a particular task, (2) proper training, and (3) effective design of equipment, procedures, and environments.

- Various theories have been proposed to explain accident causation, including accident-proneness theory (some people are more prone to accidents than others), accident-liability theory (people are prone to accidents in given situations and this proneness is not permanent), capability-demand theory (accidents increase when job demands exceed the capability of workers), adjustment-to-stress theory (accidents increase in situations with stress levels that exceed the individual's coping capabilities), arousal-alertness theory (accidents are more likely when arousal is too low or too high), and goals-freedom-alertness theory (freedom of workers to set their own goals results in high-quality performance, which reduces accidents). No single theory adequately explains all accidents and their resulting injuries; a more likely scenario is that a unique combination of factors is involved in each injury.

- Many factors contribute to accidents and injuries. Sanders and Shaw (1988) proposed a comprehensive model, termed *contributing factors in accident causation* (CFAC), that provides a framework for categorizing the many contributing factors. Categories of factors included in the model are management, physical environment, equipment design, the work itself, social and psychological environment, and workers and co-workers.

- *Risk* refers to the likelihood of injury or death associated with a particular object, task, or environment. The perception and evaluation of risk are important for determining whether an injury will occur and, if it does, the severity of the injury. Interestingly, studies indicate that while most people are quite capable of discerning the relative risk between various products (e.g., using a typewriter is less risky than riding a bicycle), their ability to estimate the absolute risk is not nearly as keen. Perception of risk may be distorted by overestimating the value of one's own expertise and experience, overemphasizing situations receiving media attention, and adopting a philosophy of "it can't happen to me."

Psychological factors are important influences before, during, and immediately following the injury and in the postinjury period, which may last for weeks, months, or even years. While the psychological factors summarized by Heil (1993) are specific to athletes, many of the factors are applicable to general injury situations as well (table 1.1). Other factors that could be added to the list include family support structures, need to work, and malingering, and there is little doubt that psychological considerations play an influential role in a comprehensive assessment of injury.

Many injuries, and certainly those that draw the most media attention, occur among athletes. The psychological profiles of highly competitive, elite athletes are in some ways different from those of the general population. The differences can be both beneficial and deleterious in dealing with the injury and the recovery process. As noted by Heil (1993), the positive psychological attributes found in many athletes are high levels of motivation, pain tolerance, goal orientation, and good physical training habits. On the negative side, athletes may experience a higher sense of loss, greater threat to their self-image, unrealistic expectations and desire for a quick recovery, and they may have higher, sport-specific demands to meet. Whether in specific populations, such as athletes, or in the general public, psychological factors play a critical role in injury and should be neither underestimated nor ignored.

Safety Professionals' Perspective

The prevention and control of injuries, while not the primary focus of this text, are nonetheless integral to a broad discussion of injury, and we would be remiss not to mention the role of safety professionals, such as safety consultants, ergonomists, safety engineers, and health and safety educators, in dealing with injury.

Injury prevention programs are typically of two types: injury control programs and health and safety education programs. One commonly referenced injury control program lists strategies that include prevention of hazard creation; modification of the hazard's rate of release from its source; protection from the hazard source; and stabilization, repair, and rehabilitation of the damaged object (Haddon & Baker 1981). The second approach seeks to reduce the incidence and severity of injury through health and safety education.

Table 1.1   Psychological Factors in Injury

Factors preceding injury	Factors associated with injury	Factors following injury
Medical history	Emotional distress	Culpability
Psychological history	Injury site	Compliance with treatment
Somatization	Pain	Perceived effectiveness
Life stress and change	Timeliness	Treatment complications
Sport stress and change	Unexpectedness	Pain
Approach of major competition		Medication use
Marginal player status		Psychological status
Overtraining		Social support
Sport-related health risk factors		Personality conflicts
		Fans and the media
		Litigation

WARNING: Hazardous to Your Health

Warning signs, it seems, are everywhere. Their purpose is to inform users of a product or people in a certain environment of the potential dangers of improper use. For any warning to be effective, it must be designed (e.g., with bright colors or flashing lights) to ensure that the person at risk senses the warning, receives the message of the warning (sensing a warning does not ensure that it will be read), and understands the warning (e.g., keep the message short, simple, and unambiguous). At a minimum, an effective warning should include the following four elements (Sanders & McCormick 1993):

- Signal word: to convey the level of risk (e.g., "danger," "caution")
- Hazard: the nature of the hazard
- Consequences: what will likely happen if the warning is not heeded
- Instructions: appropriate behavior to reduce or eliminate the hazard

Effective warnings can go a long way toward reducing the incidence of injury and death in both work and recreational situations.

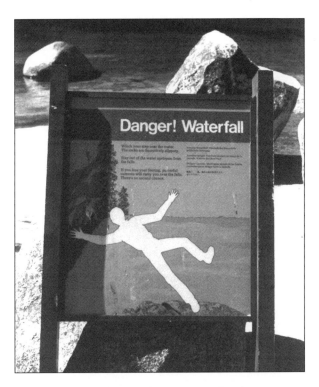

Figure 1B.2   Sign warning of potential dangers near the top of Nevada Falls in Yosemite National Park.

Neither of these approaches has been wholly successful in achieving injury prevention. This lack of success is likely due to many complex political, economic, sociological, or behavioral influences on injury prevention and control. Recent efforts to improve safety have concentrated on providing frameworks that combine elements of injury control and health education programs. For example,

Gielen (1992) notes that a comprehensive injury control program must be both effective and feasible and proposes a four-step program that includes epidemiological diagnosis, environmental and behavioral diagnosis, influencing factors diagnosis, and formulation of an intervention plan.

In any injury prevention program, at least three basic strategies are available to control or prevent injuries (Committee on Trauma Research 1985): (1) persuade (educate) those at risk of injury to alter their behavior for increased self-protection (e.g., to use helmets while cycling or to use seat belts while driving cars or flying in planes), (2) require changes in individual behavior by law or rules (e.g., enforce laws for mandatory seat belt use in cars, penalize football players who spear-tackle an opponent with the top of the helmet, require protective eyewear while playing squash), and (3) provide automatic protection by product or environmental design (e.g., air bag passive restraints in cars, multidirectional release mechanisms for ski bindings, padding for fixed goalposts, enhanced rearfoot stabilizers with shock-absorbing heel materials for running shoes).

Of these three injury prevention strategies, the third (automatic protection) is the most effective, followed by the second strategy (requiring behavioral change). Persuading is the least effective of the three. Although education about injuries is important, many injuries result less from a lack of knowledge than from failure to apply what is known. Most people will acknowledge that it is safer to wear a mask as a baseball catcher or hockey goalie, but sometimes a mask is not available or the player chooses not to wear one. Health behavior research has shown that as the amount of individual effort required to adopt a safer behavior increases, the proportion of the population that will respond by adopting the behavior decreases. For example, the more difficult or cumbersome the protective equipment is to put on, the less likely players are to use it.

The Committee on Trauma Research (1985) observed that education alone has rarely proved to be an adequate preventive strategy. The most successful attempts at changing individual behavior to prevent injuries have been when the behavior was easily observable and required by law. For example, when laws required helmet use for motorcyclists, almost all complied. But in the absence of helmet laws, only about half of motorcyclists wore a helmet (Watson, Zador, & Wilks 1980).

Interestingly, more than a decade ago the Committee on Trauma Research for the U.S. National Academy of Science (1985) reported that injury prevention for most types of recreation remains nearly unresearched. That statement is fundamentally accurate even today. More information is needed to assess the effectiveness and use of protective sports equipment and modifications, such as en-

ergy-absorbing gymnastics mats, playground surfaces, running surfaces, or gymnasium walls.

An additional fourth strategy for preventing musculoskeletal injury that should be mentioned is maintenance of flexibility and physical condition. Whether in the home, in the workplace, or in sports, individuals with better physical conditioning and flexibility are less likely to be injured and are more likely to recover faster after being injured. Indeed, one of the most important benefits of regular stretching and flexibility training may be the prevention of musculoskeletal injury. Proper flexibility training and pre-exercise stretching can reduce joint stiffness, muscle and tendon tightness, and exercise-related muscle soreness. For example, the probability of re-injuring calf muscles could be reduced to less than 1% as a result of stretching exercises (Miller 1979). On the other hand, tightness, or lack of flexibility, tends to increase the likelihood of musculoskeletal injuries.

Considering the enormous numbers and types of injuries that occur, many challenges remain for safety professionals worldwide. The obstacles cross educational, legal, scientific, political, and economic disciplines, suggesting that the most effective solutions will likely be interdisciplinary in scope.

Scientific Perspective

Among all the perspectives on injury, the one that predominates in the following chapters is a scientific perspective. As stated earlier, many different scientific disciplines have a role to play in a comprehensive understanding of injury. Anatomists, for example, study which structures and tissues are actually injured, physiologists examine the biological processes involved in tissue repair, psychologists are interested in the behavioral aspects of injury, and engineers design equipment and structures to prevent and minimize injury.

Of all the scientific disciplines, physics and its subdiscipline of mechanics are arguably most central to the study of injury. The common denominator of this area of science is energy. Indeed, energy is called the agent of injury. While thermal, electrical, magnetic, and chemical energy can cause injuries, most injuries involve mechanical energy. The fundamental relation between mechanical energy and injury highlights biomechanics as the logical discipline to study the causes and effects of human musculoskeletal injury.

In *Injury in America*, the Committee on Trauma

Research (1985) reinforced the important role of biomechanics research in the prevention of injury by arriving at the following conclusions:

- High priority should be given to research that can provide a clearer understanding of injury mechanisms.

- Quantification of the injury-related responses of critical body areas (such as the nervous system, thoracic and abdominal viscera, joints, and muscles) to mechanical forces is needed.

- High priority should be given to defining limits of human tolerance to injury, particularly with regard to segments of the population for which data are extremely limited, including children, women, and the elderly.

- Improvement in injury assessment technology is needed, including the development of methods for assessing important debilitating injuries and causes of fatality, improvement of anthropomorphic dummies, and development of computer models to predict injury in complex crash conditions.

- Organizations need to be developed to administer research on injury mechanisms and injury biomechanics, and ensure a supply of scientists trained in injury biomechanics.

Concluding Comments

Statistics show that injury is a public health problem that deserves our full attention, that it should be given greater priority, and that combined approaches to preventing and controlling injury are justified. Injury is a multifaceted problem, requiring a multidisciplinary approach to find and implement effective solutions.

Can we eliminate injury? The answer is no. Can we reduce the incidence and severity of injury? The answer is assuredly yes. Thus we embark on our exploration of the biomechanical aspects of injury, with the goals of increasing awareness of its importance to individuals and to society as a whole, and identifying ways in which biomechanics can contribute to the problem's solution.

In the next chapter we examine the fundamental structure and function of musculoskeletal tissues such as bone, cartilage, tendon, ligament, and muscle. Chapter 3 introduces and explains basic biomechanical terms and concepts that will be useful for better understanding injury. Building on that funda-

mental information, we then examine in chapter 4 how load-bearing tissues of the human body respond when forces are applied and how these tissues adapt to environmental and self-imposed forces.

We continue in the final four chapters with an exploration of mechanisms of musculoskeletal injury. We present the general concepts of injury mechanisms (chapter 5), followed by examples of injuries to the lower extremities (chapter 6), upper extremities (chapter 7), and finally to the head, neck, and trunk (chapter 8).

Condensing this information into a single text was an ambitious task, but we were convinced that armed with this basic knowledge, you will be able to better understand the processes involved in musculoskeletal injuries.

Suggested Readings

Baker, S.P., O'Neill, B., Ginsburg, M.J., & Li, G. (1992). *The Injury Fact Book*. New York: Oxford University Press.

Haddon, W., Jr., Suchman, E.A., & Klein, D. (1964). *Accident Research: Methods and Approaches*. New York: Harper & Row.

Nahum, A.M., & Melvin, J. (Eds.). (1985). *The Biomechanics of Trauma*. Norwalk, CT: Appleton-Century-Crofts.

Nahum, A.M., & Melvin, J.W. (Eds.). (1993). *Accidental Injury: Biomechanics and Prevention*. New York: Springer-Verlag.

Praemer, A., Furner, S., & Rice, D.P. (1992). *Musculoskeletal Conditions in the United States*. Park Ridge, IL: American Academy of Orthopaedic Surgeons.

Robertson, L.R. (1983). *Injuries: Causes, Control Strategies and Public Policy*. Lexington, MA: Lexington Books.

U.S. Centers for Disease Control and Prevention. (1993). Years of potential life lost before age 65— United States, 1990 and 1991. *Morbidity and Mortality Weekly Report, 42*(13).

U.S. Department of Health and Human Services. (1989). *Promoting Health/Preventing Disease, Year 2000 Objective for the Nation*. Government Printing Office, Washington, D.C.

U.S. Department of Health and Human Services. (1992). *Injury Control: Position Papers from the 3rd National Injury Control Conference*. April 22-25, 1991, Denver, CO.

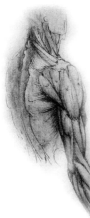

Chapter 2

Biological Tissue: Classification, Structure, and Function

The conformation of the organism, [and its] equilibrium is explained
by the interactions or balance of forces.
D'Arcy Thompson, 1917

Understanding the basic organization of tissues of the body is essential for an appreciation of normal musculoskeletal system function and of injury sequelae. As threads are woven together to form a fabric (such as a blanket), so too are cells, fibers, and other matrix components to form tissues. A tissue is an aggregation of cells and intercellular substance that together perform a specialized function.

Each tissue in the body has a specialized function and a distinctive organization. To better understand how tissues are organized and how they function, it is useful to review where they come from and how they were differentiated and formed developmentally. The following brief review of tissue embryology highlights commonalities in tissue organization and lays the groundwork for later discussions of the role of cells (e.g., mesenchymal stem cells) in the repair and healing processes of tissues of the musculoskeletal system.

Embryology: Development of the Musculoskeletal System

The following descriptions are arranged in a developmental, chronological order. The embryo stage of human development comprises the time from fertilization to week 8, and the fetal stage denotes the time from week 9 until birth. We have emphasized the development of the musculoskeletal system.

Fertilization of the egg (or oocyte) by the spermatozoa produces the zygote. By day 5 after fertilization the zygote, now referred to as the embryo, consists of a mass of about 30 to 50 cells arranged in a hollow ball shape called a blastocyst. By day 8 the blastocyst is partially implanted in the uterine wall, and by day 10 two cavities have developed within the cell mass. The primitive amniotic cavity (sac) is associated with a layer of cells called the *ectoderm* while the second cavity, the primitive yolk sac, is associated with a layer of cells called the *endoderm.* The embryo proper is the region where the endoderm and ectoderm are in contact.

The contiguous layers of cells form the bilaminar embryonic disk, which is the fundamental cellular mass that develops into the fetus. Figure 2.1 shows this stage of development and these structures of the embryo.

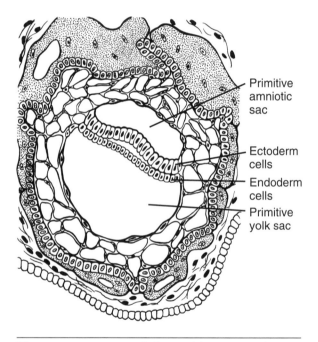

Figure 2.1   Drawing of a human blastocyst at about 12 days. The bilaminar germ cell layers are evident, as well as the primitive amniotic sac (associated with the ectoderm) and the primitive yolk sac (associated with the endoderm).

Reprinted from Langman 1969.

The first vestiges of the primitive spinal cord (notochord) are apparent by day 16 of embryonic development. Further specialization and differentiation of cells in the embryo occurs during the third week of development. At this time a third layer of cells, called the *intraembryonic mesodermal layer,* is produced. The developing mesodermal cells in-

vaginate and spread between the endodermal and ectodermal layers.

By day 20 there is evidence of the formation of distinct neural structures (plate, groove, and folds). Dorsal views of the embryo at this stage are shown in figure 2.2, a and b. Along with the neural structures, there is evidence of the first somites in figure 2.2b.

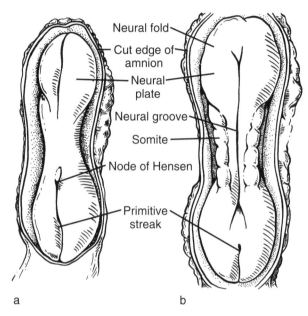

Figure 2.2   (*a*) Ectodermal (dorsal) view of a late presomite embryo (approximately 1.4 mm in length at 15 days). The amniotic sac has been removed, and the neural plate is visible. (*b*) Dorsal view of the embryo at approximately 20 days, with the emergence of the somites and the formation of a distinct neural groove and folds.

Reprinted from Langman 1969.

The somites are cuboidal bodies that form distinct surface elevations and influence the external contours of the embryo. By the beginning of week 4, the ventral and medial walls of the somites show highly proliferative activity, become polymorphous in shape, coalesce, and migrate toward the notochord. Collectively, the migrating cells are known as the sclerotome. After the sclerotome has condensed near the notochord, the remaining wall of the somite, the dorsal aspect, gives rise to a new layer of cells called the dermatome. Cells arising from the dermatome form a tissue known as the myotome, which gives rise to the musculature.

The undifferentiated cells of the sclerotome form a loosely woven tissue known as *mesenchyme* (or primitive connective tissue). Mesenchyme is the progenitor tissue of adult connective tissues, such as cartilage, ligaments, fascia, tendons, blood cells, blood vessels, skin, and bone, as well as muscle. One of the primary attributes of mesenchymal cells is their ability to differentiate into a variety of cells, thus they are pluripotent. They may become fibroblasts (associated with the formation of elastic or collagen fibers), chondroblasts (involved in the formation of cartilage matrix), or osteoblasts (associated with bone extracellular matrix).

Types of Tissues

Tissue is classified as one of four types: epithelial, nervous, muscle, and connective. The ectoderm and endoderm are primarily epithelial tissues. Most of the epithelial tissues of the body are derived from these two embryonic layers. Epithelial tissue is basically a covering (lining) tissue. It can be specialized to absorb, secrete, transport, excrete, or protect the underlying organ or tissue. Epithelial membranes consist entirely of cells and have no capillaries, but are nourished via tissue fluid from the capillaries of connective tissues. These membranes are not strong and typically are bound firmly to connective tissue separated by a thin layer of material called a basement membrane.

Epithelial tissue is subject to wear, and its cells are constantly being lost and regenerated. Structurally, the number of cells and the arrangement of the cellular layer provide the generic names of epithelial tissues. A single layer of cells is described as simple. Tissue with two or more layers of cells is stratified. In terms of cell shape, the usual categories include squamous, cuboidal, and columnar. For example, an epithelial tissue could be classified as simple cuboidal or stratified squamous. Figure 2.3 illustrates the various types of epithelial cells.

The layered or columnar arrangement of epithelial cells is mechanically weak. Epithelial tissues, however, have a prominent role in the diffusion of tissue fluid and heat and in bioelectric conduction.

Nervous tissue, a second type of tissue, develops from the ectoderm. It comprises the main parts of the nervous system, including the brain, spinal cord, peripheral nerves, nerve endings, and the sense organs. The basic unit of nervous tissue is the neuron, or nerve cell. Communication is a vital feature of nervous tissue. Inherent characteristics of nervous tissue include irritability (capacity to react to chemical or physical agents) and conductivity (ability to transmit impulses from one location to another). Nerve impulses are conducted toward the cell body by dendrites and away from the cell body

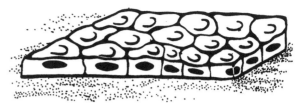

Simple squamous epithelium

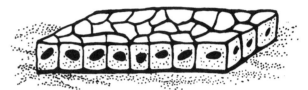

Simple cuboidal epithelium

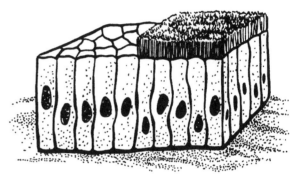

Simple columnar ciliated epithelium

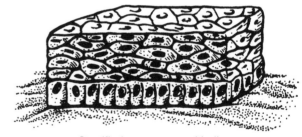

Stratified squamous epithelium

Figure 2.3 Examples of cellular shapes and arrangements of different types of epithelial tissue. Simple squamous epithelium contains platelike cells organized in a single layer that adhere closely to each other by their edges. Simple cuboidal epithelium and simple columnar epithelium appear similar on the surface as a continuous mosaic of polygons. From a side view, however, it is evident that the heights of the cells are substantially different, one being essentially a cube arrangement and the other being a much taller column. Stratified squamous epithelium consists of multiple layers, ranging from cuboidal or columnar cells to irregularly shaped polyhedral cells to superficial layers consisting of thin squamous cells.

Adapted from Fawcett 1994.

by an axon. There is only one axon per cell, but there may be many dendrites. Nerve tissue can be injured by excessive tension or compression, but its prime physiological function is not load bearing.

The third type of tissue, *muscle*, can be divided into three categories: skeletal, smooth, and cardiac. Muscle tissue is derived from the mesoderm. All three types of muscle cells perform the specialized tasks of conductivity and contractility. *Skeletal muscle* is also called striated muscle because its fibers exhibit cross striations. Skeletal muscle fibers have multinucleated cells. Skeletal muscle is under voluntary control and is enveloped in a sheath of connective tissue that blends with its tendon. Because of the contractility of skeletal muscle cells, they have a prime function of generating force to maintain posture and produce body movements.

Smooth muscle does not appear striated and generally is not considered to be under voluntary control. It is found in the walls of tubes in the arterial, intestinal, and respiratory systems. Smooth muscle is innervated by both the sympathetic and parasympathetic nerves.

Cardiac muscle displays structural and functional characteristics of both skeletal and smooth muscle. Cardiac muscle is striated in appearance but is generally considered involuntary. Cardiac muscle cells form a functional syncytium, as the cardiac tissue acts electrically as though it were a single cell.

Connective tissue is the fourth type of tissue. It too is derived from the mesoderm. It differs primarily from the other three types of tissue in the amount of extracellular substance. Cells are soft, easily deformable structures and by themselves would be unable to transmit substantial loads. The extracellular matrix that holds the connective tissues together gives it form and allows the tissue to transmit load. The ratio of cells to extracellular matrix and the composition of the matrix establish the physical characteristics of the connective tissue. The composition of the matrix can range from a relatively soft, gel-like substance (as in skin or ligament) to the rigid matrix found in bone. A primary role of the cells in bone, cartilage, tendons, and ligaments is to produce and maintain the extracellular matrix.

Connective Tissues

Connective tissues are aggregate materials consisting of cells, fibers, and other macromolecules embedded in a matrix that can also contain tissue fluid. The principal fibers in connective tissues are *collag-*

enous, reticular, and *elastic* fibers, although collagenous and reticular fibers are basically different forms of collagen (Fawcett 1986). The arrangement and packing density of fibers in connective tissues distinguishes loose connective tissue and dense connective tissue. In addition, the term *dense irregular connective tissue* is used to describe fibrous connective tissue with loosely and randomly interwoven fibers, such as fascia, and the term *dense regular connective tissue* refers to organized fibrous tissues, such as tendons, ligaments, or aponeuroses (fibrous ribbonlike membranes similar in composition to tendons).

Specialized load-bearing tissues such as bone, cartilage, tendon, and ligament (dense connective tissue) are detailed in later sections of this chapter; here we provide a description of loose connective tissues. More prevalent than dense connective tissues, four basic types of loose connective tissues persist in the adult: fibroelastic, areolar, reticular, and adipose tissues. All of these tissues contain some elastic fibers that provide extensibility to the tissues. Collagen fibers are also evident in the tissues, along with a liquid extracellular matrix that bathes the cells and fibers.

Fibroelastic tissue is a loose, woven network of fibers that encapsulates most organs. The extensibility of loose connective tissue is due to the organization of the collagen fibers. The tissue as a whole can be stretched without initially deforming the fibers. Because the collagen in loose connective tissue is configured as a mesh, the mesh is deformed first, and the fibers are aligned before the individual collagen fibers themselves are stretched. This contrasts with dense fibrous connective tissues, such as tendon, in which the collagen is arranged in parallel rows. Because the tendon collagen is already in line with the tensile load, the fibers quickly resist the applied tensile load. After a load deforms fibroelastic tissue, elastic fibers help return the stretched connective tissue back to its original position when a load is released.

Areolar tissue saturates almost every area of the body. The tissue is called areolar because there are spaces or "holes" where only fluid extracellular matrix exists. Fibroblasts and macrophages are abundant, and collagenous and some elastic and reticular fibers give limited structural strength to areolar tissue. Nonetheless, areolar tissue is a weak connective tissue and can be easily pulled apart. Reticular network fibers act as a boundary between areolar connective tissues and other structures.

Reticular tissue contains reticular fibers and some primitive cells, and thus resembles early mesenchymal tissues. The primitive cells within reticular tissue can differentiate into fibroblasts, macrophages, and even some plasma cells. Reticular tissue is found near lymph nodes and in bone marrow, liver, and spleen. Reticular fibrils are also found in many other areas of the body, such as around nerves, muscles, and blood vessels.

Adipose tissue is the fourth type of loose connective tissue. Microscopically, this tissue appears to be an aggregate of fat cells surrounded by areolar tissue. Each adipose cell has a fat droplet. Any loose connective tissue can accumulate fat, and when it predominates, the term *adipose tissue* is used. Reticular fibers enclose each fat cell, and capillaries are found between the cells. The rich vascularity is consistent with the increased metabolism of adipose tissue. It can be mobilized for use in the body when carbohydrates are not immediately available and is readily stored when not needed. Adipose tissue is commonly found around the organs in the abdominal cavity, under the skin, and in bone marrow. Adipose tissue, when present under the skin, may prevent heat dissipation and act as a cushion for the skeleton during external impacts.

Constituents of Connective Tissues

Cells, extracellular matrix (including fibers and matrix glycoproteins), and tissue fluid are the structural elements of connective tissues. The specific constituents of bone, cartilage, tendon, and ligament are discussed later in this chapter; here we present only the generic components of these tissues.

Cells. Several cell types exist within connective tissues. They are classified as either *resident* (fixed) or *migratory* (wandering) cells (Fawcett 1986). The resident cells are relatively stable within a tissue and their role is to produce and maintain the extracellular matrix.

Undifferentiated mesenchymal cells (or stem cells) are resident cells that can differentiate into a variety of connective tissue cells, including fat cells. An important characteristic of mesenchymal cells is that they can differentiate into fibroblasts, chondroblasts, or osteoblasts. Subsequently, chondroblasts and osteoblasts mature into chondrocytes and osteocytes. *Fibroblasts* are the principal cells in many fibrous connective tissues. Their function includes the formation of fibers as well as other components of extracellular matrix. Although there is some difference of opinion, generally it is agreed that the terms *fibroblast* and *fibrocyte* are synonymous. In the remainder of this text we use only the term *fibroblast* to refer to this mature cell.

The migratory cells that enter connective tissue (e.g., macrophages, monocytes, basophils, neutrophils, eosinophils, mast cells, lymphocytes, and plasma cells) travel to the tissue via the bloodstream. These cells are usually associated with the tissue's reaction to injury through the initiation and regulation of an immune response and inflammation. The numbers of these cells in connective tissues are quite variable, but two of the cells warrant further mention.

The *macrophage* contains small holes or vacuoles that can assimilate foreign material, old red blood cells, and bacteria. Because of this ability, the macrophage is part of a larger phagocytic system, the reticuloendothelial system, a major defense system in the body. *Mast cells* are relatively large cells because of their substantial amount of cytoplasm.

Fibroblast Versus Fibrocyte

Mesenchymal cells are the undifferentiated progenitors of connective tissue cells. Fawcett (1986) explains that the suffix *-blast* (derived from the Greek *blastos,* meaning germ) is frequently used to refer to the immature stages of some cell types. The term *fibroblast* has been used in the past to describe the undifferentiated stage of a fibrocyte. In turn, the term *fibrocyte* was used to indicate the relatively quiescent and mature phase of the cell's development. This is a misnomer, however. Fibroblast already means a "fiber-forming" cell. Since the mature fibroblast is the principal site of collagen and elastin biosynthesis, it is not necessary to change the name to fibrocyte when the cell becomes mature. Thus, fibroblast is the preferred term, but fibrocyte is also allowable.

The many granules in their cytoplasm are thought to contain heparin, which acts as a blood anticoagulant. Histamine (a vasodilator) and serotonin (a vasoconstrictor) may also be present in mast cells.

Extracellular Matrix.   The extracellular matrix in connective tissues is a blend of components, including protein fibers (collagen and elastin), simple and complex matrix glycoproteins, and tissue fluid. *Collagen* is the most abundant protein in the animal world and constitutes more than 30% of the total protein in the human body (Eyre 1980). Collagen is an umbrella term; there are many different forms of collagen. Collagen fibers are present in varying amounts in all types of connective tissue. The organization of collagen fibers is tissue specific and can range from a relatively random arrangement of fibers in loose connective tissue to a very organized and parallel arrangement in dense regular connective tissues such as tendon. All of the key cells of connective tissue (fibroblasts, chondroblasts, chondrocytes, osteoblasts, and osteocytes) are able to produce collagen.

Collagen fibers are proteins, or long chains of amino acids with peptide linkages. The fundamental unit of collagen is the tropocollagen molecule. The molecule is made from three spiraled polypeptide (or α) chains of about 1,000 amino acids that are intertwined to form a helix. Parallel rows of tropocollagen form microfibrils, and these microfibrils further aggregate in a parallel fashion into fibrils. Collagen fibrils are aligned into bundles to form collagen fibers. The stability of the collagen fibers can be enhanced with the formation of collagen cross links both within and between the collagen molecules. Excessive cross-linking, however, can make the collagen stiff and inextensible. Collagen is classified according to its molecular organization as type I, type II, or type III. More than 20 different types of collagen have been reported, but type I is found in skin, bone, tendon, ligament, and cornea and is the most abundant type of collagen in the body. Type II collagen is primarily found in cartilage, and type III is most abundant in loose connective tissue, the dermis of the skin, and blood vessel walls.

Elastic fibers are much more slender and extensible than collagen fibers. They can be stretched to about 150% of their original length before the fiber breaks (Fawcett 1986). Microfibrils and elastin are the two components of elastic fibers. Microfibrils are aggregated into small bundles and embedded within a relatively amorphous elastin. The chemical composition of elastin has some components that are similar to collagen.

Besides the collagen and elastic fibers, another major protein fraction of the extracellular matrix is *complex glycoproteins*. A *proteoglycan* is a protein to which are attached one or more specialized carbohydrate side chains, called glycosaminoglycans (Bray, Frank, & Miniaci 1991; Mow, Ratcliffe, & Poole 1992). Glycoproteins occupy the spaces between fibers and constitute the so-called ground substance of connective tissues. It is important to remember that these complex matrix glycoproteins are negatively charged and hydrophilic (attract water molecules). As we discuss later, these two attributes have significant effects on the mechanical behaviors of connective tissue.

In addition to proteoglycan, other specialized glycoproteins can also be found in connective tissue matrix. These are called cell-associated glycoproteins because they are important for the adhesion of cells. One type, fibronectin, plays an important role in cell migration. Also, cells involved with tissue repair can use fibronectin as a stable "handhold" during the repair process. Other types of cell-associated glycoproteins include chondronectin, which helps to stabilize the chondrocyte in its matrix, and anchorin CII, which may be important in mediating the binding of type II collagen to chondrocytes (Bray et al. 1991).

Tissue Fluid.   Tissue fluid is a filtrate of the blood and resides in the intercellular (interstitial) spaces. It aids in the transport of materials between the capillaries and cells in the extracellular matrix. The tissue fluid carries food and oxygen to the cells by diffusing through the arterial end of the capillary. Moving in the opposite direction, the fluid has two paths to remove wastes from the cell. It may either return the wastes to the venous end of the capillary for removal by the blood, or wastes may be disposed of by the lymphatic system. The latter provides channels and filtering points (lymph nodes and spleen) to cleanse the tissue fluid before it is returned to the bloodstream. If blockage occurs in the lymphatics, the tissue fluid is trapped in the intercellular spaces, and edema (tissue swelling) results.

Tissue fluid is retained in the interstitial spaces of the intertwined proteoglycans and glycosaminoglycans. The interaction of the fluid with these macromolecules gives the extracellular matrix its gel characteristics and contributes to the mechanical behavior of the tissue.

Bone

The specialized connective tissue known as bone is one of the hardest and strongest tissues in the body. The skeleton of humans and other vertebrates protects vital organs, serves as a mineral storehouse, houses bone marrow hematopoietic cells, and provides levers from which muscles control movements. Bone is a dynamic structure that perpetually remodels and responds to alterations in mechanical loads, systemic hormones, and serum calcium levels. Each of these factors is synergistically interrelated, and the specific anatomy of a bone reflects the interaction of these factors.

Bone can be studied as an organ, as a tissue, or in terms of its cells. It is important to realize that bone is a functional unit at each of these organizational levels. As an organ, bone accounts for a substantial percentage of the total body mass and is involved with metabolic processes such as hematopoiesis (formation of blood cells). Bone tissue can be classified either as cortical (also called compact) or trabecular (also called cancellous or spongy). Although cortical and trabecular bone have the same cells, their mechanical behavior and adaptive responses are different. Many types of cells are found in bone tissue, and these cells function interactively to maintain bone as a tissue and an organ.

Development of Bone.   Skeletal development begins when mesenchymal cells from the mesodermal germ layer condense. In a few bones (cranium and facial bones and, in part, the ribs, clavicle, and mandible) the cellular condensations form fibrous matrices that subsequently ossify directly (intramembranous ossification). Figure 2.4 provides a schematic representation of the stages involved in intramembranous ossification.

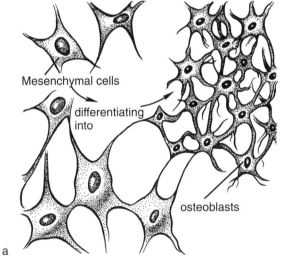

Mesenchymal cells
differentiating into
osteoblasts

a

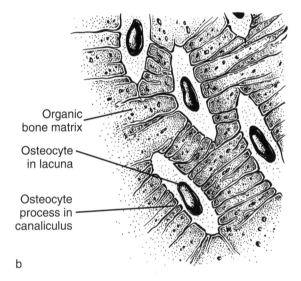

Organic bone matrix
Osteocyte in lacuna
Osteocyte process in canaliculus

b

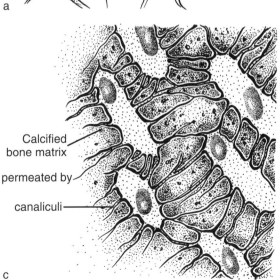

Calcified bone matrix
permeated by
canaliculi

c

Figure 2.4   Intramembranous ossification. The sequence illustrates the temporal occurrence of ossification, starting with (*a*) a differentiation of mesenchymal cells into osteoblasts. (*b*) Osteoblasts then secrete bone matrix, including type I collagen. (*c*) With the calcification of the bone extracellular matrix, distinct canaliculi are left intact to permit communication between osteocytes.

From *Ham's Histology* (9th ed.) (Fig. 12.13, p. 276) by D.H. Cormack, 1987, Philadelphia: Lippincott. Copyright 1987 by Lippincott-Raven. Adapted by permission.

In most limb and axial bones, mesenchymal condensations form a cartilaginous model (anlage) of the bones rather than proceeding directly to calcification and ossification. Figure 2.5 shows how endochondral ossification proceeds during long-bone development. At the ends of the cartilage model, the cells of zone 1 are tightly packed with little extracellular matrix. Cells of zone 2 are flattened, with their cellular axes oriented transverse to the anlage longitudinal axis. In the transition between zones 2 and 3, the chondrocytes become cuboidal in shape and develop vacuoles, indicative of active synthesis of matrix components. The cells in zone 3 have hypertrophied and are the largest of the chondrocytes. These cells rapidly produce extracellular matrix components, and in zone 4 (close to the midshaft) the new matrix begins to calcify and surround the chondrocytes. The calcification of the matrix leads to the death of the chondrocytes, and in zone 5, only large empty spaces (lacunae) remain where the chondrocytes once resided. It is in this final region where osteoid tissue is initially deposited. Circumferentially, the perichondrium surrounding zone 5 thickens and lays down a thin layer of osteoid tissue that subsequently mineralizes, forming a bony collar at the midshaft level. Vascular channels penetrate the central region and bony collar, ultimately forming the primary ossification center. Ossification proceeds quickly toward the ends to form the bone diaphysis and metaphysis.

In the epiphyseal regions the vascular channels directly invade the cartilage, which subsequently ossifies and forms secondary ossification centers. Vascular ingrowth (irruption) is an integral step in the formation of the primary and secondary ossific centers, because the blood supply ensures the arrival and subsequent differentiation of osteogenic precursor cells (Caplan 1988).

Between the bone formed by the primary and secondary ossification centers, the cartilage anlage persists as the epiphyseal (growth) plates between the shaft and ends of the long bone. The growth plate results from a compaction of the cellular zones of the cartilage anlage and thus contains analogous layers of chondrocytes. An important anatomic region within the developing long bone is the zone of Ranvier,

Zone 1. Resting (hyaline cartilage)
Zone 2. Proliferative (divide chondrocytes)
Zone 3. Hypertrophic (large chondrocytes)
Zone 4. Death of chondrocytes (calcified)
Zone 5. Ossification zone—bone tissue appears

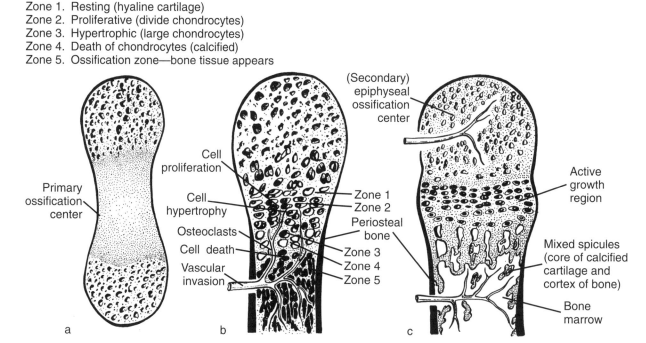

Figure 2.5 Schematic representation of endochondral ossification. (*a*) The hyaline cartilage anlage (model) with its primary ossification center. (*b*) The transitional zones (1-5), ranging from a site of cell proliferation, through hypertrophy, to cell death and ossification. (*c*) The mixed spicules (core of calcified cartilage and cortex of bone) are forming in the midshaft region, around the primary ossification center. At the epiphyseal (secondary) ossification center, there is an invagination of a vascular bud that is analogous to the vascular invasion at the primary ossification center. The active growth region is the primary site of bone accretion and thus is the primary site for long-bone growth.
Reprinted from Langman 1969.

found at the cortical margins of the growth plate toward the primary ossification center (Ogden and Grogan 1987). This complex zone is important because this is where the increase in metaphyseal diameter occurs during growth. Therefore, if trauma damages the zone of Ranvier, the normal circumferential growth of the long-bone metaphysis can be disrupted.

Longitudinal bone growth occurs through activity of the chondrocytes within three functionally distinct regions of the growth plate: the regions of growth, maturation, and transformation. The region of growth contains two types of chondrocytes. Resting cells lie close to the secondary ossification center. These cells are associated with the small arterioles and capillaries from the epiphyseal vessels. These vessels are important in transporting undifferentiated cells to add to the pool of resting cells. Away from the resting cells is an area of active cell division. In this area the cells are organized in longitudinal columns, and during a period of rapid growth the columns may account for over half the height of the growth plate (Ogden, Grogan, & Light 1987). The region of maturation is associated with chondrocytes that actively synthesize and secrete cartilaginous extracellular matrix. Cells adjacent to the region of growth are large and actively produce matrix components, whereas the cells near the ossification front become trapped in the rapidly calcifying matrix and therefore are not as active in matrix production. The third region has an area of transformation, where the cartilage matrix becomes increasingly calcified and is invaded by metaphyseal blood vessels. The irrupting vessels bring the osteoblasts necessary for formation of bone osteoid. The osteoid is rapidly mineralized to form true bony tissue.

Eventually, chondrocyte differentiation and proliferation slow in the regions of growth and maturation, allowing the bone mineralization (encroaching from the diaphyseal edge of the plate) to catch up. This unites the bone formed by the primary and secondary centers and marks the culmination of long-bone growth. This process is known as epiphyseal plate closure.

Both intramembranous and endochondral ossification can occur in the same bone. For example, the shaft of the clavicle is formed by intramembranous ossification, but a secondary ossification center develops within a cartilaginous epiphysis to form the sternal end of the bone. A primary ossification center is present in most bones at birth, but the secondary ossification center of the distal femur is the only secondary center present at birth and is often used to identify a full-term fetus. Both endochondral and intramembranous ossification processes persist postnatally, as during fracture repair (endochondral) and periosteal bone deposition (intramembranous).

Movement and its related forces during skeletal development help identify the stimuli that can influence the final skeletal form. Carter and colleagues (1987) propose that the regulation of skeletal biology by mechanical forces is accomplished by the transfer of strain energy. To this end, these researchers believe that cyclic shear stresses generated during movement accelerate the rate of chondrocytic proliferation, maturation, degeneration, and ossification that occur during endochondral ossification, whereas compressive stresses tend to retard the same sequence. Carter and colleagues propose that some of the energy imparted to the skeletal structures during movement is stored within the tissue and later released during unloading. The remaining energy is transferred to the tissue in the form of heat or a change in internal energy. This latter form of energy transfer may be an important factor in a bone's ability to recognize and respond to mechanical cues.

Extrinsic factors, such as hormones, influence the rate and extent of long-bone growth. Thyroxine, growth hormone, and testosterone can all stimulate cartilage cell differentiation in the growth plate. Estrogen exerts a greater stimulatory influence on the bony tissue while suppressing cartilage growth. The distinct influences of testosterone and estrogen may account for the differences in the timing of physeal closure between boys and girls.

Normal skeletal growth can also be interrupted by trauma or fracture. Physeal injuries account for approximately 15% of all fractures in children. Girls are more prone to physeal injury from 9 to 12 years of age, while boys are more prone between the ages of 12 to 15 years (Ogden 1990a). The periods of increased incidence parallel the times of rapid growth during which hormone-mediated changes in the growth plate cartilage may alter the response of the cartilage to mechanical stress (Muscher, Desaulles, & Schenk 1965). Most pediatric fractures are classified according to a system developed by Salter (Ogden 1990b). The system considers the location of the fracture, whether the fracture disrupts the growth plate, and the extent of the growth plate damage. Growth disturbances may result if the fracture and subsequent callus formation stimulate the premature closure of the growth plate, thereby preventing the normal longitudinal growth of the bone. Angular deformities may result if only one portion of the growth plate sustains damage while normal growth occurs in the remaining portion of the growth plate. An example of an angular deformity is demonstrated in the X ray in figure 2.6.

Components of Bone Tissue.   The three primary bone cells are osteoblasts, osteocytes, and osteoclasts. *Osteoblasts* and *osteocytes* are responsible for bone formation and are distinguished primarily by their location as opposed to their structure. The osteoblast, located on the bony surface, is the primary bone-forming cell. Once the osteoblast has produced sufficient mineralized matrix to completely surround itself, it is called an osteocyte. When the active osteoblast begins the transition to osteocyte, cell volume decreases by 30% initially, and as the metabolic activity of the osteocyte gradually decreases, cell volume also continues to decrease. The osteocyte slowly fills in its surrounding lacuna with matrix, and thus both cell and lacunar size decrease.

Neighboring osteocytes communicate with one another, and the deeper osteocytes communicate with the surface-covering osteoblasts by interconnecting processes housed within channels (canaliculi) within the extracellular matrix (refer to figure 2.4). The presence of connections between adjacent processes between bone cells suggests that the osteoblasts, osteocytes, and bone-lining cells form a functional syncytium that may play an integral role in many physiological functions, including the conversion of mechanical signals into remodeling activity and mineral movement into and out of the bone (Miller & Jee 1992).

Osteoclasts are bone-resorbing cells. Light microscopy reveals that the multinucleated osteoclasts move along the bone surface and leave behind a trail of resorbed bone that has the appearance of an etched surface. The most distinguishing feature of the osteoclast is the extensive infoldings of the cell plasma membrane that give rise to a "ruffled border." This border has important functional significance because it greatly increases the surface area along which the cell can interact with the surrounding bony matrix (Holtrop 1992).

The *extracellular bone matrix* has inorganic (mineral), organic, and fluid components. Minerals, pri-

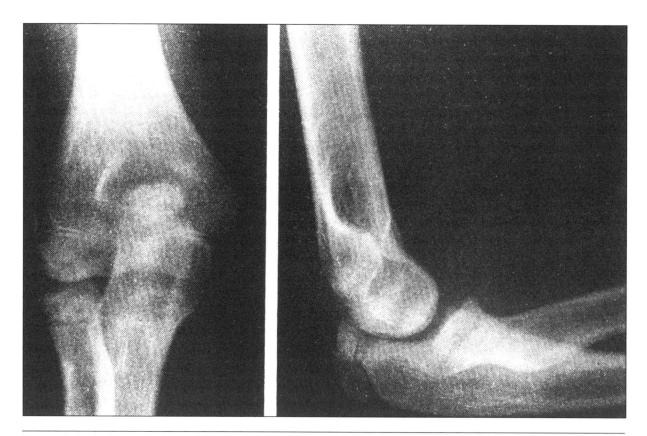

Figure 2.6   An X ray of a bone deformity resulting from a damaged growth plate.
Reprinted from Ellman 1975.

marily in the form of calcium hydroxyapatite crystals, contribute about 50% of the total bone volume. Organic components constitute 39% of the volume (95% type I collagen and 5% proteoglycans), while fluid-filled vascular channels and cellular spaces constitute the remaining volume. Bone mechanical behavior reflects a balance between the mineral and organic phases, with minerals contributing stiffness and the organic matrix adding strength to bone.

Mineral content distinguishes bone from other connective tissues and provides bone with its characteristic rigidity as well as providing a mineral storehouse. The mechanism responsible for calcification of the extracellular matrix of bone and not of other connective tissues is not completely understood, but apparently the ability to bind mineral crystallites is unique to type I collagen. Neither type II nor III collagen can bind to minerals. More than 200 noncollagenous proteins are also found within bone's extracellular matrix. In terms of concentration, however, collagen occupies the greatest portion of the matrix. Because collagen provides major structural support in connective tissues, abnormalities in collagen production can have far-reaching consequences in the ability of the skeleton to resist mechanical stresses. For example, if a genetic defect affects bone collagen formation, the bone can become very fragile and easily fractured.

Bone is richly supplied with blood vessels, including the marrow, periosteum, metaphysis, diaphysis, and epiphysis (figure 2.7). Gross, Heistad, and Marcus (1979) estimated that 11% of the cardiac output is sent to the skeleton. Blood reaches each area of the bone via extensive arterial interconnections (anastomoses) that feed a network of sinusoids (dilated venous channels). The sinusoids in turn empty into central venous channels deep within the medullary canal in long bones or a central canal in flat bones. The primary nutrient vessel enters the medullary canal via an obliquely oriented nutrient foramen. Once within the bone endosteum, the artery divides into longitudinal branches that course along the bone's length and then reenter the cortical bone. In the epiphyses, the longitudinal vessels branch into extensive arcades that supply the bony ends. Medullary vessels pierce through the cortex and anastomose with periosteal vessels to supply the outer surfaces of the cortex. Within compact bone, primary arteries and veins travel parallel to the osteonal longitudinal axes within structures called Haversian canals. Transversely oriented vessels are contained within structures called Volkmann canals.

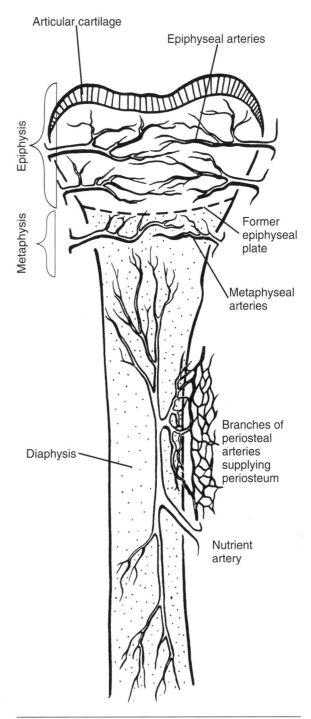

Figure 2.7 Blood supply of a mature long bone (tibia). The nutrient artery is the principal supplier of blood to the diaphysis, along with periosteal arteries of the diaphyseal regions. They account for about 90% of the blood flow within the diaphysis. The metaphyseal and epiphyseal regions of the bone are also supplied by arteries.

From *Ham's Histology* (9th ed.) (Fig. 12.39, p. 314) by D.H. Cormack, 1987, Philadelphia: Lippincott. Copyright 1987 by Lippincott-Raven. Adapted by permission.

Bone Macrostructure. Despite differences in size and mechanical properties, bone tissue is similar in all bones. As described earlier, bone can be divided at a structural level into cortical (compact) and trabecular (cancellous or spongy) bone. At a tissue level, bone may be divided into three broad categories: woven, primary, and secondary bone. These categories are described in table 2.1. *Woven bone* is laid down rapidly as a disorganized arrangement of collagen fibers and osteocytes. Although the mineral content of woven bone may be similar to that of primary and secondary bone, the disorganized pattern and generally lower proportions of noncollagenous proteins decrease the mechanical strength of woven bone compared to primary or secondary bone. Developmentally, woven bone is unique because it can be deposited de novo (without a pre-existing bone or cartilaginous model; Martin & Burr 1989). The cell-to-bone volume ratio is high in woven bone, confirming its role in providing temporary, rapid mechanical support, such as following traumatic injury. In the adult skeleton, woven bone is not usually present but can be found in a fracture callus, in areas undergoing active endochondral ossification, and in some skeletal pathologies. During maturation, primary bone systematically replaces woven bone, providing the mature skeleton with the appropriate functional stiffness.

Primary bone comprises several types of bone, each with unique morphology and function. A common factor among the types of primary bone, however, is that unlike woven bone, primary bone must replace a pre-existing structure, either a cartilaginous model or previously deposited woven bone. Primary bone is composed of multiple thin layers of bone matrix and cells organized circumferentially around the endosteal or periosteal surface of a whole bone. Vascular channels are sparse in primary bone, and therefore it can be very dense.

Primary bone is also found in cancellous bone. For example, the trabeculae (small rods) found in the vertebral bodies and in long-bone epiphyses are mostly primary bone. In this case, although vascular channels are not enclosed within the lamellar structure, the individual struts or trabeculae of cancellous bone are in intimate contact with a rich vascular supply. Because of this close proximity, cancellous bone has a very important role in mineral homeostasis because calcium stores can be mobilized quickly in response to decreased serum calcium.

Secondary bone is deposited only during remodeling and replaces pre-existing primary bone. Differences between the developmental process of primary and secondary bone imply that a different controlling mechanism may be responsible for the endosteal or periosteal deposition of primary bone versus the intracortical deposition of secondary bone during remodeling.

Cartilage

Cartilage contains the basic elements of a connective tissue, namely cells and extracellular matrix (tissue fluid and macromolecules). The relative amounts and types of matrix constituents distinguish three kinds of cartilage: hyaline, elastic, and fibrocartilage. Hyaline cartilage is the most abundant of the three. None of the cartilage types have intrinsic blood vessels, nerves, or lymph vessels. The absence of circulatory structures in cartilage makes it necessary for cartilage cells (chondrocytes) to receive their nutrients and remove metabolic waste by diffusion.

All cartilage develops from mesenchyme (primitive connective tissue). Mesenchymal cells produce

Table 2.1 Bone Macrostructure

Type of bone tissue	Deposition	Example
Woven bone	De novo	Fracture callus
Primary bone		
Lamellar	Substrate required	Trabecular bone
Plexiform	Substrate required	Bovine bone
Primary osteons	Vascular channels	Young bone
Secondary bone	Replacement of pre-existing bone	Human cortical bone

From *Structure, Function, and Adaptation of Compact Bone* (Table 2.1, p. 19) by R.B. Martin & D.B. Burr, 1989, New York: Raven Press. Copyright 1989 by Lippincott-Raven. Adapted by permission.

the extracellular matrix (including collagenous fibrils) and differentiate into chondroblasts, which are the precursors of chondrocytes. The chondrocytes, when formed, are encapsulated in caves (lacunae) in the cartilage matrix. A connective tissue membrane (perichondrium) surrounds the new cartilage. Within the perichondrium are blood and lymph vessels and nerves; nutrients leave this area to enrich the chondrocytes within the cartilage. The perichondrium also contains fibroblasts, collagen fibers, and elastic fibers.

Chondrocytes can multiply by two mechanisms. *Interstitial growth* occurs in young cartilage as the chondrocytes divide within the lacunae, forming cell nests. Younger cartilage is more flexible than

mature cartilage, and the matrix can accommodate the interstitial expansion. *Appositional growth* proceeds in the cartilage layers immediately beneath the perichondrium. The mesenchymal cells in this superficial zone develop into new cartilage cells. These, in turn, are laid between the older cells and perichondrium, and new cartilage cells produce new matrix components.

Figure 2.8a shows the distribution of cells from the surface of the perichondrium, through the chondrogenic layer immediately beneath the perichondrium (where appositional growth occurs), and on to the middle region where interstitial growth occurs within the chondrocytes. The distribution of the collagen fibers throughout this same region is

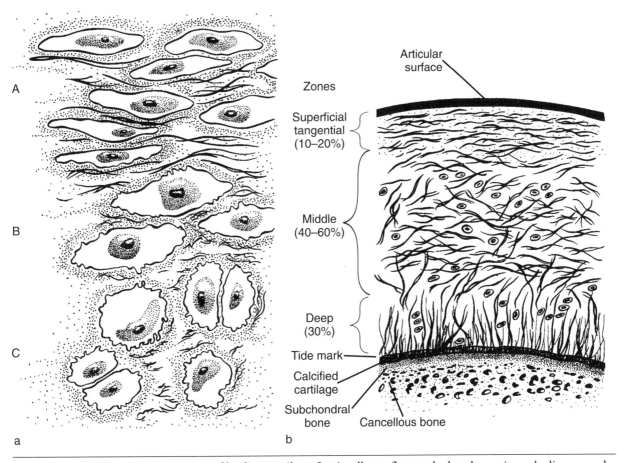

Figure 2.8 (*a*) Cellular organization of hyaline cartilage. In *A*, cells are flattened, chondrogenic, and adjacent to the perichondrium. *B* represents a continuation of the perichondrium level as cartilage cells produce extracellular matrix to distance themselves from their neighboring cells. In *C*, columns of cartilage cells are seen in lacunae. In the orientation represented in the figure, the joint surface is at the top, and the deepest part of the cartilage is at the bottom near the attachment to bone. (*b*) Collagen fiber organization in articular (hyaline) cartilage. The superficial tangential zone is at the region closest to the joint surface, and the collagen fibers are aligned tangential to the articular surface. In the middle zone, the collagen fibers are relatively random in orientation, and in the deep zone the collagen fibers are in a radial direction (with respect to the surface of the joint). The collagen fibers in the deep zone penetrate through the tide mark and into the calcified cartilage overlying the subchondral bone.

Part (*a*) reprinted from Fawcett 1994. Part (*b*) reprinted from Nordin & Frankel 1989.

illustrated in figure 2.8b. In the superficial tangential zone (perichondrium), the collagen fibers are arranged tangentially to the joint surface. In the middle 40% to 60% of the cartilage, the collagen fibers appear more randomly organized. In the deepest layer of the articular cartilage, the collagen fibers are oriented radially and penetrate into the underlying calcified cartilage to maintain a solid adhesion to the underlying bone.

Hyaline cartilage gets its name from its glassy appearance. Fetal cartilage is basically hyaline cartilage before being replaced by bone later in life. The surfaces of most of the joints, the anterior portions of the ribs, and areas of the respiratory system (e.g., trachea, nose, bronchi) are composed of hyaline cartilage. The hyaline matrix appears blue and homogeneous in the fresh state, is firm and resilient in texture, and contains collagen fibers. The collagen fibers give cartilage its tensile strength (Bray, Frank, & Miniaci 1991; Mow, Ratcliffe, & Poole 1992). The mechanical stiffness and strength throughout the cartilage depth varies with the changes in collagen fiber organization (Cohen et al. 1992). The principal collagen in hyaline cartilage is type II (90% of total collagen). The perichondrium (outer fibrous layer and interchondrogenic layer) provides the nutrients for the cartilage and surrounds all hyaline cartilage except at articular surfaces.

Cells constitute less than 10% of hyaline cartilage volume, with the principal components being macromolecules (about 20% of volume) and tissue fluid (about 70% of volume; Bray, Frank, & Miniaci 1991). The main structural macromolecule (besides type II collagen) in hyaline cartilage is proteoglycan. The integrated structure-function relations among the collagen fibers, proteoglycans, and fluid contribute to the unique mechanical behavior of articular cartilage. Figure 2.9 illustrates schematically the molecular organization of cartilage. The striated collagen fibrils are shown in a meshlike arrangement with the proteoglycans that are attached via a link protein to a hyaluronic acid molecule. The proteoglycan monomers have a three-dimensional structure that looks something like a bottle brush with a central core, or backbone protein. The remainder of the molecule (the bristles of the brush) is carbohydrates called glycosaminoglycans. This large assembly is called a proteoglycan aggregate or aggrecan. As described previously, the proteoglycans are negatively charged and are strongly hydrophilic (attract water). Many proteoglycan monomers can subsequently be joined by a link protein to a long hyaluronic acid molecule.

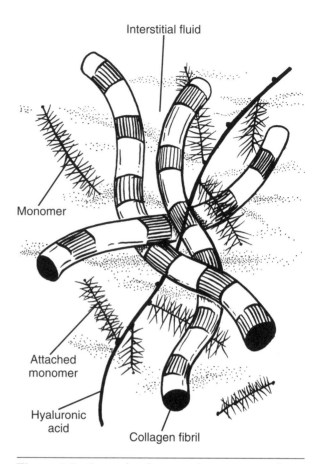

Figure 2.9 Interrelated proteoglycans, proteoglycan aggregates (aggrecan), and collagen fibrils in cartilage matrix.

Given these characteristics, you can begin to imagine the nature of the interactions between the tissue fluid, aggrecan, and collagen fibers. The hydrophilic proteoglycans tend to draw water into the matrix, and the negatively charged proteoglycans tend to repel each other. Articular cartilage wants to swell, but this expansion is resisted by the tensile restraint provided by the collagen fibrils. A dynamic interaction occurs between these matrix constituents during the loading of normal articular cartilage. Figure 2.10 illustrates the basics of this dynamic interaction. Figure 2.10a illustrates articular cartilage without any external load being applied. The cartilage is swollen with water that has been attracted by the proteoglycan, and the negative charges of the proteoglycan are repelling each other while the collagen fibers provide the restraining tensile forces to maintain the structure. In figure 2.10b an external compressive load has been applied. Now the fluid exudes from the articular cartilage, and the proteoglycan monomers and aggrecan are forced closer together. If a constant

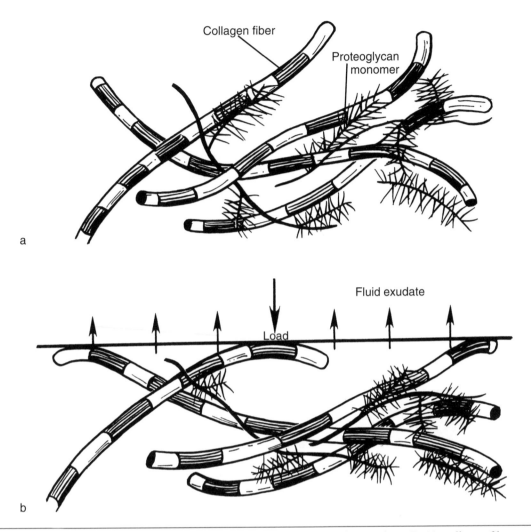

Collagen fiber

Proteoglycan monomer

a

Fluid exudate

Load

b

Figure 2.10 (*a*) Unloaded and (*b*) loaded extracellular matrix of articular cartilage. In (*a*), collagen fibers provide the tensile restraint to the swelling pressures generated by the influx of tissue fluid (assisted by the hydrophilic, negatively charged proteoglycans). In "resting" articular cartilage, there is a normal swelling pressure. In (*b*), an external load has been applied to the surface of the articular cartilage, and the matrix is being compressed. Tissue fluid exudes from the cartilage matrix, and the negatively charged proteoglycan monomers and aggrecan are being pushed closer together. For a given (constant) load, eventually a new equilibrium will be reached with the matrix in a compressed state.
Reprinted from Mankin et al. 1994.

load is applied, the cartilage will creep (slowly deform) until a new equilibrium has been reached.

In adults, chondrocytes slowly continue to produce and renew proteoglycan macromolecules. With age, however, the turnover rate of proteoglycan diminishes, and some of the proteoglycan monomers or individual glycosaminoglycans can become disconnected, which diminishes the resilience of the articular cartilage to external loads.

Elastic cartilage is found in the external ear, the epiglottis, portions of the larynx, and the Eustachian tube. As you might expect from its name, elastic cartilage possesses a great deal of flexibility. The matrix contains elastic fibers as well as collagen fibers. The matrix appears more yellow because of the higher percentage of elastic fibers and is not translucent like hyaline cartilage. Elastic cartilage is able to develop both interstitially and through appositional growth. The perichondrium is, again, a dense type of connective tissue with more elastic fibers, and the layer of cells immediately beneath the perichondrium is chondrogenic.

Fibrocartilage is strong and flexible because of its endogenous collagen fibers and is resilient due to its matrix. Fibrocartilage is found in many areas of the body, especially at stress points where friction could be problematic. It is distinct from hyaline and elastic cartilage because it contains no perichondrium.

The fibrocartilage develops much like other ordinary connective tissue: Fibroblasts produce matrix and then differentiate into chondrocytes.

Fibrocartilage is essentially a "filler" material between hyaline cartilage and other connective tissues and is found near joints, ligaments, and tendons and in the intervertebral disks. Four categories have been labeled, each with a specific function: interarticular, connecting, stratiform, and circumferential.

Interarticular fibrocartilage (meniscus) is found in the wrist and knee joints as well as in the temporomandibular joint and at the junction of the sternum and clavicle. In these joints, in which frequent movement and potential impact occurs, the fibrocartilage provides a buffer. Interarticular fibrocartilages are flattened plates that are interposed between the joint surfaces and are held in position by ligaments and tendons that connect to the edges of the fibrocartilage. The surfaces of these interarticular fibrocartilages, however, are free of connections and help to prevent friction between the moving joints. Further, the interarticular fibrocartilages act as spacers to fill the gap between the joints, improve joint geometry, and protect the surfaces of the underlying articular cartilage.

Connecting fibrocartilage occurs at limited-motion joints, such as intervertebral disks. These fibrocartilage plates allow the surfaces of the adjacent vertebral bodies to move slightly with respect to each other. (You can read more about intervertebral disks in chapter 8).

The final two varieties of fibrocartilage provide protection. Stratiform fibrocartilage forms layers over bone where tendons may be acting and can also be an integral part of the tendon surface. When a muscle contracts and a tendon is forced to slide over a bony surface, friction is minimized by interposing stratiform fibrocartilage between the bone and tendon. Circumferential fibrocartilage acts as a spacer in the joints of the hip and the shoulder (e.g., glenoid labrum). Circumferential fibrocartilage is a circular ring without a center. Thus it protects only the edge of the joints and improves the bony fit.

Tendons and Ligaments

Fibrous connective tissue can be classified into dense or loose fibrous varieties, depending on the proximity and the packing of the fibers. In turn, dense fibrous tissue can be either organized or unorganized, depending again on the fiber organization.

In organized tissue, the collagen fibers run in parallel bundles. These regularly arranged tissue types include tendons, ligaments, and aponeuroses. In all of these, the tissue is primarily composed of fibers and extracellular matrix components. Fibroblasts are the principal cells in these tissues. These tissues have great tensile strength but are able to resist stretching primarily in one direction, that is, along a tensile force generated parallel to the fiber line.

Tendons are white, collagenous flexible bands that connect muscle to bone. Figure 2.11 provides a schematic of the generic structure of a tendon. The basic building blocks of a tendon are the tropocollagen molecules. Tropocollagen molecules generally are aligned in parallel rows to form a microfibril. Subsequently the microfibrils aggregate into parallel bundles to form subfibrils and then fibrils. Fibrils are gathered into fascicles bound together by a loose connective tissue (endotendineum), which permits relative motion of the collagen fascicles and supports blood vessels, nerves, and lymphatics (Woo et al. 1994). Tendon fascicles are grouped into the tendon proper. When a tendon is relaxed (no tensile load), it takes on a crimped or wavy appearance. As a load is applied, the wavy pattern is straightened.

As is evident from the description of the collagen fiber organization in tendon, the major component of tendon is type I collagen, which accounts for about 86% of the dry weight of a tendon (Woo et al. 1994). Elastic fibers are present in small quantities in the matrix of tendons.

The surface of the tendon can be covered with an epitendineum, usually seen as a tendon sheath to act as a pulley and direct the path around sharp corners as in the flexor tendons of the hand. When tendons are not enclosed with the epitendineum and move in a relatively straight line, there is a loose areolar connective tissue (peritenon) enveloping the tendon. The peritenon contains blood vessels to serve the tendon.

The insertion of tendon into bone involves a gradual transition from tendon to fibrocartilage, to mineralized fibrocartilage, and finally to bone. Some of the collagen fibers of the tendon pass through the mineralized fibrocartilage and into the subchondral bone. These penetrating fibers are sometimes called Sharpey's fibers. An additional anchor is provided by fibers from the tendon, which blend with the bone's periosteum.

At the opposite end of the tendon, the myotendinous junction is a specialized region of longitudinal membranous infoldings that increase the surface area and reduce stress on the junction dur-

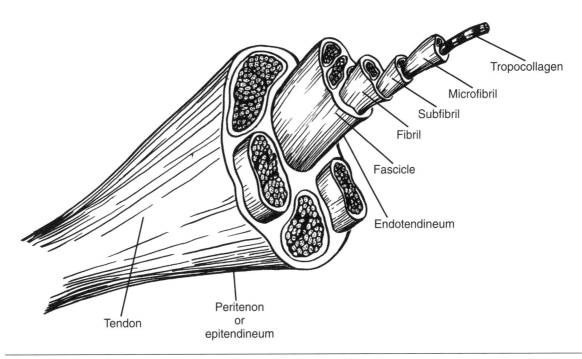

Figure 2.11 Schematic representation of the hierarchy of a tendon.

ing the contractile force transmission. The strength of an adhesive junction such as the myotendinous junction depends both on the properties of the adjoining structures and on the orientation of forces across the junction. Junctions that are loaded in shear, with the force being parallel to the membrane surface, are stronger than junctions with a large tensile component perpendicular to the membrane (Tidball 1983).

Aponeuroses are fibrous, ribbonlike membranes similar in composition to tendons. These structures are sometimes called flattened tendons. For example, the palmar aponeurosis encloses the muscles of the palm of the hand. Aponeuroses are whitish in appearance due to the presence of collagen. The fibers of aponeuroses run in a single direction and thus differ from unorganized (or irregular, dense fibrous) connective tissue (fascia).

Ligaments are dense, regular connective tissue structures that join bone to bone. The primary function of ligaments, like tendons, is to resist tensile forces along the line of the collagen fibers. Ligaments are classified and named by several different criteria. These are the criteria and examples of each: attachment sites (coracoacromial), shape (deltoid), function (capsular), position or orientation (collateral, cruciate), position relative to the joint capsule (extrinsic, intrinsic), and composition (elastic).

In general, joint ligaments have a structure that is similar to tendon, but while collagen fibril bundles in tendons are typically aligned parallel to each other (in line with the pull of the muscle), the collagen fibril bundles in ligaments may be oriented in parallel, obliquely, or even in a spiral arrangement. The geometry of the collagen fibril bundles in ligaments is specific to a ligament's function. The color of collagenous ligaments is a duller white than tendon because of the slightly greater percentage of elastic and reticular fibers found between the collagen fiber bundles.

The ligament insertion to bone is either direct or indirect (Bray, Frank, & Miniaci 1991; Woo et al. 1994). The direct attachment is comparable to the specialized collagen fibers (Sharpey's fibers) that attach tendon to bone. The indirect route is one in which the collagen fibers from the ligament blend with the periosteum of the bone.

Fibroblasts are the principal cells in ligaments, while the main fibrous component of the extracellular matrix is type I collagen (36%). Several other types of collagen are also found in ligaments. Proteoglycans are also present, although fewer than in articular cartilage. Because almost two thirds of a ligament is composed of water, the proteoglycans (which are hydrophilic) may play a role in the mechanical behavior of a ligament.

Anatomically, it is clear that joint ligaments such as those in the knee contain several types of sensory receptors (Ruffini corpuscles, Pacinian corpuscles,

Golgi tendon organs, and free-nerve endings) that are capable of providing the nervous system with information about movement, position, and pain. Nevertheless, the exact neurosensory role of ligaments and receptors in joint proprioception is controversial and continues to be studied. After reviewing a substantial amount of anatomical, neurophysiological, and mechanical data, with a particular focus on the sensory receptors of the knee joint ligaments, Johansson, Sjolander, and Sojka (1991) concluded that ligaments may provide sensory information about changes in the stiffness of muscles around the knee joint. In this way, ligaments may have an important function in regulating the stability of the knee joint.

Yellow elastic ligaments are less common in the body than collagenous ligaments. Parallel elastic fibers, which predominate in elastic ligaments, are surrounded by loose connective tissue. Elastic ligaments in humans include the vocal cords and the ligamenta flava of the vertebrae. A classic example of an elastic ligament in animals is the ligamentum nuchae of cattle that helps the animal hold up its head while grazing.

Fascia is a catch-all category that includes dense, fibrous, unorganized tissues that do not logically fall

---

Ankle Orthotics and Sprains: Mechanical Restraint or Sensory Feedback?

Inversion sprains of the ankle are common in running and jumping sports. If a person has had a previous ankle sprain, a subsequent sprain is much more likely to happen.

To reduce the number of ankle sprain injuries, taping or semirigid orthotics have been advocated. Taping has advantages and disadvantages. Although prophylactic taping can effectively reduce excessive ankle inversion before exercise, in many cases its restraint is lost during an exercise bout. Taping can also be expensive and requires a skilled individual to apply the tape. Semirigid ankle orthotics have been proposed as a substitute for taping. Few prospective studies, however, have evaluated the effectiveness of ankle orthotics for reducing or preventing ankle sprains.

Recently, researchers in South Africa completed a prospective study over a one-year soccer season (Surve et al. 1994). Adult male soccer players with a previous history of ankle sprain and those with no previous history of ankle sprain were identified. Each player was then randomly assigned to an orthotic group or to a control group (no orthotic or taping). Thus, four groups of players were studied. More than 500 players participated in this extensive study. In the study, injury was defined as any sprain that occurred during a scheduled match or practice that caused the soccer player to miss the next game or practice. Marked differences occurred among the groups during the one year of play. The principal finding was that the application of a semirigid ankle orthotic resulted in a fivefold reduction in the incidence of ankle sprains in players with a previous history of ankle sprains. The ankle orthosis, however, did not significantly alter the incidence of ankle sprains in soccer players who had never sprained their ankles before.

Why this difference? Many people suggest that the positive effects of an external support orthotic are primarily due to mechanical support that limits excessive inversion and eversion of the ankle. Nevertheless, both the previously injured and previously uninjured athletes responded differently. Only the athletes who had previously sprained their ankles received positive benefits from wearing the orthotic. Surve and colleagues (1994) suggest that proprioceptive defects can occur after an ankle sprain because of damage to sensory receptors in the ligaments of the ankle. This may lead to impaired reflex stabilization of the ankle. The application of an external orthotic may have stimulated mechanoreceptors to improve proprioceptive function of the previously injured ankle, rather than just providing mechanical support.

Loss of Knee Anterior Cruciate Ligament Can Alter Patterns of Neuromotor Control

When a person tears the anterior cruciate ligament in the knee joint so that it no longer provides a restraint on the forward motion of the tibia (with respect to the femur), the majority (75%) apparently alter their patterns of neuromotor control of muscles surrounding the knee to accommodate changes in function. Berchuck and colleagues (1990) found that when an activity such as walking requires the quadriceps to be active while the knee is flexed between 0° and 45°, the contraction of the quadriceps tends to move the proximal end of the tibia anteriorly, thereby causing strains in the anterior cruciate ligament. If a person does not have an anterior cruciate ligament, however, what can he or she do to avoid the forward motion of the tibia on the end of the femur?

In analyzing the gait of patients with anterior cruciate–deficient knees, Berchuck and colleagues (1990) reported that patients reduced contraction of their quadriceps during the stance phase of walking. They used a so-called quadriceps-avoidance gait. They also may have increased the action of the hamstring muscles to pull back on the tibia during stance, but that was not measured.

But if they avoided using the quadriceps to prevent collapse of the knee during midstance, then how did they maintain an extended knee? Why didn't their knee collapse? Apparently the patients learned to increase the amount of hip extensor activity to compensate for the reduction in the knee extensor activity. Interestingly, the patients walked with quadriceps-avoidance gait on both their ligament-deficient side and on the other (normal) knee.

These researchers suggested that after the ligament injury there is a subsequent reprogramming of the locomotor process so that excessive anterior displacement of the tibia is prevented. How this abnormal function affects the long-term outcome and the likelihood of post traumatic osteoarthritis is still unknown.

into the categories of tendon, aponeurosis, or ligament. The principal fibers in fascia are collagenous, though some elastic and reticular elements also exist. Fascia contains interwoven, meshlike, non-parallel fibers and is usually found in layers or sheaths around organs, blood vessels, bones, and cartilage, as well as in the dermis of the skin. It provides firm support for muscles. The fibers in fascia traverse in different directions and, in some cases, in different planes (as in the dermis). Because of this organization, fascia withstands stretching in many directions.

Skeletal Muscle

Skeletal muscles are the prime executors (movers) of the nervous system. Contractile proteins and a network of connective tissue are the two basic elements of muscles. Fibrous connective tissues within the muscle belly and those that blend with the tendon provide important functional stiffness, which

enhances the transmission of tension. There are significant cellular interactions that direct a muscle's physiological response, but muscle adaptation and injury are best described by considering the mechanics of a muscle's functional units.

The basic structure of skeletal muscle is diagrammatically presented in figure 2.12. From the whole-muscle level, individual muscle fibers (muscle cells) are subdivided into myofibrils, sarcomeres, and finally to actin and myosin. The connective tissue surrounding the entire muscle is called the epimysium, and the bundles of muscle fibers (fascicles) are surrounded by the perimysium. Each individual muscle fiber is surrounded by endomysium.

A skeletal muscle fiber is composed of contractile proteins called myofibrils. The myofibril is the contractile unit of muscle, with hundreds of myofibrils combining to form a single muscle fiber. Each myofibril is composed of two myofilaments: actin (thin filament) and myosin (thick filament). The myofibril has a striated appearance with transverse

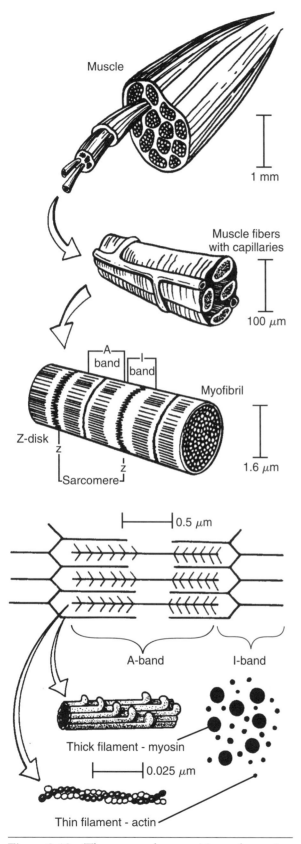

Figure 2.12 The structural composition and organization of skeletal muscle tissue.

Reprinted from di Prampero 1985.

bands of repeated units called sarcomeres. The striations are created by the overlapping of myosin and actin filaments. In the sliding filament theory of muscle contraction, muscle shortens when the myosin structure changes. The cross-bridge cycle interactions between the actin and myosin filaments allow for an increase in the overlap between the fibers and a decrease in sarcomere length. Figure 2.13 depicts the sliding filament theory of muscle contraction and shows a schematic of a relaxed and contracted sarcomere.

Figure 2.14 illustrates the four major states of interactions between myosin and actin during the cross-bridge cycle. The four states correspond to different conformations of the myosin head. Starting with state 1, the myosin binds adenosine triphosphate (ATP). In state 2 the myosin splits ATP into adenosine diphosphate (ADP) and phosphate (P) but retains both molecules in the ATPase (an enzyme) site until it attaches to actin. When it attaches (in state 3), it releases the phosphate, and the head undergoes a conformational change (called the power stroke) that shifts the actin filament and generates force. This constitutes the transition from state 3 to state 4. The head is then detached from the actin, whereby it releases ADP and binds a new ATP to start another cycle (transition from state 4 to state 1).

Muscle fibers vary in length. They can shorten to approximately one half of their resting length. Hu-

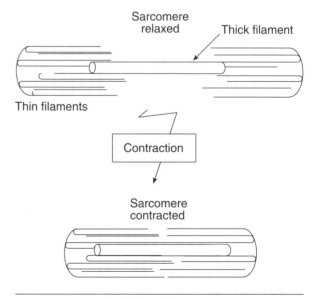

Figure 2.13 The sliding filament theory of muscle contraction. At the top is a schematic showing a relaxed sarcomere with thick and thin filaments. Below, the sarcomere is represented in a contracted state, with overlapping thick and thin filaments.

Reprinted from Alberts et al. 1989.

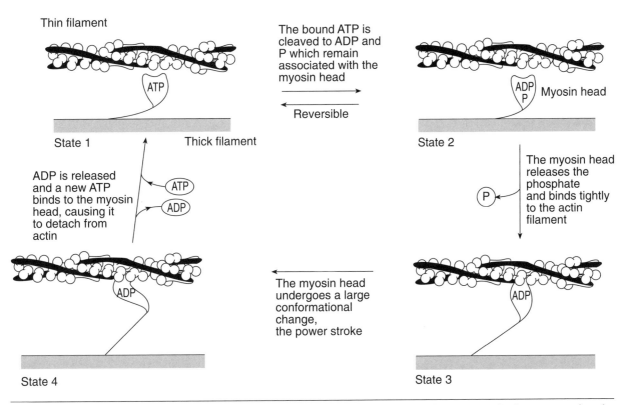

Thin filament

State 1   Thick filament

The bound ATP is cleaved to ADP and P which remain associated with the myosin head

Reversible

ADP P   Myosin head

State 2

ADP is released and a new ATP binds to the myosin head, causing it to detach from actin

ATP

ADP

The myosin head releases the phosphate and binds tightly to the actin filament

P

State 4

The myosin head undergoes a large conformational change, the power stroke

State 3

Figure 2.14   Model of the cross-bridge cycle. See text for the description of the four states, which correspond to the different confirmations of the myosin head.

Reprinted from Alberts et al. 1989.

man skeletal muscle comprises several different fiber types that have different functional characteristics. Garrett and Best (1994) provide a summary of the three different types of muscle fibers and their physiological, metabolic, and structural characteristics (table 2.2). Most muscles in the body are a mixed variety containing a combination of muscle fiber types.

Type I muscle fibers tend to have slower contrac-

tion and relaxation times and are very fatigue resistant. Their motor unit size is typically small with a high capillary density. Type II muscle fibers can be subdivided into types IIA and IIB. Type IIA fibers are fast-twitch, fast oxidative glycolytic fibers that have high contraction speeds but are relatively fatigable, with a larger motor unit size and relatively high capillary density. Type IIB muscle fibers are fast twitch and utilize glycolytic metabolic processes.

Table 2.2   Characteristics of Human Skeletal Muscle Fiber Types

	Type I	Type IIA	Type IIB
Other names	Red, slow twitch (ST) Slow oxidative (SO)	White, fast twitch (FT) Fast oxidative glycolytic (FOG)	Fast glycolytic (FG)
Speed of contraction	Slow	Fast	Fast
Strength of contraction	Low	High	High
Fatigability	Fatigue-resistant	Fatigable	Most fatigable
Aerobic capacity	High	Medium	Low
Anaerobic capacity	Low	Medium	High
Motor unit size	Small	Larger	Largest
Capillary density	High	High	Low

Adapted from Garrett & Best 1994.

Type IIB fibers are the most fatigable but have the highest contraction speeds and the greatest contraction strength. Their motor unit size is the largest of the three, but their capillary density is relatively low.

Muscle fibers with the same biochemical profiles tend to have similar force-producing characteristics. A muscle fiber shortening to one half of its length will have the same force characteristics whether it is long or short because the sarcomeres are in series. Increasing the number of muscle fibers in parallel, however, increases the effective force of the muscle.

One important aspect of muscle architecture is the angle of pennation of the muscle fibers. Longitudinal or fusiform muscles have muscle fibers lying parallel to the line of pull of the tendon. These fibers pull in a straight line, and the full magnitude of the force is directed along the tendon's line of action. The fibers of pennate muscle (uni-, bi-, or multipennate) arise at an oblique angle to the line of pull (usually considered as a straight line along the tendon). Thus, only a portion of the force generated by the contracting fiber is transmitted along the tendon. Pennation of the fibers allows the number of fibers to increase without significantly increasing the muscle's diameter. The force-producing potential of the muscle is enhanced by the increased number of fibers lying adjacent to each other (figure 2.15).

The fundamental neuromuscular unit is the motor unit (figure 2.16). Motor units consist of a motoneuron cell body located within the spinal cord, its axon, and the muscle fibers that it innervates at the motor end plates. When the neuron depolarizes, all the muscle fibers in the motor unit contract as one (all-or-none principle). Muscle tension can be increased by sending action potentials to the muscle more frequently (increasing stimulation rate) and by contracting more muscle fibers (recruiting additional motor units). Recruiting additional motor units is the more potent mechanism for developing force until the highest force levels, when increasing the firing frequency assumes a more prominent role.

In addition to the neural determinants of force, a muscle's force output also is modulated by the length of the muscle when contraction is initiated and by the velocity of contraction. Force, velocity, and length are interrelated variables that affect a muscle's mechanical response. These relationships are usually summarized as force-velocity and length-tension curves (figure 2.17). Length and velocity are not independent of each other; they are both related

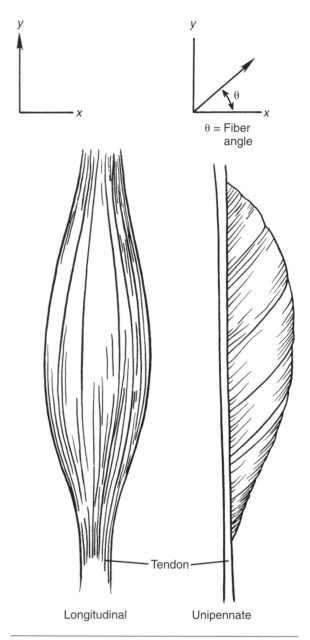

Figure 2.15 Effect of muscle fiber pennation. In this simple comparison, the effect of muscle pennation angle can be seen. In the longitudinal (fusiform) muscle, all the force generated within the muscle fiber is directed through the tendon (no horizontal x component). The advantage of this arrangement is an increased range of motion (excursion of the tendon end with respect to muscle fiber excursion). By comparison, the unipennate muscle fibers are directed at an angle with respect to the tendon. Thus, the force generated within the muscle has an x component that pulls perpendicular to the tendon, while the y component moves the tendon in the intended direction. Although only one component of the muscle fiber force is used effectively to move the tendon, the advantage of this unipennate muscle system is that an increased number of sarcomeres can be placed in parallel to increase the effective force of the muscle.

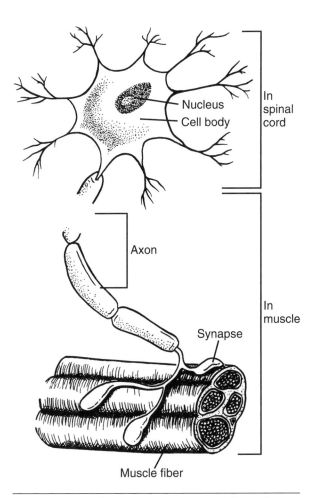

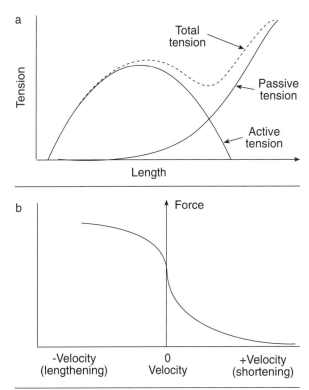

Figure 2.17   (*a*) Skeletal muscle length-tension curve and (*b*) skeletal muscle force-velocity curve.

Figure 2.16   Schematic representation of a single motor unit. A motor unit comprises the motoneuron (cell body) with its accompanying axon and the total number of muscle fibers innervated by that neuron.

From G.A. Brooks & T.D. Fahey, *Exercise Physiology: Human Bioenergetics and its Applications.* Copyright © 1985. All rights reserved. Reprinted by permission of Allyn & Bacon.

to force. The maximal tension can be generated when a muscle is forcibly lengthened while it attempts to shorten (eccentric action), and the tension declines as an active muscle shortens (concentric action). Maximal strength in rapid eccentric muscle action exceeds the maximum in isometric work, and the strength is even less in concentric muscle action.

Skeletal muscle-tendon units also have inherent passive properties that affect force output. The tension developed in a muscle-tendon unit is transmitted to the skeleton from an integrated blend of muscle cells and fibrous connective tissues. The fibrous connective tissue components within muscles include sarcoplasm, sarcolemma, and endomysium. The other major load-carrying connective tissues in the muscle-tendon unit include the tendon and the

collagen fibers that permeate the muscle belly. Some of these passive structures function in series with the active muscle cells, while others function in parallel. The terms *series-elastic component* and *parallel-elastic component* are derived from these functions. Together the two components account for the passive tension properties of muscle. These passive components can be important in muscle mechanics. As Åstrand and Rodahl (1986) note, a given tension in a muscle-tendon unit can be produced at a lower metabolic energy cost in eccentric work than in concentric muscle actions because of the mechanical energy that can be stored in the elastic components.

Activated cross-bridges within the myofibrils exhibit a resistance to stretching, thus generating an internal force that is often termed muscle stiffness. Measured as change in force per change in length, stiffness is a property of muscle believed to operate over length changes and to have functional significance during locomotion and other movements.

Arthrology

The classification of joints and joint motion (arthrology) focuses on the basic classes, types, and examples of various joints in the human body. The words *articulation* and *joint* are used synonymously

Table 2.3   Classification of Joints by Structure and Action

Kind	Class	Type — Common name	Type — Technical name	Explanation and examples
Without a joint cavity	I. Synarthrosis (immovable)	A. Fibrous	Suture*	Two bones grow together, with only a thin layer of fibrous periosteum between (e.g., suture of the skull).
	II. Amphiarthrosis (slightly movable)	B. Ligamentous	Syndesmosis*	Slight movement permitted by meager elasticity of a ligament joining two bones, which may be distinctly separated (e.g., coracoacromial "joint"; mid-radioulnar joint; mid-tibiofibular joint; anterior tibiofibular joint).
		C. Cartilaginous	Synchondrosis or symphysis	Bones are coated with hyaline cartilage, separated by a fibrocartilage disk, and joined by ligaments. Motion is allowed only by deformation of the disk (e.g., between bodies of vertebrae; symphysis pubis; between manubrium and body of sternum).
Having a joint cavity	III. Diarthrosis (freely movable)	D. Synovial 1. Gliding joint	Arthrosis or plane joint	Nonaxial. Allows gliding or twisting (e.g., intercarpal and intertarsal joints).
		2. Hinge joint	Ginglymus	Uniaxial. A concave surface glides around a convex surface, allowing flexion and extension (e.g., elbow joint).
		3. Pivot joint	Trochoid joint	Uniaxial. A rotation around a vertical or long axis is allowed (e.g., atlantoaxial joint; proximal radioulnar joint).
		4. Ellipsoid joint	Ellipsoid joint	Biaxial. An "oval" ball-and-socket joint, allowing flexion, extension, abduction, adduction, and circumduction, but not rotation (e.g., carpometacarpal [wrist] joint).
		5. Condyloid joint	Condyloid joint	Biaxial. A spheroidal ball-and-socket joint with no muscles suitably located to perform rotation, which otherwise could take place (e.g., interphalangeal joints; 2nd to 5th metacarpophalangeal joints [but not of the thumb]).
		6. Ball-and-socket joint	Spheroid, or enarthrosis	Triaxial. Spheroidal ball-and-socket allows flexion, extension, abduction, adduction, circumduction, and rotation on the long axis (e.g., shoulder and hip joints).
		7. Saddle joint	Saddle joint	Triaxial. Both bones have a saddle-shaped surface fitted into each other. Allows flexion, extension, abduction, adduction, circumduction, and slight rotation (e.g., carpometacarpal joint of the thumb).

*Some classification systems include both sutures and syndesmoses under the heading of fibrous joints. Both sutures and syndesmoses tend to ossify completely in later life, in which case the union is shown as a *synostosis*.

Reprinted from Rasch 1989.

to describe the junction of two or more bones at their sites of contact. Some joints allow free movement (e.g., hip and knee joints), while others allow little or no movement between the connecting bones (e.g., sutures of the skull). A useful classification that organizes joints by structure and action is described in table 2.3.

Joints are divided into those with and without a joint cavity. Synarthrodial (immovable) and amphiarthrodial (slightly movable) joints do not have a cavity. Diarthrodial (movable) joints typically have a joint cavity. This is the type of joint usually analyzed in movement-related injuries. For example, the knee joint is a frequently injured diarthrodial joint. A cross section of a knee joint, illustrating its many complex components, is provided in figure 2.18.

How does such a complex diarthrodial joint develop? To provide an answer to the question, we return to the description of somite-stage embryo given in the embryology section earlier in this chapter. After the appearance of the limb buds (26- to 28-day embryo), a group of mesenchymal cells coalesces within the developing limb to form a blastema (Bray, Frank, & Miniaci 1991). The blastema is the foundation material that produces the capsule, ligaments, synovial lining, and menisci of the joint. The adjoining bones at this stage are cartilage models that are undergoing endochondral ossification. At the juncture between two of these cartilage-bone models, the interzonal mesenchyme condenses and forms an articular disk (primitive joint plate). The central cavity within the developing joint emerges at about 10 weeks. This cavity ultimately becomes the synovial cavity, which will contain the synovial fluid that assists with joint lubrication.

Overall, the basic development from blastema to definable skeletal elements happens between weeks 4 to 10 in the developing human embryo. Many different factors can influence the development of joints. Movement appears to be one of the important factors and may result from the extrinsic hydrodynamic forces that act in utero or by the nascent actions of the developing skeletal muscle tissues in the limb.

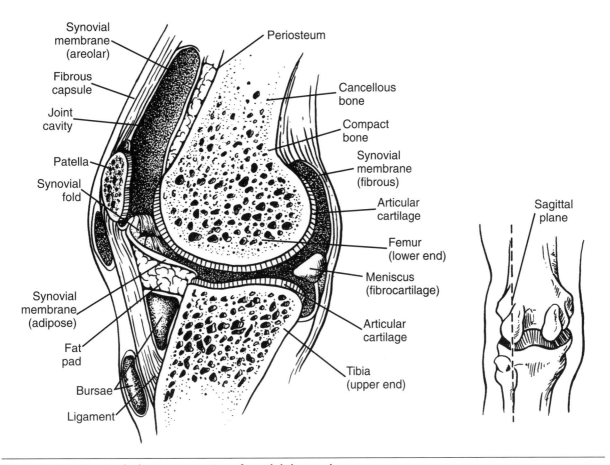

Figure 2.18 A sagittal-plane cross section of an adult human knee.

Concluding Comments

For centuries, load-transmitting connective tissues, such as bone, ligament, tendon, and articular cartilage, were viewed as inert. But in reality these tissues are dynamic and respond acutely to many physiological and mechanical stimuli—including injury. To better understand the underlying mechanisms of these tissue responses, we have provided background on the derivation, structure, and mutability of the primary tissues of the musculoskeletal system. This material was presented with broad strokes. There are excellent and extensive sources available to provide the fine details of tissue anatomy and histology, and you are encouraged to explore these details.

Suggested Readings

Embryology and Development

Iannotti, J.P., Goldstein, S., Kuhn, J.L., Lipiello, L., & Kaplan, F.S. (1994). Growth plate and bone development. In: Simon, S.R. (Ed.), *Orthopaedic Basic Science* (pp. 185-218). Park Ridge, IL: American Academy of Orthopaedic Surgeons.

Langman, J. (1969). *Medical Embryology* (2nd ed.). Baltimore: Williams & Wilkins.

Histology

Cormack, D.H. (1987). *Ham's Histology* (9th ed.). Philadelphia: Lippincott.

Fawcett, D.W. (1994). *Bloom and Fawcett: A Textbook of Histology* (12th ed.). New York: Chapman & Hall.

Bone

Currey, J.D. (1985). *The Mechanical Adaptations of Bones.* Princeton, NJ: Princeton University Press.

Hall, B.K. (Ed.). *Bone* (vols. 1-7). Boca Raton, FL: CRC Press.

Kaplan, F.S., Hayes, W.C., Keaveny, T.M., Boskey, A., Einhorn, T.A., & Iannotti, J.P. (1994). Form and function of bone. In: Simon, S.R. (Ed.), *Orthopaedic Basic Science* (pp. 127-184). Park Ridge, IL: American Academy of Orthopaedic Surgeons.

Martin, R.B., & Burr, D.B. (1989). *Structure, Function, and Adaptation of Compact Bone.* New York: Raven Press.

Cartilage

Mankin, H.J., Mow, V.C., Buckwalter, J.A., Iannotti, J.P., & Ratcliffe, A. (1994). Form and function of articular cartilage. In: Simon, S.R. (Ed.), *Orthopaedic Basic Science* (pp. 1-44). Park Ridge, IL: American Academy of Orthopaedic Surgeons.

Mow, V.C., Ratcliffe, A., & Poole, A.R. (1992). Cartilage and diarthrodial joints as paradigms for hierarchical materials and structures. *Biomaterials, 13,* 67-97.

Tendon and Ligament

Woo, S.L.-Y., An, K.-N., Arnoczky, S.P., Wayne, J.S., Fithian, D.C., & Myers, B.S. (1994). Anatomy, biology, and biomechanics of tendon, ligament, and meniscus. In: Simon, S.R. (Ed.), *Orthopaedic Basic Science* (pp. 45-87). Park Ridge, IL: American Academy of Orthopaedic Surgeons.

Skeletal Muscle

Carlson, F.D., & Wilkie, D.R. (Eds.). (1974). *Muscle Physiology.* Englewood Cliffs, NJ: Prentice Hall.

Garrett, W.E., Jr., & Best, T.M. (1994). Anatomy, physiology, and mechanics of skeletal muscle. In: Simon, S.R. (Ed.), *Orthopaedic Basic Science* (pp. 89-126). Park Ridge, IL: American Academy of Orthopaedic Surgeons.

General

Simon, S.R. (Ed.). (1994). *Orthopaedic Basic Science.* Park Ridge, IL: American Academy of Orthopaedic Surgeons.

Classic Reference

Thompson, D.W. (1961). *On Growth and Form* (abridged ed., Bonner, J.T., Ed.). Cambridge: Cambridge University Press (Originally published 1917).

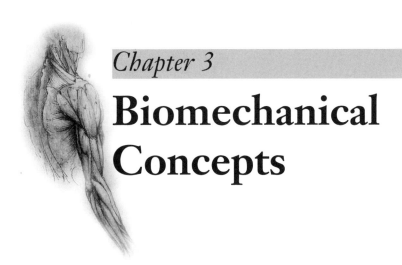

Chapter 3

Biomechanical Concepts

Mechanics is the paradise of the mathematical sciences because by means of it one comes to the fruits of mathematics.

Leonardo da Vinci (1452-1519)

Movement is essential to life. Not only do life processes such as blood circulation, respiration, and muscle contraction require motion, but activities such as walking, bending, and grasping inherently involve movement as well. Consider how the human organism seeks, consciously or not, to move. When you sit in a chair, for example, do you remain motionless? Hardly. You cross and uncross your legs, slouch, squirm, and slide to create some degree of movement. Children are perhaps the best evidence of the inherent nature of humans to move. They never seem to stop. Even as we age and "slow down," movement remains the quintessential element of our being.

In times past, movement meant survival. Those not able to move, or unable to move rapidly enough, often met with injury or death. While we no longer have to escape from predators (except on rare occasions), our ability to move can serve us well in avoiding problems that confront us (e.g., dodging an oncoming vehicle). Limited movement, such as when a person is bedridden or elects a sedentary lifestyle, can contribute to deleterious health effects such as cardiovascular disease, diabetes, and cancer. Thus our inability to move or the choice to limit movement may contribute, either directly or indirectly, to our susceptibility to musculoskeletal injury.

In mechanical terms there are two basic forms of movement: (1) *linear motion*, in which a body moves along either a straight line (rectilinear motion) or a curved line (curvilinear motion), and (2) *angular* or *rotational motion*, in which the body rotates about a fixed line (axis of rotation; figure 3.1). While there are theoretically an infinite number of axes about which a body can rotate, only a few are of interest in discussing movement of human body segments (figure 3.2).

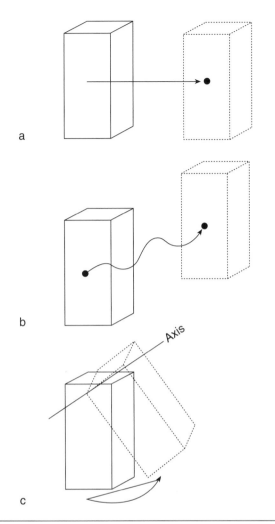

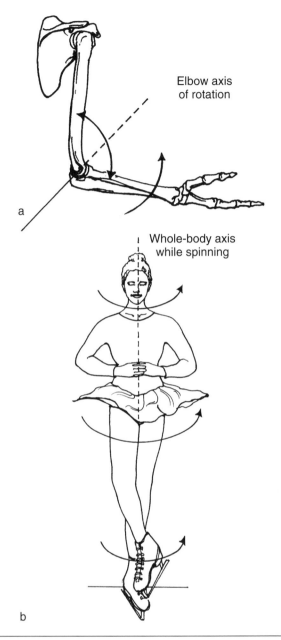

Figure 3.1 Linear and angular motion. (*a*) Rectilinear (straight line) motion. (*b*) Curvilinear motion. (*c*) Angular (rotational) motion.

Figure 3.2 Examples of anatomical axes of rotation. (*a*) Elbow flexion and extension about the elbow's axis of rotation. (*b*) Ice skater's whole body rotating about a longitudinal (vertical) axis.

Many of the movements performed by living organisms are a combination of both linear and angular motion. Consider, for example, the movement of a person's thigh during walking. There is linear motion of the entire thigh in a forward direction combined with angular motion of the thigh as it rotates about the hip joint axis in alternating phases of flexion and extension. The movement of an inanimate object can also exhibit combined motion. The flight of a basketball shot toward the rim possesses both linear motion (the curved path, or arc, of the ball) and angular motion (the backspin of the ball). As we explore the many mechanical concepts in this chapter, the notions of linear and angular motion recur often. What will emerge is an appreciation for the vast variety of movement patterns produced by this combination of two simple movement forms.

Human movement can be viewed from several perspectives. One perspective considers whether mechanical factors that produce and control movement work inside the body (*internal mechanics*) or affect the body from without (*external mechanics*). Examples of internal mechanical factors include the forces produced by muscle action and the stability provided by ligaments surrounding joints. External mechanical factors include gravity and other external forces, such as a foot striking the ground or a falling brick impacting on the top of one's head.

Another important perspective on movement involves the difference between describing a movement itself and identifying the forces involved in producing or controlling the movement. The description of movement without regard to the forces involved is known as kinematics. The assessment of movement with respect to the forces involved is called kinetics.

Kinematics

Kinematics involves five primary variables: (1) temporal characteristics of movement, (2) position or location, (3) displacement (describing what movement has occurred), (4) velocity (a measure of how fast something has moved), and (5) acceleration (an indicator of how quickly the velocity has changed). The last four variables (position, displacement, velocity, and acceleration) each can be expressed in linear or angular form, giving rise to the general descriptors of linear kinematics and angular kinematics. Keep in mind that displacement, velocity, and acceleration are all *vector* measurements, which have both magnitude and direction.

We can further assess kinematics according to whether the motion is viewed two-dimensionally (planar kinematics) or three-dimensionally (spatial kinematics). The essential terminology and formulations for planar kinematics are described in the following sections and summarized in figure 3.3.

Time

The first variable, time, provides a measure of the duration of a particular event. Noting that during a single step a person's right foot is in contact with the ground for 450 ms would be an example of a temporal kinematic measure. The duration (Δt) of force application associated with acute musculoskeletal injuries is quite short and typically lasts only a fraction of a second. This short time interval necessarily results in high loading rates. As we will see later, loading rate is an important factor in determining a tissue's mechanical response to loading.

Position

The position of a person's whole body, or a segment of the body, plays a critical role in determining the likelihood of injury. Forces applied to an arm that is hyperextended and externally rotated will cause a different injury pattern than if the arm was flexed and internally rotated at the moment of force application. Similarly, a force applied to the top of one's head when the neck is flexed will result in different injuries than if the same force is applied to the head while the neck is extended.

The position of a body segment can be described qualitatively (e.g., arm is abducted) or quantitatively (e.g., forearm is positioned with the elbow flexed 45°). The position of a specific point, or landmark, on the body can be specified quantitatively using either Cartesian (x,y) coordinates or polar (r,θ) coordinates (see figure 3.3).

Displacement

When a body moves from one location to another we measure this displacement as the straight-line distance from the starting position to the ending position. This is termed the linear displacement (Δd). A body rotating about an axis experiences angular displacement ($\Delta\theta$), which is measured as the number of degrees (or radians) of rotation (e.g., the knee flexed through an angular displacement of 35°). A direct relation exists between the linear and angular measures of displacement (figure 3.4a).

Velocity

Velocity is a measure of the time rate of displacement. The average linear velocity (v) is given by the quotient of linear displacement (Δd) divided by Δt. Angular velocity (ω) is calculated by dividing the angular displacement ($\Delta\theta$) by the change in time (Δt). A direct relation exists between the linear and angular measures of velocity (figure 3.4b).

In common usage, the terms *velocity* and *speed* often are used interchangeably. In mechanical terms, however, they have distinct—though related—meanings. Velocity is a vector quantity (magnitude and direction), while speed is a scalar (magnitude only) measure. The speed of a runner might be 5 m·s⁻¹. To transform the movement measure to velocity, we must indicate the running direction, for example, 5 m·s⁻¹ due north.

Acceleration

Acceleration measures the change in a body's velocity. Linear acceleration is measured as the change in linear velocity (Δv) divided by the change in time (Δt). Similarly, angular acceleration is the change in angular velocity ($\Delta\omega$) divided by change in time (Δt). As was the case with linear and angular velocity, a

	Linear		Angular	
	Symbol	Formula or relation	Symbol	Formula or relation
Time	t	$t_2 - t_1 = \Delta t$	t	$t_2 - t_1 = \Delta t$
Position	(x, y)	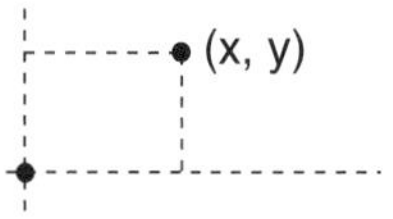	(r, θ)	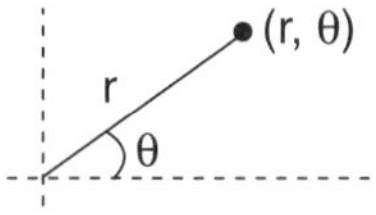
Displacement (x-direction only)	d	$d = x_2 - x_1$ $x_1 \bullet \xrightarrow[d]{} \bullet x_2$	θ	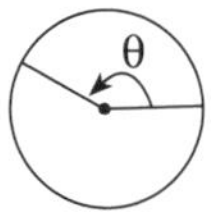
Average velocity	$\bar{v}$	$\bar{v} = \dfrac{d_2 - d_1}{t_2 - t_1} = \dfrac{\Delta d}{\Delta t}$	$\bar{\omega}$	$\bar{\omega} = \dfrac{\theta_2 - \theta_1}{t_2 - t_1} = \dfrac{\Delta \theta}{\Delta t}$
Instantaneous velocity	v	$v = \dfrac{dx}{dt} = \dot{x}$	ω	$\omega = \dfrac{d\theta}{dt} = \dot{\theta}$
Average acceleration	$\bar{a}$	$\bar{a} = \dfrac{v_2 - v_1}{t_2 - t_1} = \dfrac{\Delta v}{\Delta t}$	$\bar{\alpha}$	$\bar{\alpha} = \dfrac{\omega_2 - \omega_1}{t_2 - t_1} = \dfrac{\Delta \omega}{\Delta t}$
Instantaneous acceleration	a	$\bar{a} = \dfrac{dv}{dt} = \ddot{x}$	α	$\alpha = \dfrac{d\omega}{dt} = \ddot{\theta}$

Figure 3.3 Terminology and formulas for planar kinematics. Standard units: s (time); m (linear displacement); rad or deg (angular displacement); m·s⁻¹ (linear velocity); rad·s⁻¹ or deg·s⁻¹ (angular velocity); m·s⁻² (linear acceleration); rad·s⁻² or deg·s⁻² (angular acceleration).

direct relation exists between the linear and angular measures of acceleration (figure 3.4c). Many musculoskeletal injuries are acceleration related. Rapid acceleration or deceleration of the head, for example, can result in concussive injury to the brain.

Linear acceleration often is expressed in units of g's, where one g is the acceleration created by the earth's gravitational pull (9.81 m·s⁻²). Thus, a boxer's head that experiences 5 g's would be experiencing a force that would accelerate the head at five times the acceleration caused by the force of gravity.

Kinetics

Description is an important first step in analyzing any movement. Kinematic analyses, however, are limited to describing the spatial geometry of move-

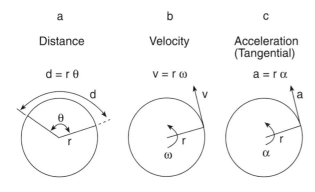

Figure 3.4 Relation between linear and angular measures. (*a*) Linear distance (=*d*) moved along the circumference of a circle (radius = *r*) equals *r*θ. (*b*) Linear velocity (=*v*) of a point on the circumference of a circle equals *r*ω. (*c*) Linear tangential acceleration (=*a*) of a point on the circumference of a circle equals *r*α. (Note: Angular measurements of θ, ω, and α in these equations must be expressed in units of radians [rad], rad·s⁻¹, and rad·s⁻², respectively).

ment without investigating the forces involved. Since force is a causal agent in movement, *kinetics* (the study of forces and their effects) is an area worthy of our consideration. The following force-related concepts are interrelated, and to consider each of them in isolation limits their applicability and our ability to analyze injury biomechanics.

Mass and Inertia

Mass is the quantity of matter and in SI units (Système international d'unités) is measured in kilograms (kg). Common sense suggests that the greater the mass, the more difficult it is to move. *Inertia*, or this resistance to being moved linearly, is defined as the property of matter by which it remains at rest or in uniform motion in a straight line (i.e., constant velocity). In order to move linearly an object that is at rest, we must overcome its inertia, or its tendency to stay where it is. An analogous concept known as the *moment of inertia* applies to angular movement. Discussion of moment of inertia requires an understanding of several other concepts, so it will be postponed until later.

Force

Force is the most fundamental element in injuries. Force is defined as the mechanical action or effect applied to a body that tends to produce acceleration. The standard unit of force is the newton (N),

defined as the force required to accelerate a 1-kg mass at 1 m per second per second in the direction of the force (1 N = 1 kg·m·s⁻²).

In preparation for a more general discussion of force, we introduce the concept of an *idealized force vector.* If we consider, for example, the forces acting on the head of the femur while a person assumes a standing posture, an infinite number of separate force vectors could be distributed over the articular surface. To analyze the effect of all these vectors would be a time-consuming task. We can create a single force vector (idealized force vector) that represents the net effect of all the other vectors, essentially idealizing the situation through simplification. What is lost in information describing the distribution of forces is gained by creating a model with a single vector from which calculations and evaluations are made. This notion of an idealized force vector is useful in many situations, as you will see shortly.

Forces inherent to injury analysis are those that act in or upon the human body. Among these are gravity (a downward force tending to accelerate objects at 9.81 m·s⁻²); the impact of the feet, hands, or body with the ground; objects impacting on the body (e.g., thrown ball, bullet); musculotendinous forces; ligament forces acting at joints; and compressive forces exerted on long bones of the lower extremities.

In injury-causing situations, seven factors combine to determine the nature of the injury, the tissue(s) injured, and the severity of the injury:

- Magnitude (How much force is applied?)
- Location (Where on the body or structure is the force applied?)
- Direction (Where is the force directed?)
- Duration (Over what time interval is the force applied?)
- Frequency (How often is the force applied?)
- Variability (Is the magnitude of the force constant or variable over the application interval?)
- Rate (How quickly is the force applied?)

Rarely does a single force act in isolation. Much more likely is the case in which multiple forces are involved. To aid in the analysis, it is useful to categorize multiple forces as force systems. Different types of force systems include linear, parallel, concurrent, and general force systems (figure 3.5, a-d). A special case of force application is a force

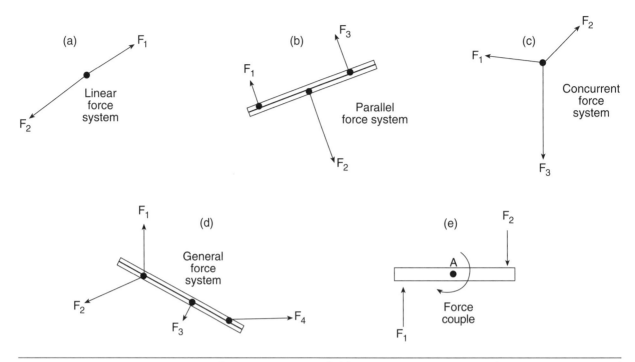

Figure 3.5 Force systems. (*a*) Linear force system. (*b*) Parallel force system. (*c*) Concurrent force system. (*d*) General force system, the designation given to a force system that does not fall under one of the classifications *a* through *c*. (*e*) Force couple; parallel and oppositely directed forces F_1 and F_2 cause rotation about axis *A*.

couple, which is composed of two oppositely directed parallel forces that tend to create rotation about an axis (figure 3.5e).

The engineering approach uses a free-body diagram for biomechanical analysis of a force system. This is simply a graphical representation of all the forces acting in the system. Figure 3.6 depicts a free-body diagram for a simple biomechanical application. Note that the effect of gravity is represented as a single vector, another example of an idealized force vector. In actuality, gravity acts upon each small element of body mass.

Center of Mass and Center of Gravity

In developing an idealized force vector, many vectors are reduced to a single one. A similar process can be applied to the mass of a body by reducing its distributed mass to a single point (point mass) that represents the entire body. Again, this type of simplification will facilitate analysis, but with some loss of information. The word *body* is taken to mean any collection of matter. It may refer to the entire human body or any collected mass (e.g., a body segment such as the thigh or upper arm, or a block of wood).

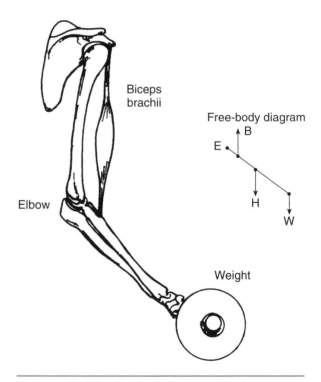

Figure 3.6 The free-body diagram (*right*) represents the forces acting on the upper extremity while holding a weight in the hand. Gravity creates force vectors for the weight (*W*) and the forearm/hand (*H*). The biceps brachii creates a muscle force represented by the vector *B*.

For any body, there exists a point, known as the *center of mass* or *center of gravity*, at which, if we concentrated the body's mass into a point mass, this point mass would move exactly the same as the body would in its distributed state. Even though there is a technical distinction between the center of gravity and the center of mass of a body, in practical terms they are located at the same point, and we therefore use the terms interchangeably.

The center of mass alternatively may be defined as the point about which a body's mass is equally distributed, acting as a balance point, as shown in figure 3.7a. It is important to realize that while the center of mass is often located within the body's boundaries (figure 3.7b), this may not always be the case (figure 3.7c).

Pressure

Since many injuries occur as a result of one object impacting on another, it is important to know how the force of impact is distributed on the surface being contacted. A sharp object contacting the skin with 300 N of force will likely have a different effect than a blunt object impacting the skin with a similar force. A general principle of injury mechanics suggests that as the area of force application is increased, the likelihood of injury decreases.

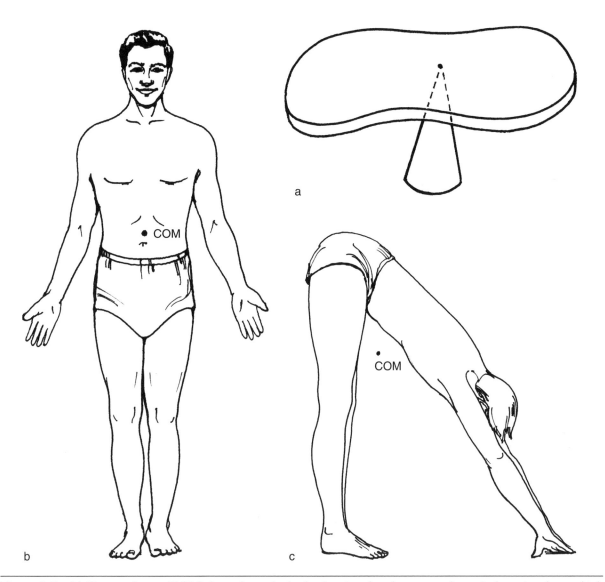

Figure 3.7   (*a*) Center of mass (COM) for an irregular body, showing that the center of mass is the point about which the body's mass is equally distributed as demonstrated by the fact that the body is able to balance on the point of a cone placed at the center of mass. (*b*) Center of mass of the human body in anatomical position. (*c*) Center of mass located outside of the body when the body assumes a piked position, as during a gymnastic maneuver or dive.

The measure of force and its distribution is *pressure*, defined as the total applied force divided by the area over which the force is applied. In equation form,

$$p = F/A \qquad (3.1)$$

where p = pressure, F = applied force, and A = area of contact. The standard unit of pressure, the pascal (Pa), is equal to a 1-N force applied to an area 1 m square (1 Pa = 1 N·m⁻²).

Moment of Force (Torque)

In the case of linear motion, force is the mechanical agent creating and controlling movement. For angular motion the agent is known as *torque* (*T*), *moment of force*, or *moment* (*M*), defined as the effect of a force that tends to cause rotation or twisting about an axis of rotation (figure 3.8).

The mathematical definition of torque and moment of force is the same; however, there is a technical difference. Torque typically refers to the twisting movement created by a force (figure 3.9a), whereas moment is related to the bending action of a force (figure 3.9b). Despite this difference, the two terms are often used interchangeably.

The magnitude of a torque is equal to the applied force times the shortest (perpendicular) distance from the axis of rotation to the line of force action. This perpendicular distance is known as the *moment arm*, *torque arm*, or *lever arm*. For a force acting at a right angle to the body being rotated, the moment arm is the distance d (figure 3.10a), and the magnitude of the moment (M) is given by this equation:

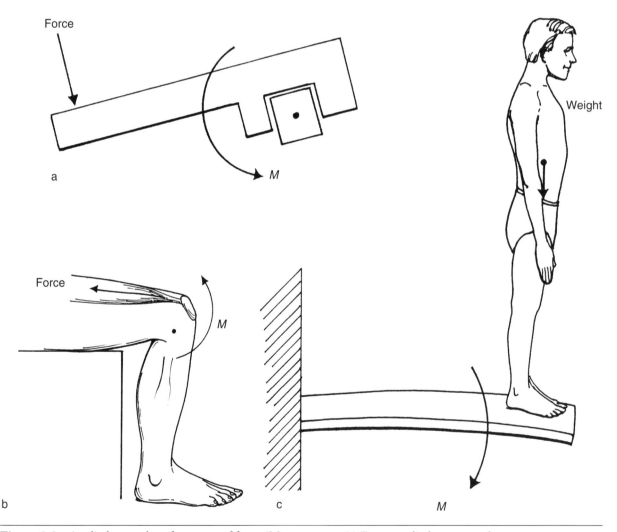

Figure 3.8 Applied examples of moment of force (M), or torque. (*a*) Force applied to a wrench creates a moment to turn a nut on a bolt. (*b*) Quadriceps muscle group creates an extensor moment about the knee joint axis. (*c*) The body weight of a diver creates a moment that bends the diving board.

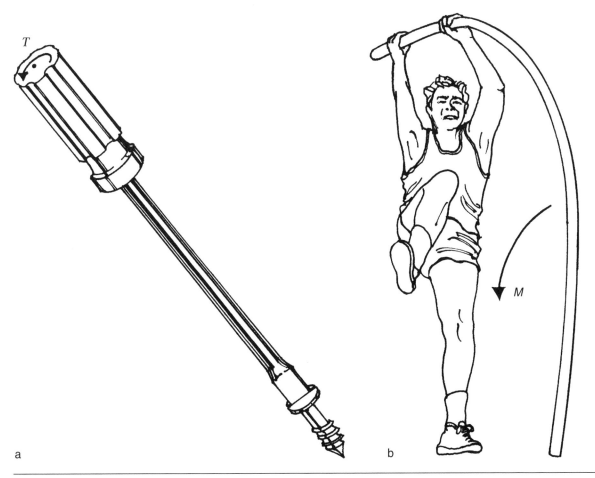

a   b

Figure 3.9 (*a*) Torque (*T*) shown by the twisting action of a screwdriver. (*b*) Moment of force (*M*) shown as the bending effect of a force on a vaulter's pole.

$$M = F \cdot d \qquad (3.2)$$

If the force *F* in figure 3.10a was 175 N, for example, and it was acting at a distance *d* of 1.2 m from the axis, the moment (torque) created would equal $F \cdot d$, or $M = 175 \text{ N} \cdot 1.2 \text{ m} = 210 \text{ N·m}$.

In cases where the force is not acting perpendicularly to the segment, the moment arm is smaller and is calculated using the appropriate trigonometric function as shown in figure 3.10b. The magnitude of the moment (*M*) in this case is

$$M = F \cdot d \cdot \sin(\beta) \quad \text{or} \quad M = F \cdot d \cdot \cos(\theta)$$
$$(3.3)$$

If the same 175-N force as in the preceding example was acting at an angle $\beta = 35°$ (as shown in figure 3.10b), the moment arm would be, $d' = d \cdot \sin(\beta) = 1.2 \text{ m} \cdot 0.574 = 0.688 \text{ m}$. The moment created now is $M = F \cdot d' = 175 \text{ N} \cdot 0.688 \text{ m} = 120.4$ N·m.

Examples of biomechanical application of torque are the biceps creating a flexion moment about the elbow, the torque created by a weighted lower leg during a knee extension exercise, and the torsional loading of the tibia in a skiing fall (figure 3.11). The standard unit of moment measurement comes from the product of the two terms: force (N) times moment arm (m). The resulting unit is a newton-meter (N·m).

Closer examination of the moment equation (3.2) reveals several general principles that are important when applying torque concepts to injury biomechanics. First, there is an obvious interaction between the force and the moment arm that directly affects the magnitude of the applied torque. To increase the moment, we have the option of (1) increasing the force while holding the moment arm constant, (2) increasing the moment arm while holding the force constant, (3) increasing both the force and the moment arm, (4) decreasing the force while increasing the moment

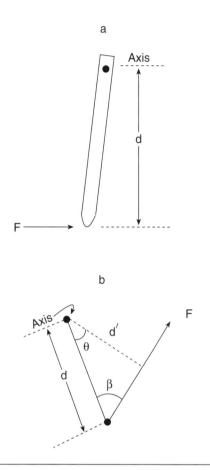

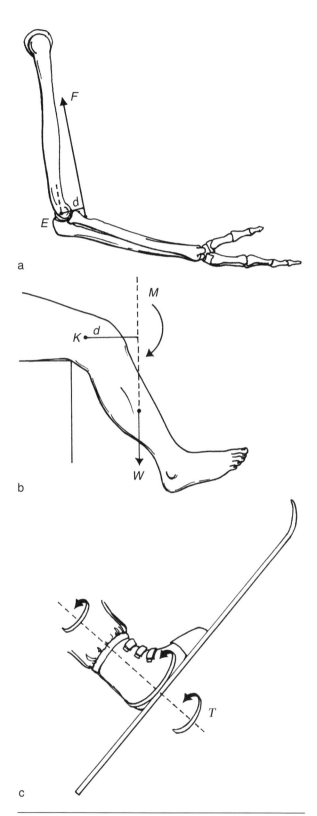

Figure 3.10 Moment (torque) arm. (*a*) When the force acts perpendicularly to the segment, the moment arm is the distance *d*. The moment is given by eq. (3.2). (*b*) When the force acts at an angle (*β*) to the segment of length *d*, the moment arm $d' = d \cdot \sin(\beta)$. The moment in this case is given by eq. (3.3).

arm more than proportionally so that the net effect is an increase in moment, or (5) decreasing the moment arm while increasing the force more than proportionally so that the net effect is again an increase in moment. To decrease the moment, we have only to reverse the logic in each of the five cases.

A second moment-related concept, while simple in statement, is powerful in its application. That is, when a force is applied through the axis of rotation, no moment is produced. This concept follows directly from the moment equation, $M = F \cdot d$, where d = moment arm. If the force passes through the axis, the moment arm is zero, hence no moment is produced. This creates the potential for a situation in which tissues are exposed to extremely high forces, but with no moment created. Compressive forces acting through the center of a vertebral body, for example, will cause no

Figure 3.11 Biomechanical examples of torque. (*a*) Flexor moment created by the biceps brachii acting at the elbow. (*b*) Moment created about the knee by gravity acting on the lower leg during a knee extension exercise. (*c*) Torque applied to a skier's leg by the twisting of the ski and boot system.

vertebral rotation and will increase the likelihood of a compressive burst fracture.

In many instances, only a portion of the applied force is involved in producing a moment. This third moment concept can be seen in the two examples depicted in figure 3.12. In the first situation (figure 3.12a), the weight attached to the foot (F_w) can be broken down into two force components: F_r, which causes rotation about the knee joint axis and is termed the rotatory component of force, and F_d, whose line of action passes through the joint axis and hence contributes nothing to the moment about the knee. F_d acts to pull the segment away from the joint axis and is thus referred to as a distraction, dislocating, or destabilizing component of force.

Similarly, in figure 3.12b the biceps force (F_b) has a rotatory component (F_r). In contrast to the previous example, however, the component (F_s) passing through the axis is directed toward the axis and hence is called a stabilizing component of force.

A fourth moment concept arises because in most real situations more than one moment is being applied to the system. The system's response is based on the net moment, or the result of adding together all the moments acting about the axis. An example of this is seen in a simple glenohumeral abduction exercise (figure 3.13). Gravity, acting on the arm and the dumbbell, creates a moment about the glenohumeral axis of rotation that tends to adduct the arm. The magnitude of this moment (M_1) is given by

$$M_1 = W_a \cdot d_a + W_b \cdot d_b \qquad (3.4)$$

where W_a = weight of the arm and hand, d_a = moment arm (distance from the glenohumeral axis of rotation to the arm's center of gravity), W_b = weight of the dumbbell, and d_b = moment arm (distance from axis to dumbbell's center of gravity). By convention, moments tending to create clockwise rotation are designated as negative (–) moments. Moments in the counterclockwise direction are positive (+). M_1 is therefore a negative moment.

If this was the only moment, the arm would immediately adduct under the effect of gravity. However, the abductor muscles acting about the glenohumeral joint create a moment that acts in the opposite direction and is termed a *countermoment* (M_2), or *countertorque*. The countermoment is a positive moment and will tend to abduct the arm. The movement that results depends on the relative magnitudes of M_1 and M_2. By adding the two moments together, we create a *net moment* (M_{net}):

$$M_{net} = M_1 + M_2 \qquad (3.5)$$

In this example we have three possible scenarios: (1) If M_1 is equal to M_2, then M_{net} = 0, and the arm remains in its horizontal position; (2) if $M_1 > M_2$, then $M_{net} < 0$, and the arm will fall (adduct); (3) if $M_1 < M_2$, then $M_{net} > 0$, and the arm will rise (abduct). The resulting movement thus depends on the net moment acting at the joint about which the movement occurs.

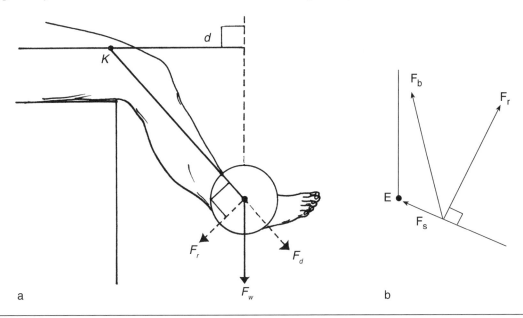

Figure 3.12   Components of force. (*a*) Rotational (F_r) and destabilizing (F_d) force components created by a weight (F_w) secured to the foot of a person performing a leg extension exercise about the knee joint axis (K). (*b*) Rotational (F_r) and stabilizing (F_s) force components created by the biceps brachii (F_b) during elbow flexion about the elbow axis (E).

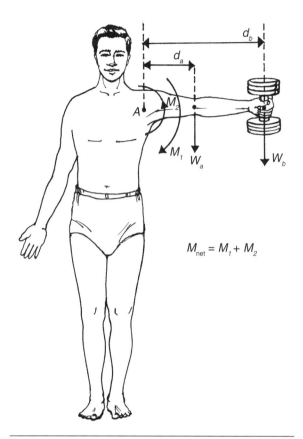

$$M_{net} = M_1 + M_2$$

Figure 3.13   Net joint moment. The net moment (M_{net}) of the combined moments created by $M_1 + M_2$. The weight of the arm (W_a) and dumbbell (W_b) combine to create an adductor moment (M_1) acting about the glenohumeral joint axis A. The force of the glenohumeral abductor muscles creates an abductor moment (M_2) to counteract M_1. (Note that M_1 acts in a clockwise direction and thus creates a negative moment. Conversely, M_2 acts counterclockwise and is positive). See text for detailed explanation.

Mass Moment of Inertia

A body at rest and with a fixed axis (e.g., a pendulum) will resist being moved rotationally, just as a body that is already rotating at a constant angular velocity (ω) will tend to maintain that angular velocity and will resist a change in velocity. The measure of this resistance to change of state is termed *mass moment of inertia* (I). Recall that the magnitude of resistance in the case of linear movement was determined by the mass of the object. In the case of angular movement, the magnitude of the resistance is determined by the mass and the mass's location with respect to the axis of rotation. For a single-point mass, the mass moment of inertia is defined as

$$I = m \cdot r^2 \qquad (3.6)$$

where m = mass of the body and r = distance from the axis of rotation to the point mass (figure 3.14). For a distributed mass, such as a limb segment, the mass moment of inertia is

$$I = \int m_i \cdot r_i^2 \qquad (3.7)$$

where m_i = mass of the ith point mass and r_i = distance of the ith point mass from the axis of rotation. As the mass is moved farther from the axis, the resistance, or mass moment of inertia, increases as a function of the square of the distance moved.

Newton's Laws of Motion

Among Sir Isaac Newton's (1642-1727) many scientific contributions, perhaps most profound and

Hip Joint Moments

Hip injuries are an unfortunate but common injury, especially in the elderly. Structural features of the hip combined with osteoporosis (low-density bone) provide a potent tandem that increases one's risk of hip fracture. Among the structural features is the relation of the femoral neck and head to the long axis of the femur. Normally, the angle between the long axis and the neck is about 120°. Abnormal angles can alter the mechanical loading of the proximal femur. In *coxa vara*, the angle is less than normal. The contrasting condition, *coxa valga*, has an angle greater than normal. When the bone is loaded, as during the stance phase of gait, compressive forces act on the femoral head. Because these forces are offset from the long axis of the femoral diaphysis, a cantilever bending occurs. This produces a moment about an axis denoted as A in figure 3B.1. In coxa vara, the moment arm (d_r) is longer than in the

(continued)

(continued)

normal condition (d_n). For a given force (F), the coxa vara moment (M_r) is greater than normal (M_n). In contrast, the deviation in coxa valga results in a shorter moment arm ($d_l < d_n$) and hence a smaller moment ($M_r > M_n > M_l$). Larger moments create greater stresses in the bony tissue. If there is an area of relative weakness, as in an osteoporotic patient, the likelihood of bone fracture increases. With this potential mechanism of injury, an older woman, for example, on occasion may "break her hip and fall," instead of the more common case in which she "falls and breaks her hip."

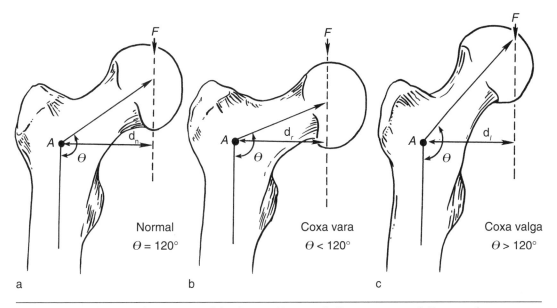

Figure 3B.1 Structural geometry of the femur: (*a*) normal, (*b*) coxa vara, and (*c*) coxa valga.

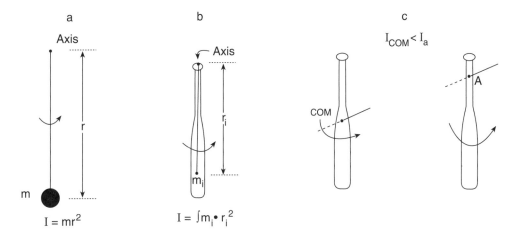

Figure 3.14 Moment of inertia. (*a*) Moment of inertia (*I*) for a point mass equals the product of the mass (*m*) and the square of the distance (*r*) from the axis to the mass [eq. (3.6)]. (*b*) A baseball bat illustrates a distributed mass with an axis shown in the handle end of the bat. The moment of inertia for a distributed mass is given by eq. (3.7). (*c*) The moment of inertia (I_{COM}) of any body (a baseball bat as shown) about an axis through its center of mass is less than the moment of inertia (I_A) for the same body about an axis at point *A* because more of the mass is farther away from the axis in the second case.

enduring are his laws of motion, which form the basis for classical mechanics.

- First law of motion: A body at rest or in uniform linear motion (moving in a straight line at a constant velocity) will tend to remain at rest or in uniform motion, unless acted upon by an external force. A body at rest or in uniform angular motion (moving about an axis at a constant angular velocity) will tend to remain at rest or in uniform motion, unless acted upon by an external torque.

- Second law of motion: A force acting on a body will produce an acceleration proportional to the force, or mathematically, $F = m \cdot a$. Angularly, a torque (T) applied to a body will produce an angular acceleration proportional to the torque, or mathematically, $T = I \cdot \alpha$ (where I = mass moment of inertia; α = angular acceleration).

- Third law of motion: For every action there is an equal and opposite reaction.

Several examples show how these laws play a role in determining the mechanisms of performance and injury (figure 3.15). A cervical whiplash mechanism during frontal impact (figure 3.15a) is simply a consequence of the first law of motion. Just prior to impact, the automobile and its seat-belted and shoulder-harnessed driver are moving at a constant velocity. At impact, the outside force abruptly decelerates the vehicle and the belted occupant's body. However, for a brief interval the head obeys the first law of motion and continues in its uniform motion (straight ahead). Resistance forces provided by neck structures rapidly decelerate the head, causing a violent flexion motion at the cervical spine. The head then rebounds into hyperextension. This flexion-extension pattern is typical of many whiplash injuries and is explained by Newton's first law.

In the second example (figure 3.15b), the weight lifter must exert considerable force in order to accelerate the bar upward. The second law of mo-

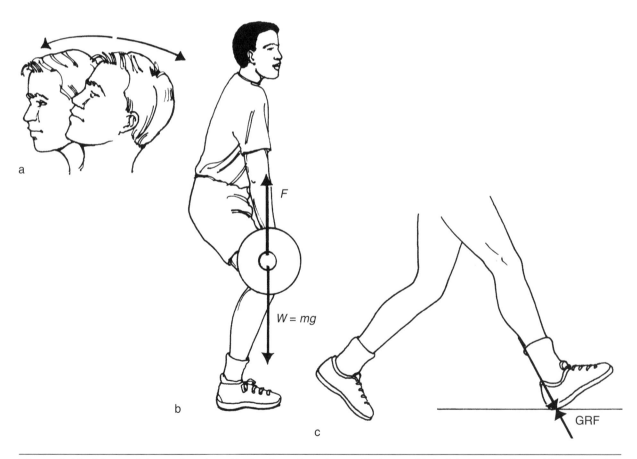

Figure 3.15   Newton's laws of motion. (*a*) First law of motion applied to a whiplash injury. (*b*) Second law of motion involved during a weight-lifting movement. F = force applied by weight lifter; W = weight; m = mass; g = acceleration due to gravity. (*c*) Third law of motion exemplified by the ground reaction force (GRF) created when a runner's foot strikes the ground.

tion determines the magnitude of the acceleration in response to the applied force, $F = m \cdot a$. More detailed application of the laws of motion allows us to estimate the forces acting at various joints throughout the body. If these forces exceed the ability of the body's structures to tolerate load, injury occurs.

In the third example (figure 3.15c), the feet of a marathon runner contact the ground many thousands of times. At each contact, Newton's third law comes into play. The force that the foot exerts on the ground is equally and oppositely resisted by the ground, giving rise to the term *ground reaction force* (GRF) to describe the forces acting on the foot by the ground. Increasing magnitude and frequency of force application increases the chances of injury, perhaps as a stress fracture.

Equilibrium

The word *equilibrium* implies a balanced condition. From a mechanical standpoint, equilibrium exists when forces and moments are balanced. In general, equilibrium exists for a body at rest or for one moving with constant linear and angular velocities; the net force and net moment acting on the body are both equal to zero. A body at rest is in a state called *static equilibrium*. In spatial terms (three-dimensional space), for a body in static equilibrium the following equations must be satisfied:

$$\Sigma F_x = 0 \qquad \Sigma F_y = 0 \qquad \Sigma F_z = 0 \qquad (3.8)$$

$$\Sigma M_x = 0 \qquad \Sigma M_y = 0 \qquad \Sigma M_z = 0 \qquad (3.9)$$

where F_x, F_y, and F_z are the forces in the x, y, and z directions, respectively, and M_x, M_y, and M_z are the moments about the x, y, and z axes, respectively.

Bodies in motion and experiencing external forces are in dynamic equilibrium, and must adhere to the following equations:

$$\Sigma F_x = m \cdot a_x \qquad \Sigma F_y = m \cdot a_y \qquad \Sigma F_z = m \cdot a_z \qquad (3.10)$$

$$\Sigma M_x = I_x \cdot \alpha_x \qquad \Sigma M_y = I_y \cdot \alpha_y \qquad \Sigma M_z = I_z \cdot \alpha_z \qquad (3.11)$$

where a_x, a_y, and a_z are the linear accelerations of the center of mass in the x, y, and z directions, respectively, and α_x, α_y, and α_z are the angular accelerations about the x, y, and z axes, respectively.

Work and Power

The term *work* is used in many ways, referring in various contexts to physical labor, physiological energy expenditure, or an employment situation. In mechanical terms, work has a specific meaning. Mechanical work is performed by a force acting through a displacement in the direction of the force. By definition, linear work (W) is equal to the product of force (F) and the displacement (d) through which the body is moved (figure 3.16a).

$$W = F \cdot d \qquad (3.12)$$

The standard (SI) unit of work is the joule (1 J = 1 N·m). If the force is not acting in the direction of motion (figure 3.16b), then only the component of force in that direction is used in calculating the work done. Figure 3.16b shows a force (F) at an angle (β) above the horizontal. In this case, the work performed is

$$W = F \cdot d \cdot \cos(\beta) \qquad (3.13)$$

where F = applied force, d = displacement, and β = angle of force above the horizontal.

In the example depicted in figure 3.16c, the work performed in lifting the barbell from point A to point B is equal to the product of the barbell's weight (W_b) and the displacement from A to B (d_{AB}). If, for example, the barbell weighed 800 N and was lifted 0.5 m, the work done would be 400 J.

In the previous example, the force was assumed constant. In real-world situations, that often is not the case. Determination of work done by a varying force becomes more involved, since it must be calculated at successive intervals. The equation becomes

$$W = \int F_x \cdot dx \qquad (3.14)$$

The calculation of work is often insufficient to completely describe the mechanics of a body's movement. In many cases, the rate of work is important. The rate of work is termed *power* (P), and linear power is defined as the rate at which work is done:

$$P = W/\Delta t \qquad (3.15)$$

where W = work performed and Δt = change in time, or the time interval over which the work was done. Power is expressed in units of watts (1 W = 1 J·s^{-1}). In the previous barbell example, a person lifting the

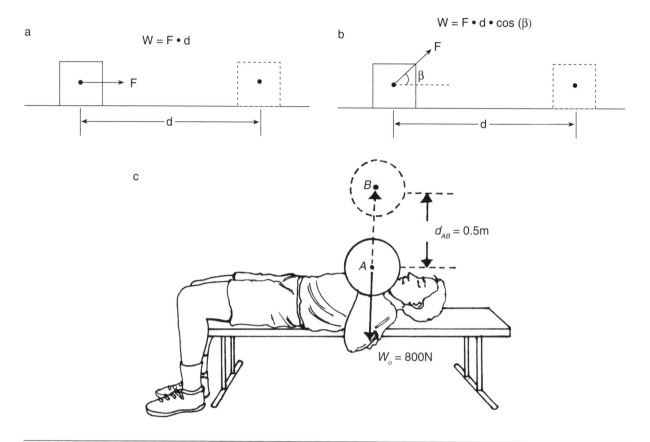

Figure 3.16   Mechanical work. (*a*) Linear work (*W*) as the product of force (*F*) and distance (*d*) in the case where the entire force acts in the direction of movement [eq. (3.12)]. (*b*) Linear work performed when only part of the force acts in the direction of movement [eq. (3.13)]. In the case shown, the force (*F*) is directed at an angle *β* above the horizontal. (*c*) A weight lifter who bench-presses 800 N through a distance of 0.5 m performs 400 J of work.

800-N barbell 0.5 m in 2 s would perform 400 J of work with a power of 200 W, while a lift done in 0.5 s would have a power of 800 W. In general, a given amount of work performed in a shorter time will have a greater power output.

Alternatively, power may be expressed as the product of force and velocity:

$$P = F \cdot v \qquad (3.16)$$

Energy

In discussing the epidemiology of injury, Robertson (1992) concludes that "mechanical energy accounts for the vast majority of severe injury." As the primary agent of injury, energy is critical to an understanding of injury biomechanics. Energy, or the capacity or ability to perform work, can assume many forms, including thermal, chemical, nuclear, electromagnetic, and mechanical. While each form of energy has the potential to cause injury, me-

chanical energy is the one most frequently involved.

The mechanical energy of a body can be classified according to its kinetic energy (motion) or its potential energy (position or deformation). Kinetic energy can be either linear or angular. These two types of kinetic energy are defined, respectively, as

$$E_k = 0.5 \cdot m \cdot v^2 \qquad E_{\angle k} = 0.5 \cdot I \cdot \omega^2 \quad (3.17)$$

where m = mass, v = linear velocity of the center of mass, I = mass moment of inertia, and ω = angular velocity.

Potential energy can take two forms. The gravitational form (potential energy of position) measures the potential to perform work as a function of the height a body is elevated above some reference level, most typically the ground. The equation describing gravitational potential energy is

$$E_p = m \cdot g \cdot h \qquad (3.18)$$

where m = mass, g = gravitational acceleration (9.81 m·s^{-2}), h = height in meters above the reference level.

The second form of potential energy is deformational (strain) energy that is stored in a body by virtue of its deformation. Common examples of strain energy include a stretched rubber band, a pole vaulter's bent pole, and a drawn bow prior to arrow release. The equation describing the amount of stored energy is dependent on the material properties of the deformable body. No single equation describes the strain energy of all bodies.

Biomechanists studying whole-body or limb segment movement dynamics often make the assumption that each of the body's segments is a rigid (i.e., nondeformable) body. When this simplifying assumption is made, there is no strain energy component in the system. In these cases, the total mechanical energy is simply the sum of the linear kinetic, angular kinetic, and positional potential energies. Consider, for example, a soccer player swinging his or her leg to kick the ball. Each of the lower-limb segments (thigh, shank, foot) possesses a continuously changing total mechanical energy. Let's focus on the shank (lower leg) to illustrate how we would calculate the total mechanical energy of a segment at a given instant. Assume that the shank has a mass of 2.6 kg and a mass moment of inertia (I) of 0.04 kg·m^2, at one point in time is rotating with an angular velocity of 7.0 rad·s^{-1}, has a center of mass (COM) that is moving at a linear velocity of 3.5 m·s^{-1}, and is positioned at a height of 0.38 m above the ground.

The total mechanical energy (TME) = linear kinetic energy + angular kinetic energy + positional potential energy. Using eqs. (3.17) and (3.18), this TME equation becomes

$$\text{TME} = E_k + E_{\angle k} + E_p = (0.5 \cdot m \cdot v^2)$$
$$+ (0.5 \cdot I \cdot \omega^2) + (m \cdot g \cdot h) \quad (3.18b)$$

where m = mass of the shank, v = linear velocity of the shank's COM, I = mass moment of inertia, ω = angular velocity, g = 9.81 m·s^{-2}, and h = height of the shank's COM. By substituting the values given, the TME for the shank at this instant is 26.6 J. Similar calculations done at successive points in time create an energy profile for the shank as a function of time and show how the energy increases and decreases (i.e., flows) throughout the kick. The same analysis can be done for the thigh and foot to create a complete mechanical energy profile of the lower extremity during a kick, or any other activity.

Momentum

In a general sense, momentum is a "quantity of motion." An old adage proffers that the bigger they are, the harder they fall. With respect to injury, this maxim is more accurately stated as the bigger and faster they are, the harder they hit. This revised maxim embodies the concept of momentum. In mechanical terms, linear momentum (p) is defined as

$$p = m \cdot v \quad (3.19)$$

where m = mass, and v = velocity of the body's center of mass. Increasing either a body's size (mass) or speed (velocity) will increase its linear momentum.

Similarly, angular momentum (L), or the "quantity of angular motion," is defined as

$$L = I \cdot \omega \quad (3.20)$$

where I = mass moment of inertia about the center of mass, and ω = angular velocity.

Two principles governing momentum and its effect are important in assessing the effects of momentum on injury. These are conservation of momentum and transfer of momentum. Each of these principles applies to both linear and angular momentum. Conservation of momentum indicates how much of a system's momentum, or quantity of motion, is conserved and how much is lost during a given time period. The more that is conserved, the greater the potential for injury.

The companion principle, transfer of momentum, is the mechanism by which momentum from one body is transferred to another. This can take many forms in the course of human movement. Transfer during a throwing motion can happen as momentum moves from a proximal segment (e.g., upper arm) to a more distal segment (e.g., lower arm, hand) as the throw progresses. Transfer of momentum can also happen between different bodies, as in the case of a football player blocking or tackling an opponent or in an automobile crash. Transfer of momentum in these cases often results in injury, when the "quantity of motion" transferred exceeds the tolerance of the tissues in one or both of the bodies. Consider a force being applied to a particular body. When the force is applied over a very short time interval, as is often the case in force-related injuries, it is referred to as an *impulsive force*.

Collisions

In many cases musculoskeletal injuries occur as a result of one object impacting on another. In athletic contests, body-body and body-ground impacts are common. In automobile crashes, multiple impacts occur between the various parts of both vehicles and occupants. In slips and falls, an impact occurs between the person and the ground. Because of their impact characteristics, all of these situations have the potential for injury. Injury can happen when the forces applied during an impact exceed the body tissue's ability to withstand the force.

A forceful impact between two or more bodies is known as a *collision*. Collisions have relatively large impact forces acting over a relatively short time interval. In every collision the contacting bodies undergo deformation; that is, their shape (configuration) changes. In some instances the deformation is negligible (e.g., a collision between two billiard balls), while in others the deformation can be considerable (e.g., a forceful blow to a person's abdomen). The deformed body may experience a plastic deformation, an elastic deformation, or a combination of both. In a *plastic deformation*, the body's change in physical configuration is permanent. In an *elastic deformation*, the body recovers from the deformation and returns to its original configuration when the force is removed. The ability of a material to return to its original shape is termed *elasticity* and is an essential characteristic of body tissues.

The nature of the collision between two bodies depends on their relative masses and velocities (both magnitude and direction) and on the material properties of the respective bodies. In theory, collisions occur along a continuum ranging from a perfectly inelastic collision at one extreme to a perfectly elastic collision at the other. In real terms, most collisions involving the human musculoskeletal system are elastoplastic in nature. The bodies deform, sometimes permanently, and there is energy transfer and loss in the collision. The greater the energy involved, the more likely injury will occur and the more severe it will be. In a perfectly inelastic collision, the bodies stick together and move together with a common velocity after impact with no loss of energy or momentum.

In elastoplastic collisions energy is lost, and the relative postcollision velocity between the two bod-

ies is decreased. To measure this loss of separation velocity, we define the concept of coefficient of restitution (e), defined as the ratio between the relative postcollision velocity (RV_{post}) and the relative precollision velocity (RV_{pre}):

$$e = RV_{post}/RV_{pre} \qquad (3.21)$$

The coefficient of restitution can range between 0 and 1. A hard rubber ball dropped onto a hard surface would have an e value near 1, indicating little energy loss. A partially deflated basketball, in contrast, would bounce very little and would have an e value much closer to 0. The material properties of the colliding bodies will determine where on the collision continuum each impact falls.

Friction

Newton's first law tells us that bodies in motion will tend to remain in motion unless acted upon by an outside force. The force may be an abrupt one, such as a collision, or it may be a force of less magnitude and greater duration, such as the force of friction. *Friction* is defined as the resistance created as a result of two bodies being in contact with one another. It acts in a direction opposite to impending or actual movement. Resistance results from microscopic irregularities, known as asperities, on the opposing surfaces. Asperities tend to adhere to each other and efforts to move the bodies result in very small resistive (shear) forces that oppose the motion.

In the simple case of a body at rest on a surface, static friction resists movement until a force, sufficient to overcome the frictional resistance, is applied. The magnitude of this static friction (f_s) is given by

$$f_s \le \mu_s \cdot N \qquad (3.22)$$

where μ_s = the coefficient of static friction, and N = the component of the contact force that is normal, or perpendicular, to the surface. In the case of a horizontal surface, N equals the weight of the body. For bodies on an inclined surface, N changes as a function of the angle of inclination, becoming less as the incline becomes steeper. As the force applied to a body at rest increases, a level is reached at which the static resistance is overcome, and the body begins to slide along the surface. Once the body begins moving, the friction decreases slightly and then is known as kinetic friction, with a kinetic coefficient of friction (μ_k):

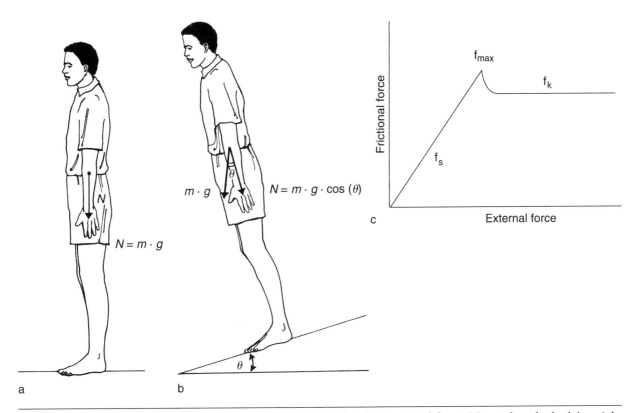

Figure 3.17 Sliding friction. (*a*) A body on a horizontal surface has a normal force (*N*) equal to the body's weight (*N = m · g*). (*b*) When placed on an inclined surface, the normal component (*N*) decreases as a function of the cosine of the angle of inclination [*N = m · g · *cos(θ)]. The result is less friction, and the body has a greater tendency to slide down the incline due to lower frictional force. (*c*) Relation between static friction and kinetic friction. For an object at rest, static friction (f_s) increases linearly to oppose the externally applied force. When maximum static friction (f_{max}) is reached, the object breaks loose and begins sliding. While sliding, kinetic friction (f_k) resists the movement.

$$f_k = \mu_k \cdot N \qquad (3.23)$$

The relation between static and kinetic friction is depicted in figure 3.17. Coefficients of sliding friction generally are between 0 and 1, where $\mu = 0$ indicates a frictionless surface.

Sliding friction plays a critical role in many injuries. A person walking on a wet, slippery surface, for example, is more likely to slip, fall, and become injured because the wet surface has a lower coefficient of friction than a dry one. Similarly, an individual navigating an icy stretch of sidewalk needs to be careful due to the very low frictional coefficient ice provides.

Another example of the prominent role friction plays is seen in the sporting world. Artificial turf was developed in the 1960s in response to inadequate outdoor playing fields in urban areas and the construction of domed stadiums. This type of playing surface withstands the harsh use and environmental conditions of outdoor fields and fulfills the need for an indoor surface where natural turf is infeasible. Considerable research has characterized the biomechanical aspects of artificial surfaces (Andreasson et al. 1986; Skovron, Levy, & Agel 1990; Nigg & Yeadon 1987). The differences in frictional characteristics between natural turf and artificial surfaces have been implicated as a major factor in injuries in soccer, tennis, and American football (Ekstrand & Nigg 1989; Nigg & Segesser 1988; Skovron, Levy, & Agel 1990). In general, surfaces with low frictional resistance are associated with fewer injuries. The typically higher friction on artificial surfaces is assumed to cause more injuries, particularly to the knee and ankle. Caution is warranted in making broad generalizations, however, since the frictional characteristics in a given situation are determined by the interactive effect of many factors such as shoe type, surface wear, type of sport, weather conditions, and the athlete's individual anthropometrics (e.g., height, weight), experience, and skill level.

When an automobile or bicycle is moving, the tires are in contact with the road surface. If tires are prevented from rotating (e.g., when one slams on the brakes), the vehicle slides along the road. In this case, sliding friction comes into play. Most of the time, however, the wheels are free to rotate and the vehicle rolls along. Even in rolling movement, friction is present. This rolling resistance is not as obvious as sliding resistance, because rolling resistance is much lower, often by a factor of 100 to 1,000 times. The actual value of resistance depends on the material properties of the body and surface, and on the normal force acting between them.

In some cases friction works to our advantage. In fact, we would be unable to walk or run without friction acting between our shoes and the ground. Too much friction, however, may contribute to injury. High levels of friction lead to abrupt deceleration, which causes high force levels and extreme loading of body tissue structures.

Our examples so far have focused on friction acting on the body. Friction also plays an important role within the human body. During normal limb movements, for instance, the friction in joints is extremely low, allowing for freedom of movement with minimal resistance. Details of this low joint friction are presented in the section on joint mechanics to follow.

Fluid Mechanics

Fluid mechanics is the branch of mechanics dealing with the properties and behavior of gases and liquids and assumes an important role in our framework for considering human biomechanics. Areas as diverse as performance biomechanics (study of human mechanical function), biotribology (study of the friction, lubrication, and wear of diarthrodial joints), tissue biomechanics (study of mechanical response of tissues), and hemodynamics (study of blood circulation) all rely on the basic principles of fluid mechanics.

We live and operate in various fluid environments, with air as the principal gas and water as the predominant liquid. The temperature, density, and composition of each fluid contributes to its mechanical properties. We will consider these mechanical properties in two broad categories: fluid flow and fluid resistance. Fluid flow refers to the characteristics of a fluid, whether liquid or gas, that allow it to move and govern the nature of this movement. Blood circulating through a coronary artery is an example of fluid flow. Fluids also provide resistance, such as the resistance we might experience while running into a head wind or swimming in a pool. Both flow and resistance are critical to our understanding of body function and tissue response and are intrinsically related to the biomechanics of injury.

Fluid Mechanics of Atherosclerosis

Normal physiological function depends on the efficient transport provided by the cardiovascular system. Compromise of this system's efficiency can have harmful, even fatal, consequences. Normal, healthy vessels allow for smooth, unobstructed blood flow with minimal resistance. Fatty buildup (plaque) on vessel walls signals the onset of atherosclerosis. As the amount of atherosclerotic plaque increases, the vessel wall becomes rougher and more irregular, and the vessel cavity (lumen) is occluded and therefore narrows.

These changes can have serious physiological consequences as a result of the mechanical changes that accompany plaque accumulation. Roughened arterial walls increase the turbulence of the blood's flow, increasing resistance (as seen in hypertension). The narrowing of the lumen also increases the resistance to flow. The increase in resistance can be dramatic for even small degrees of narrowing. A reduction in radius of one-half normal, for example, produces a 16-fold increase in resistance. The heart, which must pump much harder to force the blood through the narrowed passage, is at risk for serious and deleterious long-term effects.

The injury that atherosclerosis inflicts on vessel walls can have catastrophic consequences if left untreated. For example, when a piece of plaque becomes dislodged from an arterial wall and blocks blood flow, the situation can become life threatening. Such a blockage in a coronary artery is termed a myocardial infarction, or heart attack.

Fluid Flow

Fluid flow can exhibit many movement patterns. Laminar flow is characterized by a smooth, essentially parallel pattern of movement. Turbulent flow exhibits a more chaotic pattern of flow, characterized by areas of turbulence (eddies) and multidirectional movement. Arterial blood flow provides us with a good example of these differences. Factors contributing to turbulent flow include the roughness (degree of irregularity) of the surface over which the fluid is flowing, the diameter of the vessel through which the fluid flows, and the speed of flow.

Fluid Resistance

Fluid resistance takes many forms, some of which are advantageous and others that may be detrimental. Examples of the positive effects of fluid resistance include *buoyant forces* (according to Archimedes' principle), which allow a person to float in water; *lift forces* (as seen in aerodynamics), which assist in keeping an object in flight; and *Magnus forces*, which affect the trajectories of objects spinning through the air. Negative effects of fluid resistance are evident in the extra physiological work expenditure required by a cyclist moving into the wind or by the severe and unpredictable forces acting on an airplane during a storm.

The resistance produced by fluids may be considered "fluid friction" and is termed viscosity. *Viscosity* is the property of a fluid that enables it to develop and maintain a resistance to flow dependent on the flow's velocity (rate of flow). This viscous effect and its dependence on the velocity can be seen in a familiar example. When you move your hand slowly through water, the resistance is minimal. Increasing the speed of movement markedly increases the resistance.

Since all biological tissues have a fluid component, it stands to reason that tissue response to mechanical loading will include a viscous component. For example, the response of tendon and ligament to being stretched will vary depending on the rate of stretch created by the applied load. The details of this response are considered later.

Joint Mechanics

Hundreds of articulations (joints) in the human body are responsible for allowing movements. Since many injuries occur to joint structures, a study of their mechanical characteristics is essential to our discussion of injury biomechanics. No two joints are the same in structural terms; each has its own distinct combination of tissues, tissue configuration, and movement potential. This variety of joint structure and function results in many complex injuries, which we explore in subsequent chapters.

Description of Joint Motion

Movement analysis depends on proper description of the joint motions that constitute each movement pattern. By convention, joint motions are defined with respect to anatomical position. In anatomical position, the body is referenced according to three mutually orthogonal planes: the sagittal plane, frontal plane, and transverse plane (figure 3.18). Primary

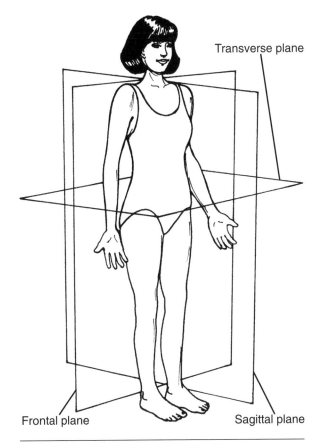

Figure 3.18 Three primary movement planes shown for a person standing in anatomical position. These planes are the transverse (horizontal), frontal (coronal), and sagittal planes. These names are given to any plane parallel to the ones shown. The sagittal plane that bisects the body is sometimes referred to as the midsagittal or median plane.

Table 3.1   Summary of Joint Motions and Planes of Action

Joint	Joint motion	Plane of action*
Hip	Flexion/extension	Sagittal
	Abduction/adduction	Frontal
	Internal/external rotation	Transverse
Knee	Flexion/extension	Sagittal
Ankle	Plantarflexion/dorsiflexion	Sagittal
Shoulder	Flexion/extension	Sagittal
	Abduction/adduction	Frontal
	Internal/external rotation	Transverse
	Horizontal flexion/extension	Transverse
Elbow	Flexion/extension	Sagittal
Radioulnar	Forearm pronation/supination	Transverse
Intervertebral spine	Spinal flexion/extension	Sagittal
	Spinal lateral flexion	Frontal
	Spinal rotation	Transverse

*Planes for movement made from anatomical position.

joint motion typically occurs in one of these movement planes. For example, knee flexion in anatomical position occurs in the sagittal plane, glenohumeral abduction occurs in the frontal plane, and hip internal (medial) rotation occurs in the transverse plane (table 3.1).

Joint Mobility and Stability

Each joint in the body has a *range of motion* (ROM) throughout which the joint normally operates. This ROM determines a joint's mobility. The magnitude of allowable ROM is both joint specific and person specific. Joints with an ability to move in more than one plane have ROMs specific to each particular plane of movement. Note that ROMs vary considerably from one person to another, and thus individual measurement is the surest method of determining accurate joint ROMs (table 3.2). Intrinsically related to ROM is the notion of joint stability, defined as "the ability of a joint to maintain an appropriate functional position throughout its range of motion" (Burstein & Wright 1994, 63).

Injuries often occur when a joint exceeds its normal ROM, as when an elbow hyperextends, which raises the question of what determines normal ROM. In general, joint ROM is determined by the combined effects of (1) the shape of the articular surfaces and their geometric interaction (de-

gree of bony fit), (2) the restraint provided by ligaments, joint capsule, and other periarticular structures, and (3) the action of muscles around the joint. When the limits imposed by these stabilizing factors are exceeded, normal ROM is violated, and the tissues may experience injury-producing forces.

One way of viewing joint stability is the joint's ability to resist dislocation. Stable joints have a high resistance to dislocation. Unstable joints tend to dislocate more easily. In general, joints can be classified along a mobility-stability continuum, which specifies that joints that have a tight bony fit or numerous ligamentous and other supporting structures or that are surrounded by large muscle groups will be very stable and relatively immobile. Joints with a loose bony fit, limited extrinsic support, or minimal surrounding musculature tend to be very mobile and unstable. One exception to this categorization is the hip joint, which is both very mobile—with large ROM potential in all three primary planes—and very stable, as seen by the rarity of its dislocation.

Lever Systems

Most motion at the major joints results from the body's structures acting as a system of levers. A lever is a rigid structure, fixed at a single point, to which two forces are applied at two different points. One of the forces is commonly referred to as the *resistance*

Table 3.2 Average Ranges of Joint Motion*

Joint	Joint motion	ROM (degrees)
Hip	Flexion	90-125
	Hyperextension	10-30
	Abduction	40-45
	Adduction	10-30
	Internal rotation	35-45
	External rotation	45-50
Knee	Flexion	120-150
Ankle	Plantarflexion	20-45
	Dorsiflexion	15-30
Shoulder	Flexion	130-180
	Hyperextension	30-80
	Abduction	170-180
	Adduction	50
	Internal rotation**	60-90
	External rotation**	70-90
	Horizontal flexion**	135
	Horizontal extension**	45
Elbow	Flexion	140-160
Radioulnar	Forearm pronation (from midposition)	80-90
	Forearm supination (from midposition)	80-90
Cervical spine	Flexion	40-60
	Hyperextension	40-75
	Lateral flexion	40-45
	Rotation	50-80
Thoracolumbar spine	Flexion	45-75
	Hyperextension	20-35
	Lateral flexion	25-35
	Rotation	30-45

*Range of motion (ROM) for movements made from anatomical position (unless otherwise noted). Averages reported in the literature vary, sometimes considerably, depending on method of measurement and population measured. Values above are representative of the ranges of reported maximum ROM.

**Movement from abducted position.

force (R), the other termed the *applied* or *effort force* (F). The fixed point, known as the pivot or fulcrum, is the point about which the lever rotates. In the human body these three components are typically an externally applied force (R), a muscle force (F), and a joint axis of rotation (A), such as when lifting a weight.

These lever system components may be spatially related to one another in three different configurations, giving rise to three classes of levers. Distinctions among the classes are determined by the location of each component relative to the other

two (figure 3.19). In a first-class lever, the pivot-point axis (A) is located between the resistance (R) and the force (F). A second-class lever has R located between F and A, while a third-class lever has F between R and A. Joints in the human body are predominantly third-class levers (figure 3.19d), with some first-class levers (figure 3.19e) and few second-class lever systems.

The lever systems in the human body provide two important functions. First, they increase the effect of an applied force, because the applied force and the resisting force have different moment arms,

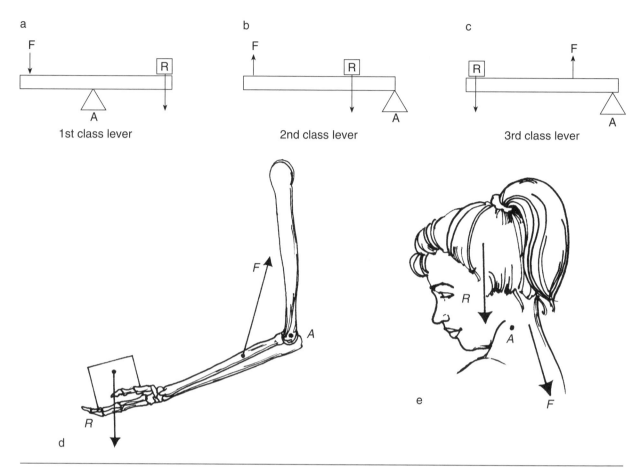

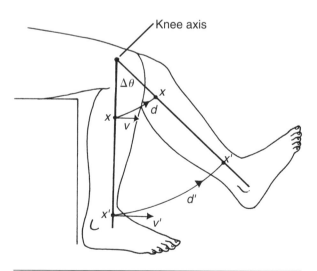

Figure 3.19 Lever systems. Simple lever systems comprise three elements: an axis (*A*), effort force (*F*), and resistance (*R*). (*a*) First-class lever system. (*b*) Second-class lever system. (*c*) Third-class lever system. (*d*) Biceps brachii acting about the elbow joint as a third-class lever system. (*e*) Extensors of the head and neck acting as a first-class lever system to counteract the tendency of the weight of the head to flex the cervical spine.

in the same way that a leverage advantage is gained in using a bar to pry a large rock loose from the ground. In a first-class lever, for example, increasing the moment arm on the side of the applied force increases the effective force seen on the other side of the pivot point.

The second function of levers is to increase the effective speed (or velocity) of movement. During knee extension (figure 3.20), a given angular displacement ($\Delta\theta$) produces different linear displacements of points *x* and *x'* on the lower leg. Similarly, if the knee is extended at a constant angular velocity (ω), the linear velocity of point *x'* will be greater than that of *x*. Thus, by increasing the lever arm distance from *x* to *x'*, we have increased the linear velocity of movement. The human body makes effective use of both the force and speed advantages provided by lever systems in accomplishing the many tasks it performs on a daily basis. As expected, these force and speed enhancements play a role in injury occurrence and prevention as well.

Figure 3.20 Knee extensor mechanism acting as a lever system. For a given angular displacement ($\Delta\theta$), the curvilinear displacement (*d'*) for point *x'* will be greater than the displacement (*d*) for point *x*. Similarly, for a given angular velocity (ω), the linear velocity (*v'*) for point *x'* exceeds the velocity (*v*) of point *x*.

Moment of Force (Torque) and Joint Motion

We defined torque, or moment of force, as the effect of a force tending to cause rotation about an axis. With respect to joint function, moments created by the action of skeletal muscles are the essential element in controlling joint motion. Figure 3.21 depicts moment production at a joint. The muscle force F is acting at a perpendicular distance (moment arm = d) from the joint axis E, producing a moment $M = F \cdot d$. In static situations such as this, calculation of the moment is straightforward.

In real-life cases involving joint motion, the calculation becomes much more complex. Consider each component of the moment calculation. The magnitude of muscle force F typically varies and is determined by a combination of factors including the muscle's length, velocity, level of neural activation, and fatigue, along with the external resistance that the system is experiencing. Instantaneous changes in any or all of these factors directly influence the amount of muscle force produced.

As the joint moves throughout its range, the musculotendinous line of action (i.e., its direction of pull) changes continuously, thus affecting the moment arm distance. Because joints in the human body are not perfect hinge joints, the location of the axis of rotation relative to the bony structures at any instant in time (instantaneous joint center) changes as well (figure 3.22). These changes in muscle force, line of action, and moment arm result in a continuously varying moment of force.

The asymmetry of joint motion that accounts for the movement of the instantaneous joint center motion (figure 3.22) is caused by a combination of three basic movements: rotation, sliding, and rolling (figure 3.23). In rotation, the motion is purely angular, with rotation about a fixed axis (figure 3.23a). Sliding joint motion occurs when one articulating surface moves linearly relative to the other (figure 3.23b). Rolling results in angular joint movement combined with linear displacement of the axis of rotation (figure 3.23c).

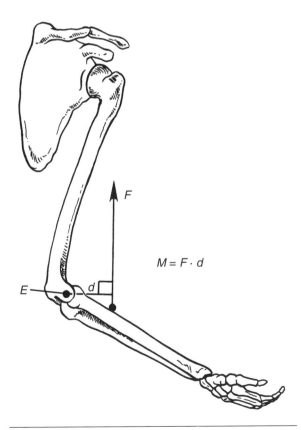

Figure 3.21 Biceps brachii muscle force (F) with a moment arm (d) producing a moment of force (M) about the elbow joint axis (E).

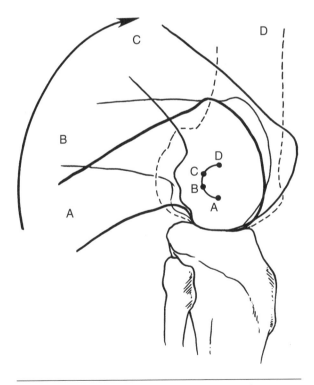

Figure 3.22 Instantaneous joint center of rotation. Structural asymmetries result in movement of the instantaneous joint center with respect to the bones constituting the joint. Movement of the instantaneous joint center is shown for the knee as the joint extends from a flexed position (A) to full extension (D).

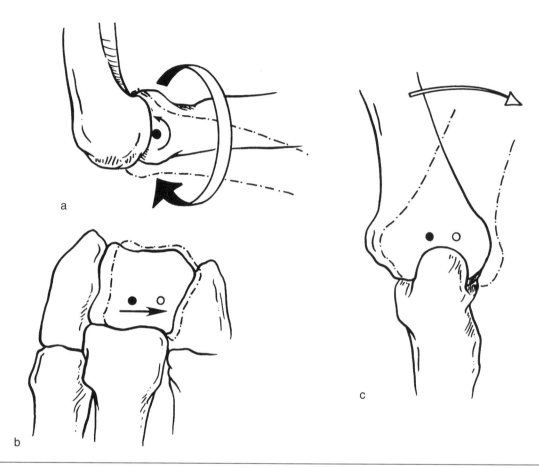

Figure 3.23 Components of joint motion: (*a*) rotation, (*b*) sliding, and (*c*) rolling.

Joint Reaction Force Versus Bone-on-Bone Forces

Forces experienced by articular surfaces during activities can be of considerable magnitude, such as those occurring at the knee during running or jumping. Repeated high-force loading may lead to joint injuries (e.g., meniscal tears, articular cartilage degeneration). Actual measurement of these forces can be a complex undertaking, and thus mathematical models (discussed in more detail later in this chapter) are often used to estimate these joint loads. The net effect of muscle and other forces acting across a joint is called the *joint reaction force* (JRF). Exemplar JRFs are depicted in figure 3.24. Calculation of actual bone-on-bone forces is more complex than this depiction (Winter 1990).

Joint Lubrication

Diarthrodial (synovial) joints contain synovial fluid that serves lubricative, shock absorptive, and nutritive functions. In its lubricative role, synovial fluid reduces friction in the joint to extremely low levels.

This minimal friction plays an important part in the durability (i.e., lack of wear) of normal articular cartilage. The lubrication mechanisms acting in synovial joints are complex and not completely understood. These mechanisms are detailed in chapter 4.

Material Mechanics

Our discussion so far has focused on the movement of bodies and the causal agents affecting those movements. We have concentrated on external mechanics or the effect of external forces on the movement of bodies. In this section we shift our attention to the internal mechanics of structures, focusing on the internal response of materials to externally applied loads.

Rigid-Body Mechanics and Deformable Solids

In previous sections we considered bodies as if they were rigid structures whose size and shape do not change when loads are applied. This approach, known

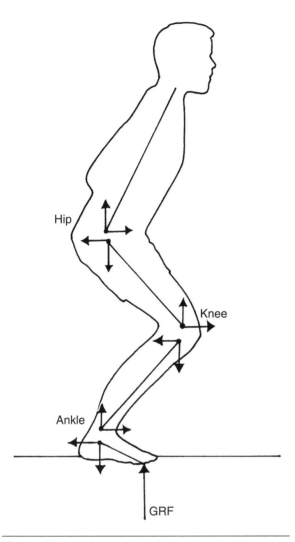

Figure 3.24 Joint reaction forces. Equal and opposite joint reaction forces (in accordance with Newton's third law) act at the ankle, knee, and hip joints in a squatting position with each joint in a flexed position.

as rigid-body mechanics, is useful when examining movement characteristics. Rigid-body formulations make certain assumptions about the body, including nondeformability, fixed center of mass, and homogeneity of the composite material. Although biological tissues are in fact deformable, viewing body segments as rigid bodies is a reasonable approximation in fields of inquiry such as movement mechanics. In examining the biomechanics of injury, however, we also need to explore the mechanics of deformable solids since often the injury mechanism results in considerable tissue deformation.

Material Properties

Biological materials such as tissues exhibit many properties that influence the material's response to

loading and hence the likelihood and severity of injury. Among these properties are the material's size, shape, area, volume, and mass. Additional properties derived from these fundamental ones include density (ratio of mass to volume) and centroid (center of mass). The tissue's structural constituents and form, discussed in the previous chapter, are also important factors in describing tissue mechanical response.

Stress and Strain

Any tissue, when loaded, develops an internal resistance to the external load. In the case of a small rubber band, this resistance is minimal. In contrast, the resistance is considerable for a steel bar. This internal resistance to an axial load is common to all materials and in mechanics is called stress (σ). Axial, or normal, stresses are categorized as either compressive stress (i.e., resistance to being pushed together) or tensile stress (i.e., resistance to being pulled apart). The magnitude of the normal stress is

$$\sigma = F/A \qquad (3.24)$$

where F = the magnitude of axial load, and A = the cross-sectional area over which the load is distributed.

Those forces acting parallel, or tangential, to the applied load create shear stress (τ):

$$\tau = F/A \qquad (3.25)$$

The standard (SI) unit of stress is the pascal (Pa), defined as 1 N distributed over one square meter (1 Pa = 1 N·m^{-2}).

Materials change their shape, though sometimes imperceptibly, when subjected to external loads. This change in shape is termed deformation and is measured by the mechanical strain (ε). When the material elongates due to a tensile load, we have tensile strain. Similarly, axial compression results in a compressive strain, and a shear load causes a shear strain (figure 3.25). Strain may be measured as absolute strain, but more commonly is expressed as relative strain. Deformation is measured in terms of dimensions prior to loading. For example, consider an unloaded tissue of length 50 mm. A tension load causes an elongation of 3 mm. This simple case has an absolute strain of 3 mm, and a relative strain of 3 mm/50 mm, expressed as a percentage: 6% strain.

A direct relation exists between stress and strain, and the consequences of this relation in a tissue determine its susceptibility to injury. Compressively

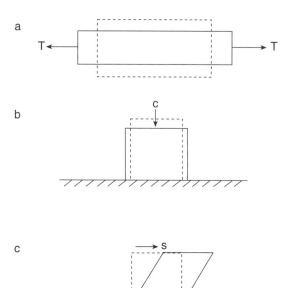

Figure 3.25 Mechanical strain. External loads change the shape of a material. This deformation, or strain, can manifest as (*a*) an elongation, or tensile strain, (*b*) a compression, or compressive strain, or (*c*) an angulation, or shear strain.

loaded bone, for example, develops high resistance while deforming very little. Skin, in contrast, deforms considerably more at substantially lower forces. The strain responses of tendon, ligament, and cartilage fall somewhere between these two. Plotting stress as a function of strain (figure 3.26a) allows us to visualize the σ/ε relation. The figure shows linear σ/ε curves for two materials labeled A and B. A closer look at the curves reveals several important relations. For a given stress (σ_o), material B exhibits more strain than material A which is evident as $\varepsilon_B > \varepsilon_A$. Conversely, for a given strain (ε_o), material A develops a greater stress than material B, as demonstrated by $\sigma_A > \sigma_B$ (figure 3.26b).

The stress-strain (σ/ε) relation can be summarized in a single measure as the ratio of the two values. This σ/ε ratio defines the material's stiffness. The stiffness value is denoted by E. The opposite, or inverse, of stiffness is known as compliance. Stiff materials such as bone have a steeply sloped σ/ε curve and a high E value. More compliant materials such as skin have flatter σ/ε slopes and lower E values.

Thus far we have considered only the linear σ/ε relation. Linear materials are said to operate according to Hooke's law, which posits that the stress and strain are linearly related; that is, the resulting

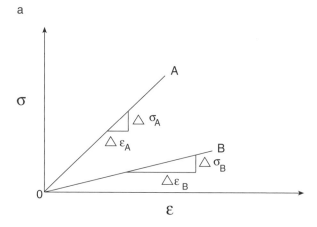

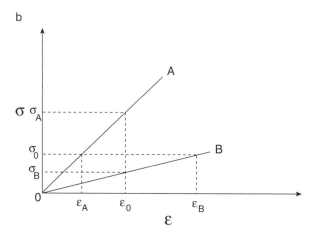

Figure 3.26 Relation between mechanical stress (σ) and strain (ε). (*a*) Linear stress-strain (σ/ε) curves for two materials. The slope ($\Delta\sigma/\Delta\varepsilon$) of each line measures each material's stiffness (i.e., A is stiffer than B). (*b*) The relative stiffness of the materials determines their response to loading. For a given stress level (σ_o), material B shows more strain than material A (i.e., B is more compliant than A).

strain is proportional to the developed stress. Mathematically, Hooke's law is expressed by

$$\sigma = E \cdot \varepsilon \qquad (3.26)$$

The mechanical response of biological tissues typically is not linear throughout its physiological range, due largely to the nonlinear characteristics of the tissue's fluid component.

Uniaxial Loading

Recall from earlier discussion the seven factors involved in force application. These factors (magnitude, location, direction, duration, frequency, variability, and rate of force application) are fundamental determinants of loading response. We focus now on the actual loading of tissue by first considering uniaxial loading, the simplest form of force application. Uniaxial loading refers to forces applied along a single line, typically along a primary axis of the structure. For any uniaxially loaded material, the location and direction of the force will determine which of the three basic types of loading is present. These three types, *compression* (compressive load), *tension* (tensile load), and *shear* (shear load), are depicted in figure 3.25. Tension loads tend to pull the ends apart (figure 3.25a). Compressive loads tend to push the ends of a body together (figure 3.25b). And shear loads tend to produce horizontal sliding of one layer over another (figure 3.25c). As the magnitude of an applied load increases, the tissue eventually is unable to withstand the loading and fails (i.e., tears apart). The level of force (load) at which failure occurs is the tissue's ultimate strength. This concept of ultimate strength has obvious implications as we look at the failure characteristics of tissue in injury situations.

We noted that the direction of force application is an essential factor. A homogeneous material will respond the same irrespective of the direction of loading. Biological tissues are generally not homogeneous (i.e., their structure varies throughout the body), and as a result the loading response is dependent on the direction of load. A material exhibiting this direction-dependent response is anisotropic. As an example, consider a long bone experiencing uniaxial compression. The ultimate strength for a compressive load along the longitudinal axis is much greater than the ultimate strength directed perpendicular to the long axis, largely a result of the bone's structure.

Biological tissues can exhibit linear behavior through certain loading ranges but typically are nonlinear through other parts of their physiological range. Such nonlinearities result in a generalized σ/ε curve (figure 3.27a). We will apply this curve to specific tissues in the following chapter, explaining at this point only general aspects of the curve.

Consider a tissue experiencing a gradually increasing tensile load. At low loads, with commensurate low stress levels, the σ/ε response is linear (hookean). The proportional response continues until point B. At stresses above σ_B, the response becomes nonlinear. Point B is therefore known as the linear, or proportional, limit. As the stress continues to increase, we reach point C, known as the elastic limit. At stresses below σ_C, the material is

elastic (i.e., returns to its original shape when the load is removed). Above σ_C, the material is no longer elastic and experiences permanent, or plastic, deformation. This plastic deformation is shown in figure 3.27b. When the load is removed, stress decreases, and the material shortens. Since we have exceeded the elastic limit, the tissue is no longer able to return to its original shape (point A). Instead, it shortens to a length at point P. The difference between points A and P is the amount of plastic deformation, or permanent set.

Point D is approached as stress continues to increase. This is known as the yield point, at which there begins a brief region of relatively large strain

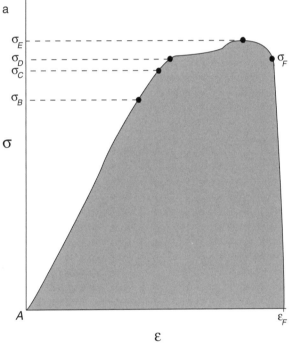

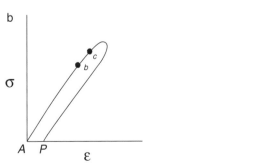

Figure 3.27 Generalized stress-strain (σ/ε) curve for biological tissues. (*a*) Stress-strain relation (described in text); energy to failure is measured by the area under the σ/ε curve (shaded area). (*b*) Permanent set (AP) created by stress exceeding the elastic limit at point C.

for little increase in stress. This yielding phenomenon is characteristic of many biological tissues. Further increase in stress eventually brings the material to its ultimate stress (σ_E) and failure begins to occur. Because the failure of some tissues is not instantaneous, the actual completion of failure may occur at a stress level below σ_E, at what is termed the rupture point (F) at a stress level of σ_F. Note that the actual σ/ε curves for specific tissues vary in their response characteristics and may not exactly mirror the curve presented in figure 3.27. Detailed discussion of the differences for bone, cartilage, tendon, and ligament will be presented in chapter 4. Two other important mechanical parameters shown in figure 3.27 are the

energy to failure, a measure of the strain energy stored by the tissue prior to failure, and the elongation or deformation to failure (ε_F), a measure of how much the tissue has deformed up to the point of failure.

When a compressive load is imposed on a ball (figure 3.28a), a compressive strain results, which compresses the ball in the direction of the load. At the same time, an accompanying deformation occurs perpendicular to the axial load. This deformation is a tensile strain, and the ball in this example gets wider. This simple case is an example of Poisson's effect, which says that when a body is subjected to a uniaxial load and its dimension decreases in the axial direction, its perpendicular, or

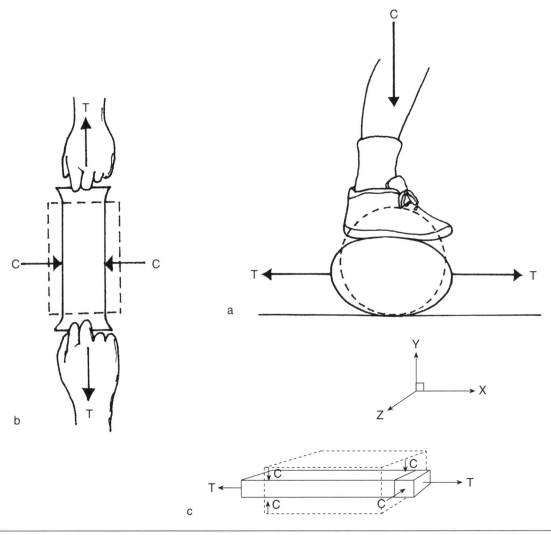

Figure 3.28 Poisson's effect. (*a*) An applied compressive load causes tensile stress and strain perpendicular to the imposed load. (*b*) An applied tensile load results in compressive stress and strain perpendicular to the applied load. (*c*) Poisson's effect shown for a three-dimensional case in which tension (*T*) is applied in the *x* direction and causes contraction in the *y* and *z* directions. Dashed lines indicate conformation prior to loading. Solid lines indicate conformation while loaded.

transverse, dimension increases. Poisson's effect applies in the opposite sense as well: A body experiencing a tensile load shows an increase in its axial dimension and a decrease in its transverse dimension (figure 3.28b). The quantitative measure of this effect is given by Poisson's ratio (ν):

$$\nu = -(\varepsilon_t / \varepsilon_a) \qquad (3.27)$$

where ε_t = transverse strain, and ε_a = axial strain.

Similar to the two-dimensional case just presented, Poisson's effect also occurs in three-dimensional space, with transverse strains occurring in two directions in response to a uniaxial load in the third direction (figure 3.28c).

Multiaxial Loading

We have considered only the simple case of uniaxial loading. In many real-life situations, however, the forces applied to a body are multidimensional, and hence a study of multiaxial loading and its effects is essential. An analysis of multiaxial loading uses the same stress and strain concepts just discussed and extends them into two- and three-dimensional space. Though the biaxial and triaxial responses are illustrated for tensile loading only, note that the concepts are equally applicable to compressive loading and to force vectors with reversed orientation, and that the following formulations are for linearly elastic materials.

Biaxial (Two-Dimensional) Loading Responses

Consider a three-dimensional body (figure 3.29) with sides of length x', y', and z' that is subjected to axial forces F_x and F_y. The stresses produced in the x and y directions are

$$\sigma_x = F_x/A_x = F_x/(y' \cdot z')$$
$$\text{and} \qquad \sigma_y = F_y/A_y = F_y/(x' \cdot z') \qquad (3.28)$$

The x direction stress (σ_x) will, according to Poisson's effect, produce deformation in all three directions. The elongation in the x direction and contraction in the y and z directions are shown in figure 3.29b. By applying eqs. 3.26 and 3.27, we obtain x and y direction strains due to σ_x:

x direction: $\qquad \varepsilon_{x_{\sigma x}} = \sigma_x/E \qquad (3.29)$

y direction: $\qquad \varepsilon_{y_{\sigma x}} = -\nu \cdot \varepsilon_{x_{\sigma x}} = -\nu \cdot (\sigma_x/E) \qquad (3.30)$

We similarly obtain y and x direction strains due to σ_y:

y direction: $\qquad \varepsilon_{y_{\sigma y}} = \sigma_y/E \qquad (3.31)$

x direction: $\qquad \varepsilon_{x_{\sigma y}} = -\nu \cdot \varepsilon_{y_{\sigma y}} = -\nu \cdot (\sigma_y/E) \qquad (3.32)$

To obtain the combined effect of σ_x and σ_y, we simply add the strain effects just calculated. The net strains in the x and y directions are then

$$\varepsilon_x = \varepsilon_{x_{\sigma x}} + \varepsilon_{x_{\sigma y}} = \sigma_x/E - \nu \cdot (\sigma_y/E) \qquad (3.33)$$

$$\varepsilon_y = \varepsilon_{y_{\sigma y}} + \varepsilon_{y_{\sigma x}} = \sigma_y/E - \nu \cdot (\sigma_x/E) \qquad (3.34)$$

We have presented two normal stresses, σ_x and σ_y. As previously described, a tangential, or shear, stress (τ) is also created. In the case of biaxial loading, shear stress (τ_{xy}) is created as shown in figure 3.30a.

Triaxial (Three-Dimensional) Loading Responses

The addition of a third axial force in the z direction complicates the conceptual model only slightly,

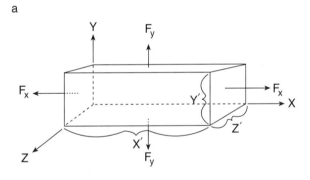

a

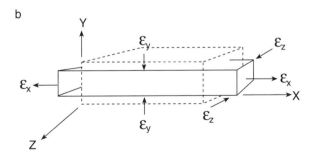

b

Figure 3.29 Biaxial loading. (*a*) Applied forces in the x and y directions (F_x and F_y, respectively) load the material biaxially. (*b*) Elongation caused by F_x and the resulting perpendicular contraction in the y and z directions. Dashed lines indicate conformation prior to loading. Solid lines indicate conformation while loaded.

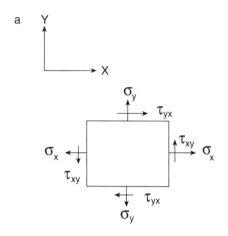

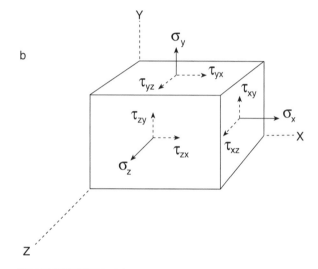

Figure 3.30   Shear stresses in response to biaxial and triaxial loading. (*a*) Shear stress (τ_{xy}) created by biaxial loading. Due to equilibrium conditions $\tau_{xy} = \tau_{yx}$. (*b*) Tensile stresses (σ_x, σ_y, σ_z), shown as solid vectors, result in shear stresses (τ_{xy}, τ_{yz}, τ_{zx}), depicted as broken-line vectors. Note that equilibrium constraints dictate that $\tau_{xy} = \tau_{yx}$, $\tau_{yz} = \tau_{zy}$, and $\tau_{zx} = \tau_{xz}$.

while the mathematical aspects of the model become quite involved. Focusing on the conceptual application (figure 3.31), we now have

- F_x, which creates $\sigma_x = F_x/(y' \cdot z')$ and produces elongation in the x direction and contraction in the y and z directions
- F_y, which creates $\sigma_y = F_y/(x' \cdot z')$ and produces elongation in the y direction and contraction in the x and z directions
- F_z, which creates $\sigma_z = F_z/(x' \cdot y')$ and produces elongation in the z direction and contraction in the x and y directions

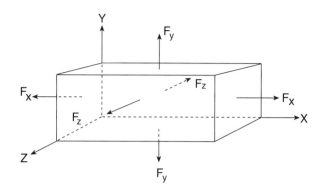

Figure 3.31   Triaxial loading. Applied forces in the x, y, and z directions (F_x, F_y, and F_z, respectively) load the material triaxially.

The equations for resultant strains seen in triaxial loading are

$$\varepsilon_x = (1/E) \cdot [\sigma_x - \nu \cdot (\sigma_y + \sigma_z)] \qquad (3.35)$$

$$\varepsilon_y = (1/E) \cdot [\sigma_y - \nu \cdot (\sigma_x + \sigma_z)] \qquad (3.36)$$

$$\varepsilon_z = (1/E) \cdot [\sigma_z - \nu \cdot (\sigma_x + \sigma_y)] \qquad (3.37)$$

The shear stresses (τ_{xy}, τ_{yz}, τ_{zx}) produced in triaxial loading are shown in figure 3.30b.

The axial loading we have discussed so far is one of three primary types of loading. Two other types occur frequently in the human body, and a brief description of their mechanical characteristics will aid in our subsequent discussions of injury mechanisms. These two loading conditions are bending and torsion.

Bending

Any structure that is relatively long and slender (e.g., long bone) may be considered in mechanical terms as a beam. Any force, force component, or moment acting perpendicular to the longitudinal axis of such a beam will tend to deflect, or bend, the beam and create normal and shearing stresses in any cross section.

In any bending situation the material on the concave (inner) surface of the structure experiences compressive stress, while that on the convex (outer) surface is subject to tensile stress (figure 3.32a). These tensile and compressive stresses are maximal at the outer surfaces of the beam, with the material closer to the neutral axis experiencing less stress than at the surfaces. The line along which neither compressive or tensile stress exists is known as the neutral axis.

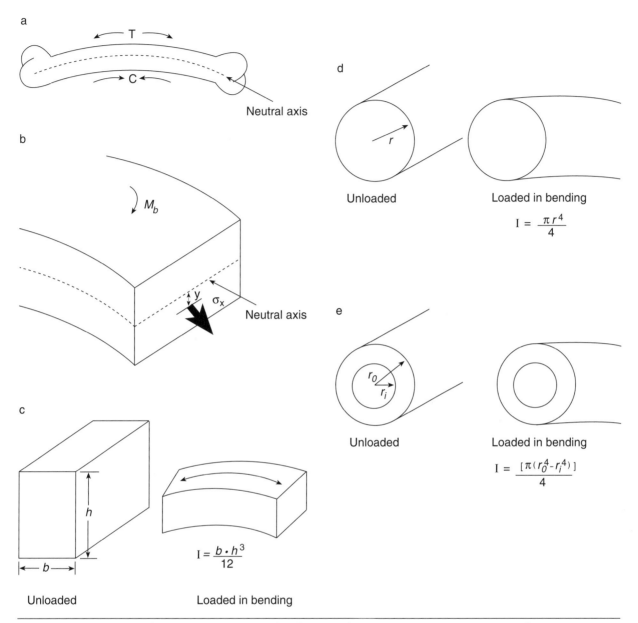

Figure 3.32 (*a*) Material stresses in response to bending. Bending creates compressive stress on the concave (inner) surface and tensile stress on the convex (outer) surface. Maximal stress occurs at the surfaces, with lower stress levels toward the center of the bent object. A neutral axis exists along which there are no tensile or compressive stresses present. (*b*) Bending moment. A beam subjected to a bending moment ($=M_b$) develops a normal stress (σ_x) as given by eq. (3.38). (*c*) The area moment of inertia for a rectangular cross section depends on the height ($=b$) and base ($=b$) dimensions of the cross section. (*d*) The area moment of inertia for a solid cylinder depends on the radius ($=r$). (*e*) For a hollowed cylinder (tube), the area moment of inertia depends on the outer radius ($=r_o$) and the inner radius ($=r_i$).

Each force acting on the beam may create a moment in the beam. The sum of these moments is referred to as the bending moment (M_b), which creates different stress levels in the beam that vary with the distance from the neutral axis. At a distance y from the neutral axis (figure 3.32b), a normal stress (σ_x) is created with a value given by

$$\sigma_x = (M_b \cdot y)/I \qquad (3.38)$$

where M_b = bending moment, y = distance from neutral axis, and I = area moment of inertia of the cross-sectional area about the neutral axis. The area moment of inertia (I) value depends on the cross-sectional shape of the structure. The area moment

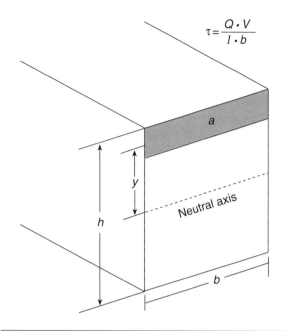

$$\tau = \frac{Q \cdot V}{I \cdot b}$$

Figure 3.33 Shear stress in response to bending. The magnitude of the shear stress (τ) is given by eq. (3.39). V = vertical shear force (obtained from a shear force diagram or from static analysis), Q = area moment (calculated as the product of the shaded area a and the distance y from the neutral axis to the centroid of area a), I = moment of inertia of the total cross section (see figure 3.32c), and b = width of cross section.

of inertia for common shapes is depicted in figures 3.32c-e.

In instances when shear forces are acting on a beam, shear stresses are created that are maximal at the neutral axis and zero at the surfaces (figure 3.33). The magnitude of this shear stress (τ) is given by

$$\tau = (Q \cdot V)/(I \cdot b) \qquad (3.39)$$

where Q = the first moment of the area about the neutral axis, V = shear force, I = area moment of inertia, and b = width of the cross section.

Two common bending modes seen in biomechanical cases are three-point bending and four-point bending (figure 3.34, a and b). As examples, a boot-top skiing injury mechanism illustrates three-point bending (figure 3.34c), while muscle forces acting on a long bone may produce a four-point bending situation (figure 3.34d). The mechanical differences between these two modes as is seen in their failure characteristics are important for considering injury mechanisms. In three-point bending, failure occurs at the middle point of force

application (figure 3.35a). In contrast, failure in four-point bending occurs at the weakest point between the two inner forces, and not necessarily at the midpoint (figure 3.35b).

Another type of loading is cantilever bending, in which a force offset from the longitudinal axis creates both compression and bending. Cantilever bending occurs in a loaded femur when compressive forces are applied to the femoral head, creating a bending moment in the diaphyseal shaft of the bone (figure 3.36).

Torsion

Any twisting action applied to a structure results in torsional loading, as seen in the simple example of unscrewing a lid from its jar. The torsion concepts are generally applicable to both cylindrical and noncylindrical structures. Due to the complex mathematics necessary to explain the nature of torsional loads applied to noncylindrical structures, we restrict our mathematical formulations to solid, circular shafts. The following torsion formulations are based on assumptions of tissue isotropy, linear elasticity, and structural homogeneity.

Earlier we presented two types of moment of inertia: mass moment of inertia (resistance to rotation of a body about a fixed axis) and area moment of inertia (resistance to bending of a beam about its neutral axis). A third form of angular resistance is involved when torsional loads are applied to a body. The internal stresses developed in response to the torsional loading produce resistance to the applied torque. This resistance to torsional loading about the longitudinal axis is termed polar moment of inertia (J), and its magnitude for a solid shaft (figure 3.37a) is

$$J = (\pi \cdot r^4)/2 \qquad (3.40)$$

where r = radius of the shaft. For a hollow cylindrical shaft (figure 3.37b), such as a long bone, the polar moment of inertia (J) is

$$J = [\pi \cdot (r_o^4 - r_i^4)]/2 \qquad (3.41)$$

where r_o = outer radius of the shaft, and r_i = inner radius.

Torsion creates stresses throughout the shaft with the magnitude of shear stress (τ) being a function of shaft length, applied torque (T), and polar moment of inertia (figure 3.38a), expressed as

$$\tau = (T \cdot r)/J \qquad (3.42)$$

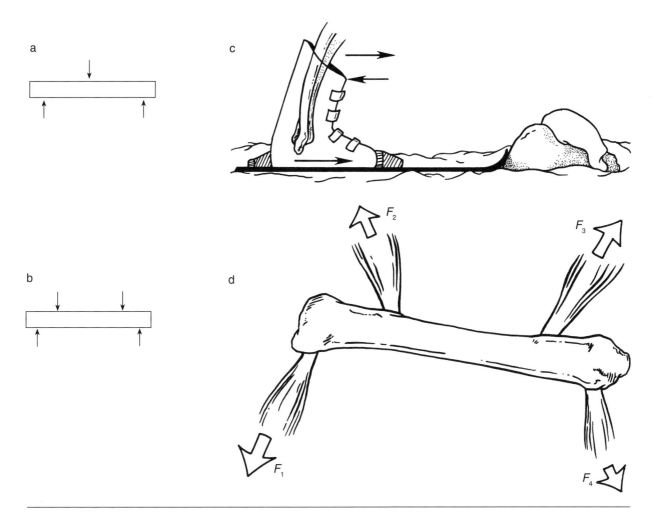

Figure 3.34 Three- and four-point bending. (*a*) Three-point bending caused by the action of three parallel forces. The middle force is in the direction opposite to the outer two forces. (*b*) Four-point bending caused by two pairs of parallel forces. The inner pair is in the direction opposite to the outer pair. (*c*) Skiing boot-top fracture exemplifies three-point bending. (*d*) Muscle force system exemplifying four-point bending.

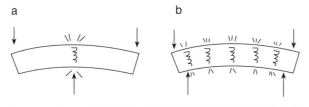

Figure 3.35 Failure due to bending. (*a*) Failure (fracture) caused by three-point bending occurs at the point of middle force application. (*b*) In four-point bending, failure (fracture) occurs at the weakest point between the two inner forces, not necessarily at the midpoint.

The resulting shear strain (γ) is shown in figure 3.38b. The ratio of shear stress (τ) to shear strain (γ) is called the shear modulus of elasticity (G):

$$G = \tau / \gamma \qquad (3.43)$$

The angle of twist (θ) shown in figure 3.38c is given by

$$\theta = (T \cdot l)/(G \cdot J) \qquad (3.44)$$

where T = applied torque, l = shaft length, G = shear modulus of elasticity, and J = polar moment of inertia.

Several important generalizations emerge from an examination of torsional loading:

- The larger the radius of the shaft, the more resistance it creates and the more difficult it is to deform.

- The stiffer the material being loaded, the harder it is to deform in torsion.

- In addition to shear stress, torsion produces normal stresses (tensile and compressive) in the

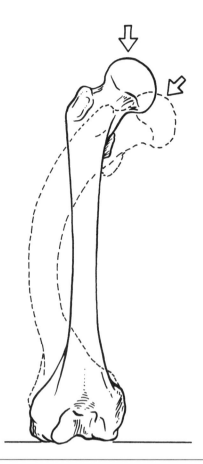

Figure 3.36 Cantilever bending. Compressive loading offset from the longitudinal axis creates a combined loading situation (compression and bending) known as cantilever bending. Solid lines indicate conformation prior to loading. Dashed lines indicate conformation while loaded.

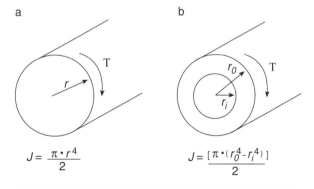

a

b

$$J = \frac{\pi \cdot r^4}{2}$$

$$J = \frac{[\pi \cdot (r_0^4 - r_i^4)]}{2}$$

Figure 3.37 Polar moment of inertia. Resistance to an applied torque, measured by the polar moment of inertia, for (*a*) a solid shaft and (*b*) a hollow cylindrical shaft.

form of helical stress trajectories (figure 3.39a). These stresses are maximal at the outer surfaces and may result in spiral failure lines (figure 3.39b).

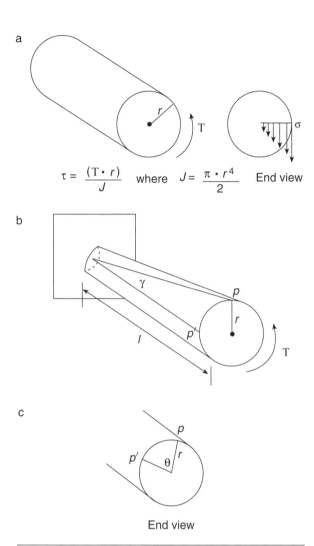

a

$$\tau = \frac{(T \cdot r)}{J} \quad \text{where} \quad J = \frac{\pi \cdot r^4}{2} \quad \text{End view}$$

b

c

End view

Figure 3.38 Torsional loading. (*a*) Shear stress (τ) developed in response to torsional loading (T) [eq. (3.42)] where r is the radius of the cylinder and J is the polar moment of inertia. (*b*) Shear strain (γ) created by torsional loading. (*c*) Angle of twist (θ).

Viscoelasticity

As noted in the discussion of fluid mechanics, the mechanical response of a material depends on its constituent matter, which in the case of biological tissues generally has a fluid component. This viscous element provides resistance to flow and affects the stress-strain (σ/ε) relation in viscoelastic tissues. The stress response is a function of both the strain and the strain rate ($\dot{\varepsilon}$). In viscoelastic tissues an increasing strain rate increases the slope of the σ/ε curve and hence the stiffness of the material.

Purely elastic (i.e., nonviscous) materials subjected to load will deform according to their particular σ/ε relationship and store energy in the process. When the load is removed, the stored

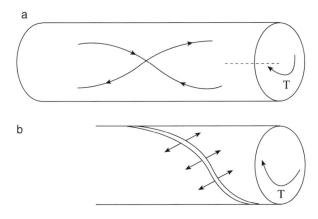

Figure 3.39   Helical stress trajectories. (*a*) Applied torque (*T*) creates helical (spiral) stress lines. (*b*) When the stresses exceed the material's threshold, tensile failure occurs along the helical stress trajectories. This fracture pattern is seen in spiral fractures of long bones.

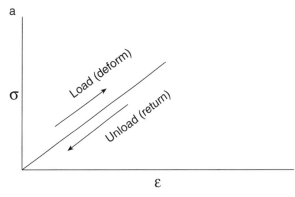

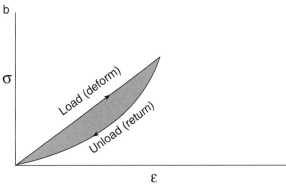

Figure 3.40   (*a*) Purely elastic materials return along the same σ/ε path and therefore lose no energy. (*b*) Viscoelastic materials exhibit a delayed return response (hysteresis) and lose energy (heat) during the deformation-return cycle. The shaded area within the hysteresis loop is a measure of the energy loss.

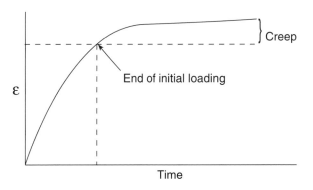

Figure 3.41   Mechanical creep in response to constant load. After an initial deformation while the load is initially applied, the material further deforms (creeps) to an asymptotic value while under constant load.

strain energy is returned, and the tissue returns to its original shape with no energy loss by retracing the σ/ε path traversed during loading (figure 3.40a).

Viscoelastic tissues, in contrast, lose energy to heat during deformation, and the return following unloading is retarded, resulting in a return path different from the initial path during loading (figure 3.40b). The rate of elastic return is determined by the material properties, in particular the amount of viscous resistance. Materials that quickly return to their original shape are termed resilient; those that return more slowly exhibit a dampened response. The area enclosed by the loading-unloading paths (shaded area in figure 3.40b) is called the hysteresis loop and represents the energy lost during the loading-unloading cycle.

Viscous effects also are responsible for two common, time-dependent phenomena associated with biological tissues. The first of these, creep response, is seen when a tissue is subjected to a constant load. At initial loading, the tissue deforms rapidly until the specified constant force level is reached. Instead of maintaining this deformation under the constant load, the tissue continues to deform, or creep, as it approaches an asymptotic deformation plateau (figure 3.41).

The second phenomenon, seen in viscoelastic tissues subjected to constant deformation, is the stress-relaxation response. A tissue stretched (or compressed) to a given length and then held at that length, develops an initial resistance, or stress. While being maintained at the constant deformation, the stress decreases, or "relaxes," as shown in figure 3.42a.

The creep and stress-relaxation responses are also strain rate dependent. This is shown for the stress-relaxation curve in figure 3.42b. With increased strain rate ($\dot{\varepsilon}_2$) the tissue is stiffer (i.e., steeper σ/ε slope), and the peak stress (σ_{max}) is higher and occurs sooner than with the slower strain rate ($\dot{\varepsilon}_1$).

a

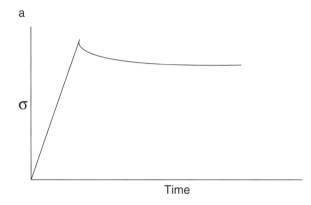

b

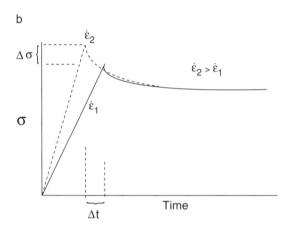

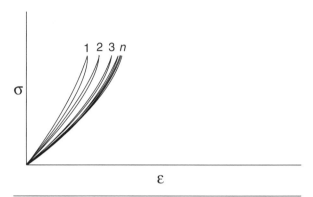

Figure 3.43 Initial-cycle or first-cycle effect. Schematic representation of the different σ/ε responses seen in early loading cycles compared with later cycles when the response settles into a steady-state pattern.

Figure 3.42 (*a*) Stress-relaxation in response to constant deformation. The initial deformation elicits a stress (σ) response. Once the material reaches and maintains its constant deformation, the stress decreases (relaxes) to a constant level. (*b*) The effect of strain rate on the stress-relaxation response. At the higher strain rate ($\dot{\varepsilon}_2$), the maximum stress is greater by $\Delta\sigma$ and reaches this peak stress earlier (by Δt).

Material Fatigue and Failure

Materials, including biological tissues, subjected to repeated loads above a certain threshold experience material fatigue and exhibit a decreased ability to withstand applied forces. Continued loading of a fatiguing material leads to eventual material failure. The number of loading cycles required prior to failure may range from a few, as in the case of repeatedly bending a paper clip, to many millions.

An important fatigue-related concept, known as the initial-cycle or first-cycle effect, implies that the mechanical response seen in initial loading cycles may differ from the response seen during later loading cycles. This effect is shown in the σ/ε relationships depicted in figure 3.43. We see a gradual shift in tissue behavior from the initial

cycles to later ones. Reasons for this shift include temperature fluctuation, fluid shift, and viscous response characteristics.

The susceptibility to tissue failure is determined in large part by how the stresses generated in response to loads are distributed throughout the material. If the stress is equally distributed, as in a smooth, homogenous solid, there is less chance of failure. If the stress is concentrated at a specific location, the likelihood of failure at that point increases. Stress concentration tends to occur at locations of discontinuity within the tissue. These discontinuities create stress risers, or points of focused stress. Examples of stress risers include abrupt tissue interfaces (e.g., osteotendinous junction), fracture sites, and bone screw insertion points (figure 3.44).

The material response prior to failure can vary considerably. Some materials (e.g., glass, bone) deform very little prior to failure and are classified as brittle. Other materials (e.g., putty, elastic ligament) undergo considerable deformation before failing and are called ductile. Caution must be taken not to confuse the strength of a material with its brittleness or ductility. Brittle materials, for example, may possess high strength (e.g., steel) or may fail quite easily (e.g., chalk).

Three mechanical theories have been proposed to explain the failure behavior of materials: (1) maximal normal stress, (2) maximal shear stress, and (3) maximal energy of distortion (Nash 1994). The second theory (maximal shear stress) appears valid for brittle materials, while the first and third theories appear to explain failures in ductile materials.

Regardless of the theory used to explain material failure, the critical point is that failure in biological

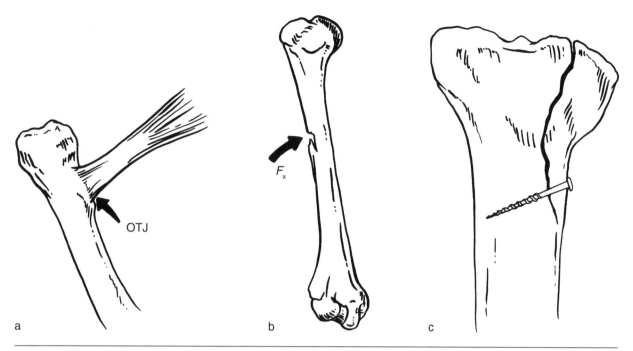

Figure 3.44 Stress risers. Discontinuities in a material's substance serve to concentrate stresses at the site of discontinuity and increase the risk of failure at that site. Stress risers at (*a*) osteotendinous junction (OTJ), (*b*) bone fracture site, and (*c*) site of surgically implanted bone screw.

tissues is closely associated with severe injury. Greater insight into a tissue's mechanical behavior may lead to more specific strategies to control or reduce injury.

Biomechanical Modeling and Simulation

In general, a *model* is defined as a representation of one or more of an object's or system's characteristics. One of the primary goals of modeling is to improve, often through idealization and simplification, our understanding of the system or phenomenon being studied. Virtually every field of endeavor uses models in some way. Engineers and architects construct miniaturized versions of machines and buildings prior to constructing the real structure; economists create elaborate models to represent how the financial markets behave; psychologists construct models of human behavior. Simulations are intrinsically related to models, so much so that the two terms often and erroneously are used interchangeably. The distinction is that a model comprises the equations describing the system, while a simulation is the process of using the validated model to perform experiments to address questions related to a system and its operation.

Model Types

Biomechanical models typically exist in one of two forms: a physical model or a mathematical (or computer) model. Many of these models have the potential to provide valuable insights into the mechanisms of injury. Physical models in biomechanics are perhaps best exemplified by crash-test dummies, which have generated valuable data to improve vehicle occupant safety.

The biomechanics literature is replete with examples of computer models. These models use mathematics in the form of equations as the language of expression to characterize aspects of the system being modeled. In biomechanics, mathematical models have addressed movements such as walking, running, jumping, and throwing, along with more sport-specific movement patterns found in swimming, diving, track and field events, gymnastics, ice skating, golf, and other sports. Recent biomechanical models have probed areas as diverse as muscle force production, meniscal dysfunction, arterial hemodynamics, prosthetic design, and foot placement during gait.

Why choose to develop a model over other means of investigation, such as direct experimentation? First, mathematical models prove useful in situations that are not easily duplicated in real life. For obvious reasons, studies involving collisions or injuries are not tenable using human subjects. Computer models provide a means of manipulating potential injury conditions without risk. Second, models allow investigators to make changes in a system that could not be accomplished readily by an organism operating in a real environment. A human running, for example, would be unable to modulate his or her performance to produce specific changes in ground reaction forces at each step. A model of the runner, however, could easily produce these forces through appropriate inputs and can be used to predict the response of the system across a range of values. The third major reason is time. Time-consuming direct experimental paradigms can be simulated in a fraction of the time. The continuing development of sophisticated mathematical models in the past two decades parallels the development of computing power. The speed and calculation power afforded by computers allow the implementation of complex models that in the past would have been computationally intractable.

Model Selection Criteria

Once the decision is made to create a model of a device, object, or system, the next step in the process

Crash-Test Dummies Are No Dummies!

Anthropometric models, commonly known as crash-test dummies, are much more than friendly reminders for us to buckle our seat belts. The data they provide about the body's response in collision has proved invaluable in making automobiles safer. Countless lives have been saved through the innovations these "dummies" have pioneered. State-of-the-art versions are much more than lifeless masses; current models employ sophisticated instrumentation that allows measurement of body velocities, accelerations, impact forces, and much more. The effective designs of current passive restraint systems, air bags, crumple zones, side-impact reinforcements, collapsing steering columns, and safety windshields are in large part products of information generated from crash-test dummies.

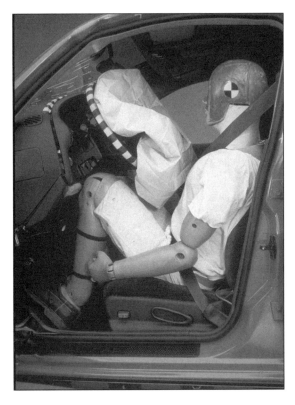

Figure 3B.2 Crash-test dummy.
Reprinted from Insurance Institute for Highway Safety.

(continued)

(continued)

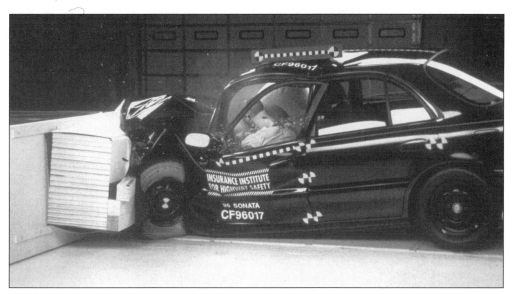

Figure 3B.3 Automobile crash using crash-test dummy.
Reprinted from Insurance Institute for Highway Safety.

involves selecting the most appropriate type or class of model. Proper selection of model type depends largely on the questions being posed. An important caveat is that model complexity is directly related to the difficulty of model formulation and interpretation.

Biomechanical model selection relies on many considerations, including those outlined in the following discussion. These criteria are not mutually exclusive, but rather are complementary in refining the selection process to identify the best model for a given problem. The human body can be studied at many structural levels, ranging from molecular to whole body. The questions being addressed by the model dictate whether the model is a molecular, cellular, tissue, organ, segmental, or whole-body formulation.

Body tissues are subjected to external loads and will deform to varying extents. Thus, different structural types can be modeled. Tissues experiencing measurable deformation are best modeled using a deformable-body model. Tissues exhibiting negligible deformation or bodies assumed to be nondeformable (e.g., limb segments) can be represented by a rigid-body model. Structures considered without regard to their molecular characteristics are best examined using a continuum mechanical model. A contrasting view of a structure according to its component parts is best considered with a discrete-element, or finite-element model.

The level of system motion determines whether the appropriate model is a static model (e.g., assessing the loads on the low back while in a bent-over position), a quasi-static model (e.g., patellofemoral joint loads during a slow squat), or a dynamic model (e.g., ankle joint moments during a vertical jump).

Most human body functions are inherently nonlinear across their physiological ranges. Thus, even though linear models are easier to formulate and manipulate, more complex nonlinear models often are the models of choice. The complexity of the process being modeled dictates the level of mathematical sophistication required for its formulation. Some simple systems may only require algebraic calculations for their solution, but complex systems may be assessable only through advanced mathematics. Another aspect affecting model selection is whether the system is fully determined (i.e., deterministic model) or comprises functions based on certain probability behaviors (i.e., stochastic model).

Activities involving movement in a single plane, or primarily in a single plane (e.g., walking), can be represented by a two-dimensional, or planar, model. Most human movements, however, occur in multiple planes and require a more complex three-dimensional, or spatial, model.

If actual forces and moments (i.e., kinetics) are measured and used in a model to predict the details of movement (kinematics), we have a forward, or direct solution, approach. In contrast, using measured kinematics (velocities and accelerations) to predict the kinetics (forces and moments) is referred to as an inverse solution approach. This second approach, sometimes called inverse dynamics, is useful when the movement characteristics are measurable, but measuring the actual forces or moments is either very difficult or impossible. Inverse dynamics models are commonly used, for example, to estimate the internal forces and moments at joints. Direct measurement of muscle forces and joint torques is difficult at best, and inverse dynamics techniques provide a non-invasive means of calculating these values.

As noted earlier, all models are simplifications of the actual situation being modeled. Simplification, however, does not necessarily imply simplicity. Even with simplification, models can become quite complex, and with available computer processing power increasing exponentially, there is a temptation to create extremely complex models. How complex a model is needed? Hubbard provides us with sage advice: "Always begin with the simplest possible model which captures the essence of the task being studied" (Hubbard 1993, 55).

Elements of a model are often idealized representations of real-life variables, in much the same way as an idealized force vector is representative of many force vectors. In idealizing a system component, however, some information is lost about its actual functional properties. The ability of a model or simulation to achieve its purpose is only as good as the data that it receives as input. The usefulness of the model's output is directly related to the fidelity of the input data.

A stable model can maintain its validity over an appropriate range of values and conditions. The predictive ability, and therefore the usefulness, of any model is related to the accuracy to which variables can be specified over a range of values. The critical issue becomes, How well does the model predict values between known data points (interpolative ability) and beyond the ranges of known values (extrapolative ability)?

Biomechanical modeling is a useful tool for exploring many areas of human function, particularly in describing and evaluating human movement. The potential of modeling in assessing the biomechanics of injury has yet to reach its full potential and holds much promise. With increasingly available technological capabilities, care must be taken to maintain focus on the physiological processes of interest and not to become mesmerized by mathematical sophistication.

Our discussions of tissue structure (chapter 2) and material mechanics (this chapter) have highlighted the viscoelastic nature of tissues such as bone, tendon, ligament, and cartilage. The details of these tissues' mechanical characteristics are presented in chapter 4, but it is instructive at this point to examine the viscoelastic properties of tissue in an example modeling application.

Rheological Models

Rheology is the study of the deformation and flow of matter. Given that body tissues all have a fluid component and therefore have flowlike characteristics, we introduce the concept of a rheological model, which has been used extensively to examine the mechanical behavior of human tissues.

Rheological models of tissue interrelate the stress (σ), strain (ε), and strain rate ($\dot{\varepsilon}$) of biological tissues. They employ three basic model components that, while having no direct association to actual tissue structural elements, allow us to examine tissue response to loading. These three model components are the linear spring, the dashpot, and the frictional element (figure 3.45). In normal situations, internal friction is negligible compared with other forces and so is often omitted from rheological models of biological tissues.

The linear spring represents the elastic properties of the tissue, assuming that the material deforms and returns to its original shape linearly with respect to the applied force and the deformation. The relationship between the spring's stress (σ) and strain (ε) is given by eq. (3.26), where E is Young's modulus, or stiffness of the material.

The fluid component of biological tissues dictates a loading response that is strain rate dependent. The dashpot models this viscous contribution to the overall response. If the fluid's stress–strain rate response is linear, the fluid is termed a Newtonian fluid. The following equation indicates the dashpot's linear relationship:

$$\sigma = \eta \cdot \dot{\varepsilon} \qquad (3.45)$$

where η = the proportionality coefficient relating stress and strain rate.

Researchers can use linear springs (or nonlinear springs) and dashpots as building blocks in constructing composite models with the goal of

Finite-Element Modeling

The finite-element (FE) method originated in the mid-1950s as a tool to assist engineers in the design of structures. The FE approach often requires lengthy and complex calculations and therefore became tractable only with the advances in computer technology. Originally, its use was restricted to experts specializing in FE methods who used large, mainframe computers to solve problems. As computer size decreased and speed increased, FE methods became more accessible to nonspecialists via commercially available FE program packages. Originally used in aerospace engineering (primarily by NASA), FE methods gradually found their way into other areas of structural analysis in mechanical and civil engineering. In recent years biomechanists have found finite-element modeling to be a valuable tool for investigating a wide range of biological problems, such as designing better artificial hip joints.

What is finite-element modeling? Basically, FE makes use of simple shapes, known as elements (building blocks), which are assembled to form complex geometrical structures. The elements are connected at points known as nodes. In a model, a finite number of elements (or shapes) are connected at nodes to form a mathematical representation of a structure such as bone. As forces are applied to the model or as the model is deformed, elaborate equations predict the structure's stress and strain responses to loading. The complexity of a finite-element model is determined by the imagination of its creator, the level of mathematical sophistication, and computing power.

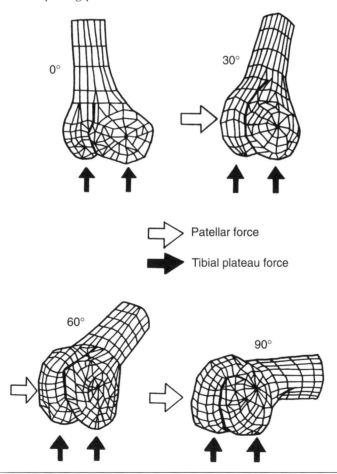

Figure 3B.4 Finite-element model of the distal femur.
Reprinted from Nambu et al. 1991.

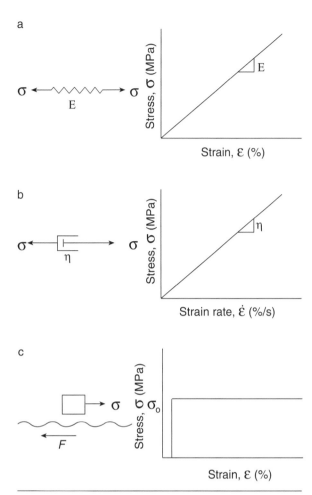

Figure 3.45 Rheological model components: (*a*) spring, (*b*) dashpot, and (*c*) frictional element.

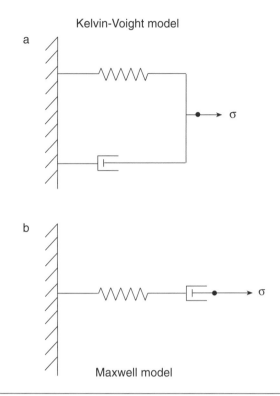

Kelvin-Voight model

Maxwell model

Figure 3.46 Rheological models. (*a*) Kelvin-Voight model, with spring and dashpot in parallel. (*b*) Maxwell model, with spring and dashpot in series.

accurately predicting the response of real tissues. Two standard combinations of linear spring and dashpot are the Kelvin-Voight model (spring and dashpot in parallel) and the Maxwell model (spring and dashpot in series). These models and their loading responses are shown in figure 3.46. Neither of these models is directly applicable for modeling tissue behavior, but combining them with other components produces models with good predictive abilities. A simple, standard solid model and a more complex model are depicted in figure 3.47. By varying the coefficients E_i and η, the models can be fine-tuned to provide an accurate representation of the tissue's response to loading.

Concluding Comments

Many of the mechanical concepts presented in this chapter will be used as we explore tissue biomech-

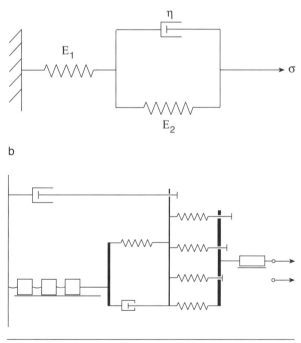

Figure 3.47 Examples of rheological models. (*a*) Standard solid model. (*b*) Complex model.
Reprinted from Viidik 1968.

anics and injury mechanisms in the following chapters. Keep in mind that while the information was divided into separate parts for presentation, the concepts are interrelated in complex and fascinating ways. One of the essential challenges in studying the biomechanics of injury is to identify the salient aspects of movement, fluid, joint, and material mechanics and blend them into an understandable and useful context.

Suggested Readings

Enoka, R.M. (1994). *Neuromechanical Basis of Kinesiology* (2nd ed.). Champaign, IL: Human Kinetics.

Green, M., & Nokes, L.D.M. (1988). *Engineering Theory in Orthopaedics.* New York: Halsted Press.

Hall, S.J. (1995). *Basic Biomechanics* (2nd ed.). St. Louis: Mosby.

Hamill, J., & Knutzen, K. (1995). *Biomechanical Basis of Human Movement.* Baltimore: Williams & Wilkins.

Hay, J.G. (1993). *The Biomechanics of Sports Techniques* (4th ed.). Englewood Cliffs, NJ: Prentice Hall.

Jackson, J.J., & Wirtz, H.G. (1983). *Elementary Statics and Strength of Materials.* New York: McGraw-Hill.

Kane, T.R., & Levinson, D.A. (1985). *Dynamics: Theory and Application.* New York: McGraw-Hill.

Luttgens, K., Deutsch, H., & Hamilton, N. (1992). *Kinesiology: Scientific Basis of Human Motion* (8th ed.). Dubuque, IA: Brown & Benchmark.

Morecki, A. (Ed.). (1987). *Biomechanics of Engineering: Modelling, Simulation, Control.* New York: Springer-Verlag.

Mow, V.C., Flatow, E.L, & Foster, R.J. (1994). Biomechanics. In: Simon, S.R. (Ed.), *Orthopaedic Basic Science.* Park Ridge, IL: American Academy of Orthopaedic Surgeons.

Nahum, A.M., & Melvin, J.W. (Eds.). (1993). *Accidental Injury: Biomechanics and Prevention.* New York: Springer-Verlag.

Nordin, M., & Frankel, V.H. (1989). *Basic Biomechanics of the Musculoskeletal System* (2nd ed.). Philadelphia: Lea & Febiger.

Norkin, C.C., & Levangie, P.K. (1992). *Joint Structure and Function: A Comprehensive Analysis* (2nd ed.). Philadelphia: Davis.

Simon, S.R. (Ed.). (1994). *Orthopaedic Basic Science.* Park Ridge, IL: American Academy of Orthopaedic Surgeons.

Spiegel, L., & Limbrunner, G.F. (1994). *Applied Statics and Strength of Materials.* New York: Merrill.

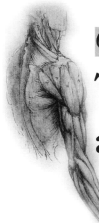

Chapter 4

Tissue Biomechanics and Adaptation

The form . . . of matter . . . and the changes of form which are apparent in . . .
its growth . . . are due to the action of force(s).
D'Arcy Thompson, 1917

Building on the tissue anatomy presented in chapter 2 and the biomechanical principles detailed in chapter 3, in this chapter we review the viscoelastic behaviors and adaptive responses of the tissues of the human musculoskeletal system (bone, articular cartilage, tendon, ligament, and skeletal muscle). These tissues exhibit complex mechanical behaviors, such as stress relaxation at constant strain, creep at constant stress, hysteresis under cyclic loading, strain-rate dependency, and cyclic stress fatigue. Skeletal muscle, in addition to these passive phenomena, also has active force, length, and velocity properties that are unique and synergistic. Information about the mechanical properties and behaviors of musculoskeletal tissues has been gathered using in vitro, in situ, and in vivo methods.

The adaptive capabilities of musculoskeletal tissues are as important to understanding injury as is tissue biomechanical function. Although homeostasis is a basic tenet of physiology, when we examine that tenet more closely, the actual situation is closer to a continually changing equilibrium—tissues in the body are constantly adapting. Adaptation is a natural, form-function interaction and can be defined as the "modification of an organism or its parts that makes it more fit for existence under the conditions of its environment" (Mish 1984).

Bone Biomechanics

Throughout the life span, dramatic changes and adaptations occur in bone, cartilage, tendon, ligament, and muscle. Factors such as physical activity, immobilization with a cast or brace, or

In Vitro, in Situ, or in Vivo?

It is essential to test and accurately measure mechanical properties to understand tissue function and responses, but the act of measuring, in itself, can change a tissue's behavior. The dilemma facing scientists who study the properties of biological tissues is highlighted by these two quotes:

> [T]he most likely way, therefore, to get any insight into the nature of those parts of creation which come within our observation, must in all reason be to number, weigh and measure.
>
> S. Hales, 1727

> Error is all around us and creeps in at the least opportunity. Every method is imperfect.
>
> C.J.H. Nicolle, 1932

Methodological approaches exist to study the full range of joints, tissues, or tissue constituents, and these fall broadly into three categories: in vitro, in situ, and in vivo. Each successive category gets closer to measuring tissue behaviors as they exist in the body—although each method has advantages and disadvantages.

In vitro literally means "within a glass," but in the generic sense *in vitro* connotes testing done in an artificial environment. The range of specimens (from whole bones to cells) are usually immersed in a physiological buffer solution maintained at body temperature, but the environment is artificial, and the test is therefore in vitro.

One advantage of in vitro tests is that *direct measurements* can be taken. One disadvantage, however, is that the in vitro method is invasive—a tissue or its cells are removed from the body and their normal environment. The isolated cells no longer have their native chemical and physical connections to the surrounding tissues and fluids.

In situ means "in its normal place," or confined to the site of origin, and one advantage of in situ preparations is that some elements of the natural environment are preserved in the testing. Notably, much of the information available on skeletal muscle properties has been gathered through in situ techniques. During in situ experiments to record skeletal muscle contractions, a muscle's natural blood supply can be maintained, as well as the terminal nerve-muscle interface. The orientation of the muscle with respect to its bony attachments can be maintained, and the muscle temperature can be kept within the physiological range. Though this method is closer to natural, nonetheless components of the test environment are still "artificial." The properties are determined under constrained conditions and not in the freely moving organism.

In vivo indicates that the testing is done within the living body, and ideally this approach would appear to be the best. However, obtaining accurate in vivo data is very challenging technically. Even if the data are recorded successfully, the transducers that are implanted can affect the measurements being taken. Furthermore, ethical concerns must be addressed, especially when trying to measure responses of musculoskeletal tissues in humans. A few investigators have recorded muscle-tendon forces (Gregor et al. 1991) or bone strains (Burr et al. 1995) in humans, but the great majority of in vivo experiments involving musculoskeletal tissues have been done with animal models.

changes in diet can profoundly affect the quality and quantity of load-bearing connective tissues. Here, for each musculoskeletal tissue, we first review the biomechanical properties and then summarize the tissue's adaptive capabilities.

Compact (Cortical) Bone

The mechanical behavior of compact (cortical) bone can be assessed in a variety of ways. The method of testing should be selected to approximate most closely the loading situation that the structure experiences in the body. Because bone is usually loaded multiaxially, it is difficult to test each condition in which bone is loaded. With simplifying assumptions, compact bone is treated as an elastic beam of uniform dimension and tested in three- or four-point bending, or a sample of bone of known dimension is machined out of a larger piece and tested in uniaxial compression or tension.

In a typical bending test (figure 4.1), as the bone is initially loaded, the load-deformation curve is concave toward the load axis. As the load increases, load and deformation increase in a relatively linear fashion, obeying Hooke's law. The slope of this linear region is related to the bone's flexural rigidity, a measure of bending stiffness. The *proportional limit* marks the end of the linear region. In compact bone the proportional limit and the elastic limit are usually closely related. The *elastic limit* demarcates the transition from bone's elastic behavior into its plastic region. As the response of bone moves into the region of *plastic deformation*, smaller and smaller increases in load will produce greater and greater increases in deformation. If the applied load is removed just after the transition to plastic deformation (but before maximal and failure loads are reached), the bone does not return to its original (preloaded) configuration. Instead, the bone takes on a permanent set: It remains bent.

Flexural rigidity, load behaviors, and energy (area under a load-deformation curve) are structural properties of the bone. Further, if the geometry (shape) of the bone sample is known, then the material properties of the bone can be calculated. *Material* refers to the mechanical quality of the bone. The elastic modulus and stresses (force per unit area) at the proportional limit and at the maximal and failure points are examples of the bone's material properties.

The distinction between structural and material properties is easily recognized by considering the diaphyses of a femur and a phalange. The obviously larger femoral diaphysis is able to carry substantially greater loads than the smaller phalange, and thus the structural properties (e.g., maximal load and bending stiffness) of the femur will be much greater than the phalange. Nonetheless, the compact bone within the femur and phalange could have very similar composition, and thus, if their differences in size were removed (normalized), the material properties of the two bones may be very similar (e.g., maximal stress, calculated as force per unit area).

The preceding discussion of the importance of

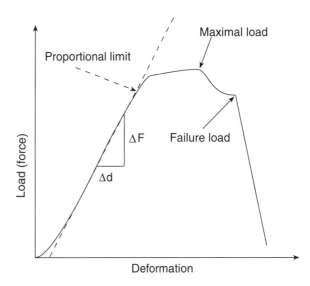

Figure 4.1 Example of a load-deformation curve from a sample of cortical bone that is being tested in three-point bending. The initial region of the load-deformation curve is nonlinear, but then a primary linear response develops until the proportional limit is reached. Up to the elastic limit (which is close to the proportional limit in cortical bone), the bone tissue behaves elastically. When the elastic limit is exceeded, plastic deformation occurs, until maximal load is reached. Catastrophic failure of the sample happens after or at the same time as maximal load. In three-point bending the flexural rigidity of the bone is calculated as $(L^3/48) \cdot (F/d)$, where L is equal to the distance between the two supporting points on which the bone rests and (F/d) is the slope of the force-deformation curve in the linear region. Flexural rigidity itself is the product of the elastic modulus (E) and the cross-sectional area moment of inertia (I) of the sample.

bone shape and geometry leads us to consider how the area moment of inertia (I) influences the structural properties of bone during bending. But before using a bone example, try the following thought experiment. Imagine that you are standing on a 2-m-long oak plank that is 5 cm thick and 30 cm wide. The board is supported only at its two ends; if you stand at midlength, the board is being loaded in three-point bending. When you stand on the flat (30-cm) side of the board, you will definitely bend the board as it sags under your weight. If, however, you rotate the board 90° so you balance on the 5-cm edge, the sag will be much less, and the board will be much stiffer.

This potent effect of bone cross-sectional geometry can be seen in the three scenarios illustrated in figure 4.2. Assume that you are testing tubular long bones of three different cross-sectional shapes in three-point bending. Examples I and II have the same periosteal diameter, but example I has marrow core, while example II has no marrow core (a solid bone). Example III has a slightly larger periosteal diameter of 2.5 cm and a relatively large marrow core (a thin-walled, tubular bone). As seen in the table in figure 4.2, these shape differences generate pronounced differences in area moment of inertia and bending behaviors. The bone cross-sectional areas for examples I (2.95 cm²) and II (3.14 cm²) are more than 65% greater than the cross-sectional area of the large tubular bone shown in example III (1.77 cm²). At the same time, because the area moment of inertia [cf. figure 3.32] is related to the amount of bone and the distribution of the bone about the bending axis, the thin-walled, tubular

bone (example III) has an area moment of inertia that is substantially greater (> 40%) than either example I or II. Thus, if the same bending load was applied to each of the bones, at least 14% more stress would be developed within both the smaller tubular bone (example I) and the solid bone (example II) than in the large tubular bone (example III).

Changing the ratio of the periosteal-to-endosteal diameters provides a creative way to increase the bending stiffness of a long bone without necessarily adding large amounts of bone mass. The theoretical implications and potential optimization of the structural features of the wall thickness of tubular bones were explored in a fascinating paper by Currey and Alexander (1985).

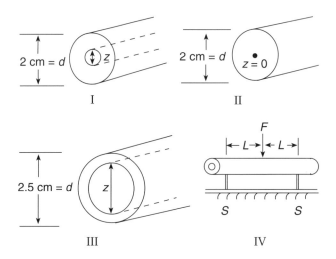

Figure 4.2   Cross-sectional geometry affects bone bending behavior. In examples I, II, and III, d is the periosteal (outside) diameter, and z is the endosteal (core) diameter of the long bone. IV depicts three-point-bending loads being applied to the bone samples. F is the applied force, and S marks the positions of the two supports under the bone sample. The distance between the applied force F and each support S is L. In examples I and III (tubular bone of different dimensions), area = $\pi \cdot (d^2 - z^2)/4$, and area moment of inertia $(I) = \pi \cdot (d^4 - z^4)/64$. In example II (solid bone, no endosteal [marrow] cavity), area = $\pi \cdot d^2/4$, and area moment of inertia $(I) = \pi \cdot d^4/64$. For examples I, II, and III during three-point bending (see IV), the stress (σ) developed in the bone is $\sigma = MC/I$, where M = moment, C = distance from the center of the cross section to the periosteal surface (a radius), and I = area moment of inertia of the cross section. $M = (F/2) \cdot L$, where F = 20 N, and L = 20 cm.

	Example I	Example II	Example III
Periosteal diameter (d), cm	2.00	2.00	2.50
Endosteal diameter (z), cm	0.50	0.00	2.00
Bone area (A), cm²	2.95	3.14	1.77
Area moment of inertia (I), cm⁴	0.78	0.79	1.13
Force (F), N	20.0	20.0	20.0
Stress ($\sigma = MC/I$), N/cm²	256	253	221

What If Bones Were Solid Beams Rather Than Thin-Walled Tubes?

Two renowned biologists, John Currey and McNeill Alexander (1985), hypothesized that the mechanical design of tubular long bones suggests that there may be an optimal ratio of the diameter of thin-walled bones to their cortical thickness. It is generally accepted that the tubular structure of most limb bones ensures that they will be lighter without sacrificing strength or stiffness. But does this notion hold across a wide range of species?

In assessing "optimum," Currey and Alexander considered the counterbalancing of relative bone mass against structural properties, such as yield (or fatigue) strength, ultimate (or impact) strength, and stiffness. By measuring the limb bones of a substantial array (56 species) of extant and some extinct mammals, birds, and reptiles, they came up with intriguing results showing why tubular, marrow-filled bones appear to be an effective design for bones that undergo substantial bending loads—such as the bones of limbs.

They calculated the ratio of cross-sectional radius (C) to the thickness of the bone cortical shell (t). Currey and Alexander predicted that if marrow-filled bones were basically tubular structures of minimal mass and optimal strength, then the C/t ratio would be 2.3. By comparison, if stiffness was the criterion for bone design, then C/t would be 3.9. Using the measurements of actual limb bones, they found that the median C/t ratio for terrestrial mammals was about 2.0—close to the predicted optimal values for impact loading and ultimate strength. Nonetheless, a spectrum of experimental results emerged from their analysis. For example, the manatee (*Trichechus manatus,* an aquatic mammal) has a solid humerus ($C/t = 1.0$), and the elephant (*Loxodonta africana*) has solid metacarpals. On the other hand, the humerus of a bat (*Pipistrellus* sp.) had thinner walls than most mammals ($C/t = 3.7$).

The extinct *Pteranadon,* with its huge wing span—presumably used for soaring and gliding on wind currents—had astonishingly thin-walled but very large-diameter wing bones that would be particularly well designed if minimal mass was vital. The *Pteranadon* humerus, for example, had a C/t value of 20.0. It was the only animal with C/t values greater than 7.7. At the other end of the spectrum, alligators have a femoral C/t value of 1.3—the walls of their femurs are very thick with a small marrow cavity.

To get another view of the effects of the different-sized tubular bones, compare the three long bones (examples I, II, and III in figure 4.2) for which we contrasted cross-sectional geometry and stresses in three-point bending. In the following table, we provide values for their cross-sectional radius (C), cortical thickness (t), and the ratio C/t. The larger-diameter and thinner-walled bone (example III) has the much larger C/t ratio.

Table 4B.1

	Example I*	Example II*	Example III*
Radius (C), cm	1.00	1.00	1.25
Cortex thickness (t), cm	0.75	1.00	0.25
Radius/thickness (C/t)	1.33	1.00	5.00

*See figure 4.2 for sketches and dimensions of these long bones.

Interestingly, chickens trained by running on a treadmill also demonstrate a shift toward Currey and Alexander's predicted ultimate (and impact) strength optimal C/t for a weight-bearing limb bone (Loitz & Zernicke 1992; Matsuda et al. 1986). The adult roosters were

(continued)

(continued)

exercised on a treadmill for 1 h/d, 5 d/wk for 9 wk, at 70% to 75% predicted maximal aerobic capacity (Loitz & Zernicke 1992) and had an average *C/t* of 2.3 in their tarsometatarsal bones—precisely the values predicted by Currey and Alexander (1985).

Why is this important? Consider the following. Currey calculated that when a horse gallops at 54 km/h, about 50% of its power is used to accelerate and decelerate the bones of its limbs. Thus, a 10% decrease in limb bone mass would generate a 5% savings of power. This savings could be significant either in the context of natural selection (escape from a predator) or even in a thoroughbred horse race.

Extensive data on the material properties of cortical bones of many different species (including human) were reported by Yamada (1973). Besides a wide assortment of human cortical bones (e.g., femur, tibia, fibula, humerus, radius, ulna), bone samples from a range of animals were also tested (e.g., horses, cattle, wild boars, deer, ostriches). Yamada noted that the average ultimate tensile stress for the long bones of limbs from humans 20 to 39 years of age ranged between 120 and 150 MPa. Later studies (Martin & Burr 1989) of the ultimate tensile stress in cortical bone have been in the same general range (e.g., 108-130 MPa). In terms of ultimate compressive stress, the human femur had the greatest value (up to 166 MPa in persons 20-39 years of age), followed by the tibia, then the humerus, with the lowest values in the fibula, ulna, and radius—although even those three bones had an average ultimate compressive stress greater than 115 MPa. In comparison to human cortical bone, the mechanical properties of compact bone from a host of species have been studied extensively (Currey 1979, 1985, 1988a, 1988b, 1990).

Currey's comparative osteological results have shown that a bone's calcium content and porosity

Comparative Properties of Bone

From his perspective as a biologist, John Currey views the structure-function relation of bones as it relates to natural selection. For example, in 1979 he assessed the mechanical properties of three types of bones with very different functions and consequently very different mechanical properties—a deer's (*Cervus elaphus*) antler, a cow's (*Bos taurus*) femur, and a fin whale's (*Balaenoptera physalus*) tympanic bulla. Using machined specimens, Currey tested the bones' work of fracture during bending, bending strength, and modulus of elasticity in bending. The *work of fracture* is the amount of mechanical work needed to propagate a crack through the bone and is a measure of a bone's resistance to impact loading.

The principal function of the red deer's antlers is for display and dueling, and *impact strength* is probably an important property for winning the fight. Currey found a high "impact resistance" in the antlers, but a concomitantly low elastic modulus and relatively low bending strength.

The fin whale's tympanic bulla, in contrast, had the highest mineral content and highest elastic modulus of the three bones, and he described the bulla as "quite rocklike to handle" and about the size of your fist. As you might expect, like the auditory ossicles in your own ear, the tympanic bulla of the fin whale is securely protected in the skull from the outside world. Stiffness (high modulus) would be a very important property to ensure that sound waves are transmitted with fidelity for accurate hearing. The fracture strength of the fin whale's bulla therefore is less important, and there is a natural blend of form and function in this bone. The cow's femur, on the other hand, has an elastic modulus, impact strength, and bending strength that are all rather high but not extreme.

can explain about 80% of the variation seen in a bone's elastic modulus (stiffness). Sampling 28 bones from 17 different species of mammals, birds, and reptiles, Currey (1988a) reported that bone's maximal strain and the mechanical work under the stress-strain curve are sharply decreased with excessive mineralization.

Compact bone is an *anisotropic* material, and as such, bone's elastic modulus and strength depend on the orientation of the collagen-mineral matrix with respect to the loading direction. As with a piece of wood, bone has a "grain" associated with its structure. If you apply a compressive load along the long axis of a piece of wood or bone (in line with its grain), the piece of wood or bone has a much greater elastic modulus and strength than if you applied the load at right angles to the long axis (perpendicular to the grain). In contrast, if you apply loads from any direction to an *isotropic* metal (e.g., stainless steel), the elastic modulus and strength are the same in all directions.

Poisson's ratio (ν) is the other parameter used to characterize a bone's elastic behavior. This effect was illustrated in chapter 3, figure 3.28, and mathematically defined in eq. (3.27). The ratio ν is the negative of the strain transverse to the load divided by the strain of bone in line with the applied load. Bone has a relatively high Poisson's ratio ($\nu \leq 0.6$), much higher than found in metals.

Cortical bone is considered to be tough because it is able to absorb a great deal of mechanical energy before it fractures. Bone is also a relatively ductile material. If a metal is ductile, it can be hammered into thin sheets without breaking. A gold nugget, for example, can be flattened into a wafer-thin foil and thus is considered to be very ductile. Bone, of course, is not as ductile, but it can be deformed (to some extent) without fracture. The opposite of ductile is brittle. With increasing age, bones have a tendency to become less ductile and more brittle, less stiff, and more fragile.

Finally, compact bone is viscoelastic. That is, it exhibits strain-rate sensitivity, creep behavior, hysteresis, and fatigue. Indeed, some of the mechanical properties of cortical bone are very sensitive to differing strain rates. As a bone is loaded more and more rapidly, its ultimate strength increases at a faster rate than does its elastic modulus. *Fatigue* is the loss of strength and stiffness that occurs in materials subjected to repeated cyclic loads. Although bone can withstand substantial stresses when loaded only once, as the number of cyclic loads increases, the ability of a bone to withstand the stress decreases exponentially. In bone, fatigue has been attributed to microscopic cracks that develop within and between the osteons (Martin & Burr 1989). In healthy bone, if damage is not excessive, remodeling resorbs the material around microcracks, and new bone is deposited. If the damage is excessive, however, and the normal remodeling process cannot keep up with the repair, macroscopic failure (fractures) can happen.

When mechanical properties of a material such as bone are compromised, it can be said that the material is "damaged." Using a new type of microscopy, Zioupos and Currey (1994) have been able to visualize the three-dimensional distributions of microcracks in cortical bone. Because microcracks usually develop within the interior of compact bone, they are hard to see in situ. But Zioupos and Currey used a laser-scanning confocal microscope to take "optical sections" through a translucent piece of bone. By focusing the microscope at a given depth within the bone, an image can be digitized. Then through step-by-step refocusing, images can be made at successive layers of the tissue. The thin, sequential sections are then digitally reconstructed to give a three-dimensional picture of the tissue and its components. Zioupos and Currey loaded small strips of bovine compact bone and examined the microcracks that developed. They were satisfied that the microcracks were not caused by machining artifacts and that the cracks were associated with regions of high strain (stress). The microstructure (grain) of the bone affected the propagation of the microcracks within the bone, and microcracks were most likely to occur in the most highly mineralized parts of the bone.

Why are these microcracks significant? As we know, bone has both an elastic and a plastic response. In the plastic region, with decreasing load levels during continuous and cyclic loading, there is an increasing amount of deformation—the bone becomes "damaged" and increasingly compliant. Dispersed microcracks may weaken bone and decrease its structural stiffness. Clinically, the accumulation of fatigue microdamage may produce a stress fracture—an injury not uncommon for athletes such as ballet dancers, gymnasts, basketball players, and long-distance runners, who place highly repetitive, cyclic loads on their weight-bearing bones.

Trabecular (Cancellous) Bone

The lattice-work organization of trabecular bone is quite diverse, and the apparent density and architecture of trabecular bone have potent, nonlinear effects on the elastic modulus and strength. The elastic modulus of trabecular bone can vary from 10 to 2,000 MPa, in contrast to cortical bone with an elastic modulus around 13 to 17 GPa.

The "spaces" in trabecular bone are typically filled with marrow, which can play an important part in the load-bearing capabilities of trabecular bone. If the bone marrow is left in specimens of trabecular bone during impact-speed tests, the strength and elastic modulus are dramatically greater than if the marrow is removed before the test. The enhancing effect of the marrow is minimal, however, at typical physiological rates of loading. Nevertheless, with or without the marrow, trabecular bone exhibits viscoelastic effects because its fundamental building block is viscoelastic lamellar bone (as exists in compact bone).

Bone Adaptation

Bone is a dynamic tissue that usually is exquisitely adapted to the multiple internal factors (e.g., systemic calcium or hormone levels) and external factors (e.g., mechanical loads) that can affect the structure, composition, and quantity of bone. Events that signal change in bone are generally classified as either modeling or remodeling. *Modeling* is the addition (formation) of new bone, whereas *remodeling* involves resorption and (re)formation of bone. Differences between modeling and remodeling of bone are summarized in table 4.1. Modeling can happen at different rates and is a continuous process that can occur on any bony surface to produce a net gain in bone. During modeling, osteoclasts and osteoblasts are not active along the

same surface; resorption can occur along one cortex while deposition occurs along another. The specific stimulus that initiates modeling remains unclear. Modeling happens mainly during the growing years. The ability of bone to adapt to mechanical loading is greater during growth than after maturity, but limited modeling can still occur after skeletal maturation (Bailey, Faulkner, & McKay 1996).

Remodeling is the resorption and replacement of existing bone. Skeletal remodeling can trigger a release of mineral stored in the bone in response to a low serum calcium level, to repair skeletal microdamage, or to balance mechanical and mass needs of the skeleton (Kahn & Parfitt 1992). The sequence of remodeling events can be remembered as ARF: activation, resorption, formation. The first step in remodeling is activation of osteoclasts to resorb existing bone. New bone is deposited by osteoblasts that follow the resorptive front of osteoclasts. Deposition of new bone takes three times longer than resorption. This translates into a 1-wk time lapse between the resorption and formation (Martin & Burr 1989).

Lanyon (1987) described functional remodeling as an "interpretation and purposeful reaction" to a bone's strain state, allowing for adaptation to both increased and decreased strains. "Functional strains are both the objective and the stimulus for the process of adaptive modeling and remodeling" (Lanyon 1987, 1084). Rubin and Lanyon (1985) proposed that if functional strains are too high, the incidence of damage and probability of failure increase. If strains are too low, the metabolic cost of maintaining the unnecessary bone mass is high, and bone therefore is resorbed. Thus, functional strain appears to be a relevant parameter to control. The question remains, however, as to which attribute, or combination of attributes, of strain (magnitude,

Table 4.1   Summary of Modeling-Remodeling Differences

	Modeling	Remodeling
Timing	Continuous	Cyclical (ARF)*
Resorption and formation surfaces	Different	Same
Surfaces affected	100%	20%
Activation	Not required	Required
Balance	Net gain	Net loss
Coupling of formation & resorption	Systemic? (No ARF)	Local

*ARF = Activation-resorption-formation.

From "The cellular basis of bone remodeling: The quantum concept reexamined in light of recent advances in the cell biology of bone" by A.M. Parfitt, 1984, *Calcified Tissue International, 36* (p. S38). Adapted by permission.

rate of application, distribution, or gradient) the bone has the greatest sensitivity.

Another remodeling theory related to mechanical use of the bone suggests that remodeling is stimulated by fatigue damage that may happen during physical activity. In bone, fatigue (loss of strength and stiffness that occurs in materials subjected to repeated cyclic loads) has been attributed to the microscopic cracks that develop within and between the osteons (Martin & Burr 1989). In healthy bone, if the damage is not excessive, remodeling resorbs the material around the crack, and new bone is deposited. If the damage is excessive and normal remodeling cannot keep up with the repair demands, macroscopic failure and fracture may result.

Development, Maturation, and Aging

Much of the accumulated information about the relation between bone growth and bone mineral

How Much Is Too Much?

Whether it is during puberty with its rapid bone growth or during menopause with its precipitous loss of bone, sex hormones have a potent effect on bone health. For females, estrogen is important in building or maintaining the skeleton, and it is becoming apparent that highly intensive training by young female athletes can lead to deleterious consequences on the skeleton as a result of disturbances in normal menstrual cycles.

In sports such as gymnastics, ballet, running, and figure skating, there are numerous examples of young female athletes who experience no menstruation (amenorrhea) or only intermittent and irregular menstruation (oligomenorrhea) as a consequence of altered hormone levels. With the lower estrogen levels that accompany amenorrhea and oligomenorrhea, these young athletes may not achieve a peak bone mass as great as they would have if they had experienced normal levels of estrogen. When this is coupled with calorie-restricted diets to reduce body weight, there is a further danger of slipping into what is termed the *female athlete triad,* namely eating disorders, disrupted hormone levels, and increased risk of poor bone quantity and quality. A comparison of the vertebral mineral mass of amenorrheic elite athletes and cohorts with normal menstrual function found that the amenorrheic athletes had up to 25% less mineral mass than the normal women, suggesting that estrogen deprivation has a powerful effect on trabecular mineral mass (Marcus et al. 1985).

Not only are these young female athletes at potentially greater risk of osteoporosis in later years, but they can also have a likelihood of developing stress fractures in their late teens and early 20s (Zernicke et al. 1994). Among the multiple factors that could contribute to lower-extremity stress fractures in elite intercollegiate runners, one of the most significant predictors of who did and who did not sustain a stress fracture was how much time elapsed between beginning serious, high-intensity training and the runner's first menses. Those runners who had been training in earnest longer before their first menses (and with the heavy training, that first menses may also have been delayed) had a significantly greater chance of having a stress fracture while they were running at the intercollegiate level.

Interestingly, high-intensity and high-impact loading activities (even though they may disrupt normal hormonal balance in young females) may partially counterbalance the full effects of the menstrual disturbances (Bailey, Faulkner, & McKay 1996). For example, Robinson and colleagues (1995) report that despite the finding that 47% of the young female gymnasts they studied were either oligo- or amenorrheic, these gymnasts had greater bone mineral density than either a cohort of runners or control females with normal menses. Bailey and colleagues (1996, 256) conclude that the data suggest that high-impact loading activities in female athletes with disrupted menstrual function have a "sparing effect at weight-bearing sites but not to the same extent at non-weight-bearing sites."

acquisition is summarized in figure 4.3. While undoubtedly a wealth of bone modeling and growth occurs in both axial and appendicular (limb) skeleton during childhood until the pubertal growth period, the differences between sexes in bone mineral content (BMC) are negligible. At about 13 years of age, the bone mineral content for boys and girls diverges, with boys having a greater rate of gain than girls (figure 4.3).

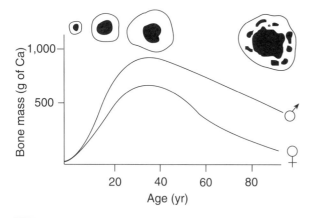

Figure 4.3 Relation among bone mass, age, and sex. The ordinate, bone mass, is represented by the total grams of calcium (Ca) in the skeleton.

Adapted from Kaplan et al. 1994.

Usually about one year after the peak rate of longitudinal growth (peak height velocity, PHV), the peak rate of gain in BMC occurs (figure 4.4). Peak gains in BMC occur at about 13 years for girls and about 14.4 years for boys. Thus, in the year between the time of PHV and the rapid gain in BMC, there is a period of relative bone weakness with a greater chance of fracture. Growth and sex hormones are mainly responsible for the rapid increases in BMC (Bailey, Faulkner, & McKay 1996).

As longitudinal growth begins to slow toward late adolescence, about 90% of adult bone mineral content has already been deposited. Maximal BMC is attained between 20 and 30 years of age. Furthermore, it seems that bone mineral content or bone mineral density does not increase after the age of 30 for men or women. At skeletal maturity, men have greater BMC than women, and most of that difference is because of the men's thicker cortical bone.

By the fifth decade, bone mass begins to decline. Both men and women lose cortical bone at about the same rate, but women lose trabecular bone much more rapidly than men—especially when women enter menopause. Between the ages of 40 and 50,

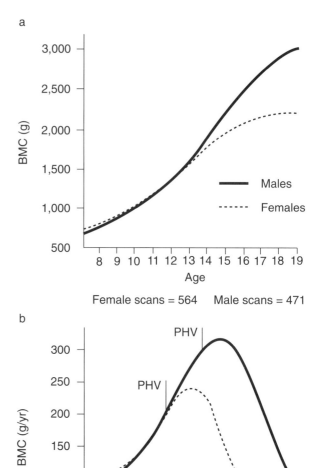

Female scans = 564   Male scans = 471

Figure 4.4 (*a*) Total body bone mineral content (BMC) and (*b*) BMC rate-of-gain curves for males and females. In (*b*), peak rate of change in height (peak height velocity, PHV) is shown for both the boys and girls in this cross-sectional sample. BMC (*a*) is given in total grams of mineral in the body, while the BMC rate-of-gain curve (*b*) is in grams per year.

Reprinted from Bailey, Faulkner, & McKay 1996.

men will generally lose up to 0.75% of total bone mass yearly, while women can lose bone at more than twice that rate. In the few years immediately following menopause, the yearly rate of bone loss in some women can be as much as 3% (Kaplan et al. 1994).

Reaching maximal bone mass in adolescence and early adulthood, therefore, is crucial for reducing the effects of bone loss and mitigating fracture risk later in life. Suggestions for optimizing bone mineral acquisition during the growing years include making a lifelong commitment to weight-bearing physical activity at an early age; engaging in a variety of vigorous daily activities of short duration as opposed to prolonged repetitive activity; doing activities that increase muscle strength and work all large muscle groups; and avoiding periods of immobility (Bailey, Faulkner, & McKay 1996).

On the other end of the spectrum are aging and osteoporosis. Typically, cortical bone becomes weaker and slightly more brittle with increasing age (Martin & Burr 1989). Most of these changes are associated with remodeling, and manifest as age-dependent alterations in bone geometry, size, and number of osteons. A negative balance between bone resorption and formation (frequently, excessive resorption) is the basic mechanism associated with many age-related bone diseases. Generally, advancing age is associated with increased bone porosity.

Osteoporosis is a disease marked by reduced bone mineral mass and changes in bone geometry, leading to an increased probability of fractures, primarily of the hip, spine, and wrist. Progressive loss of bone mass can be a function of the normal aging process, or it can be caused by other disease processes. Further, the amount of bone mass at one site is not necessarily correlated with bone mass at other sites in the body. Finally, many individuals are unaware of the existence of osteoporosis, particularly at the early stages. A longitudinal study on aging in the United States reported the prevalence of osteoporosis and hip fractures in individuals 70 years of age and older (table 4.2). These estimates are based on self-reports and are not confirmed through radiological detection; therefore, the true prevalence may be over- or underestimated.

Both men and women experience some loss of bone mass as part of normal aging, but osteoporosis progresses much more rapidly in postmenopausal women. After the age of 30, men typically lose bone mass at approximately the same rate for the remainder of their lives. In women, however, the loss of bone increases significantly for about five years after menopause and then slows to a more gradual loss. Just after menopause the rate of bone mass loss is up to 10 times faster than in men of the same age (Christiansen 1992). Therapeutic interventions and exercise have been proposed to slow the rapid loss of bone in postmenopausal women. In premenopausal, adult women the rates of bone formation and bone resorption are approximately equal, calcium balance is maintained, and there is no effective loss of bone mass. After menopause, however, bone resorption outpaces formation, which in turn produces a calcium imbalance and a net loss of bone. One of the goals of osteoporosis prevention is to maintain or to restore bone resorption and formation rates to premenopausal levels. Various preventive and therapeutic agents, such as hormone replacement therapy, calcitonin, bisphosphonates, and vitamin D metabolites, are currently being used and investigated in the prevention and treatment of osteoporosis.

Table 4.2   Prevalence of Self-Reported Osteoporosis and Hip Fracture in People 70 Years of Age and Older (United States, 1984)

Type of impairment	(Rate per 100 people)		
	Osteoporosis	Hip fracture	Either condition
Total (70 yrs and older)	3.7	4.5	7.7
70-79 yrs	3.5	3.2	6.2
80 yrs and older	4.3	8.0	11.6
Male (70 yrs and older)	0.6	2.7	3.3
70-79 yrs	0.7	1.9	2.5
80 yrs and older	0.4	5.5	5.9
Female (70 yrs and older)	5.7	5.6	10.5
70-79 yrs	5.5	4.0	8.8
80 yrs and older	6.2	9.2	14.4

*Source of data: U.S. National Center for Health Statistics, Longitudinal Study on Aging
Adapted from Praemer, Furner, & Rice 1992.

Regular exercise may have a positive effect on bone mass. Trabecular bone density may be increased as a result of exercise that specifically loads the affected bones in postmenopausal women, but the effects are site specific. Which exercise best promotes bone density is still unknown. Running, jogging, and walking are the types of exercise usually prescribed to ameliorate bone loss related to menopause, and exercise with higher loads at specific sites may provide a greater osteogenic response (Snow-Harter & Marcus 1991).

Nutrition

Nutrition has potent effects on bone growth and remodeling and therefore on bone quality and mechanical properties. Very briefly, we discuss a few of the nutritional factors that can influence bone quality and quantity: calcium, vitamin D, protein, fats, and sugar.

Normally, the body's bone-mineral balance is exquisitely regulated by the synergistic actions of vitamin D metabolites, parathyroid hormone, and calcitonin—substances that influence the dietary absorption of calcium, bone mineral resorption and deposition, and the renal secretion and resorption of calcium and phosphorus. Of the total-body calcium, about 99% is found in the skeleton, with the remaining 1% circulating in the extracellular fluid (Kaplan et al. 1994). Calcium compounds constitute more than half of the mass of bone. Because calcium is excreted throughout the day, adequate calcium intake is vital for bone health. Bones with diminished bone mineral content are less stiff and consequently may be more prone to fractures.

Vitamin D, dietary protein, phosphorus, fiber, and fats all can affect calcium absorption. Vitamin D is a fat-soluble molecule that can be stored in body fat. Stores of vitamin D primarily depend on the amount of time the skin is exposed to the sun and on the size of the exposed area. A relatively small fraction of the body's vitamin D stores comes from the diet. Vitamin D helps to increase calcium absorption from the intestinal tract; thus, a person deficient in vitamin D poorly absorbs dietary calcium (Toss 1992).

Dietary protein has a significant effect on urinary calcium handling (Heaney 1988). Protein deficiency can lead to decreased levels of calcium in the urine (hypocalciuria) and reduced calcium absorption in the intestine (Orwoll et al. 1992). Conversely, excessive dietary protein can result in greater renal calcium loss and the development of negative calcium balance (Heaney & Recker 1982). Protein deficiency has been implicated in the genesis of osteopenia (reduced bone mass) in malnourished humans (Garn & Kangas 1981) and animals (Ferretti et al. 1988).

For optimal bone health, excessive ingestion of saturated fats and refined sugar should be avoided because both can have negative effects on the body's ability to absorb calcium. High levels of dietary fatty acids reduce the amount of dietary calcium absorbed in the intestine and thereby lead to lower calcium levels in bones (Atteh & Leeson 1984).

Is Exercise Enough?

Snow-Harter and Marcus (1991) state that the efficacy of exercise in preventing and treating osteoporosis still remains unknown. Nevertheless, they summarize what is known by answering the following questions (p. 381):

1. Can exercise maximize peak bone mass?

2. Can exercise forestall or reduce age-related bone losses?

3. Does exercise enhance bone mineral density in people with existing osteoporosis?

4. Can exercise supersede estrogen replacement therapy during the postmenopausal years?

With reasonable qualifications, the answer is yes to the first three questions, but the answer to the fourth question is no. To date, there is no basis to state that exercise alone is as effective as estrogen replacement for maintaining bone mass and reducing the fracture risk for postmenopausal women.

Use Versus Disuse

Exercise and physical activity can stimulate bone remodeling, but how exercise affects the skeleton is a profoundly complex problem. Exercise intensity, skeletal maturity, type of bones (trabecular or cortical), and anatomical location (axial or extremity bones) can all influence the response of specific bones to exercise (Loitz & Zernicke 1992).

The following five points summarize current knowledge of the relationship between physical activity and bone mass. (1) Growing bone responds to low or moderate exercise through significant addition of new cortical and trabecular bone, with periosteal expansion and endocortical contraction. (2) A threshold of activity exists above which some bones respond negatively by suppressing normal growth and modeling activity. (3) Moderate to intense physical training can generate modest increases (1%-3%) in bone mineral content (BMC) in men and premenopausal women; in young adults very strenuous training may increase BMC of the tibia by up to 11% and its bone density by 7%. Some evidence shows that exercise can also add bone mass to the postmenopausal skeleton, although the amounts are modest and site specific: After one to two years of intensive exercise, increases as high as 5% to 8% can be found, but usually less than 2%. (4) The long-term benefits of exercise are retained only by continuing to exercise. (5) The amount of bone mass that can be achieved appears to depend primarily on the initial bone mass, suggesting that individuals with extremely low initial bone mass may have more to gain from exercise than those with moderately reduced bone mass (Forwood & Burr 1993).

In the adult skeleton, regular prolonged exercise can generally increase the skeletal mass (Dalen & Olsson 1974; Pirnay et al. 1987), cortical thickness (Jones et al. 1977; Woo et al. 1981), and bone mineral content (Krolner et al. 1983). If, for example, a person participated in a sport such as tennis for many years, greater bone density would be expected in the radius and the ulna of the dominant arm. But are there "thresholds" above which there is a diminishing return in adding new bone in

Are There Exercise "Thresholds"?

MacDougall and colleagues (1992) at McMaster University investigated the relation between the amount of running and bone mineral mass in adult male runners. Using dual-photon absorptiometry, they examined the bone density of the trunk, spine, pelvis, thighs, and lower legs of 22 sedentary controls and 53 runners who were selected according to their running mileage. The runners were grouped by their weekly mileage as follows: 5-10, 15-20, 25-30, 40-55, and 60-75 mi/wk. The ages (20-45 years old) and dietary habits of the runners were similar. In this cross-sectional study the researchers found no significant differences in bone density measurements, except in the lower legs. The bone mineral density of the lower legs of the runners in the 15-20 mi/wk group was significantly greater than that of the control or 5-10 mi/wk groups. Interestingly, the researchers found no further increase in bone mineral density in the lower legs of runners who covered more than 20 mi/wk. Indeed, there was a tendency for decreased bone mineral density for runners who covered 60-75 mi/wk. These high-mileage runners had bone mineral density that was no different from that of the sedentary controls.

These data suggest that the amount of running may influence bone mineral density and bone thickness in weight-bearing bones but that there also may be a threshold effect for these adaptations—both at the high and low ends of the loading spectrum. Other investigators have found similar lower bone mineral densities in the vertebrae (Bilanin, Blanchard, & Russek-Cohen 1989) and the legs (Ormerod, McDougall, & Webber 1988) of very high-mileage male runners compared with normal subjects and weight lifters. In the aggregate, these studies suggest that there is an upper limit for exercise beyond which bone mechanical integrity may stop increasing and actually decrease.

response to greater and greater exercise? One facet of the answer to that question is examined in the sidebar on page 99.

Disuse-related changes in bone are commonly associated with bed rest, immobilization, or space flight. Without normal loading, resorption substantially increases and deposition of bone decreases. In some cases, bone resorption can dramatically increase in a very short period of time (Loitz-Ramage & Zernicke 1996).

In humans, the adverse effects of reduced loading on bone have been highlighted by the substantial skeletal degeneration and calcium loss that can occur in space flight. It appears that the loss of bone density may not be as dramatic in the non-weight-bearing bones (e.g., radius and ulna) but that weight-bearing trabecular bones (e.g., calcaneus) are particularly sensitive to the lack of normal loads experienced during microgravity (Rambaut & Goode 1985).

Because disuse changes are dramatic and immobilization may be necessary in some instances, the question of whether disuse-related changes are reversed by remobilization is important. To examine this issue, a study by a group from Finland (Tuukkanen et al. 1991) reported the effects of 1 or 3 wk of immobilization followed by 3 wk of remobilization in rats. The researchers examined the tibia and the femur; after 3 wk of immobilization the bone ash weights decreased up to 12% compared with nonimmobilized controls. After a period of remobilization, the tibia recovered 62% of its mineral mass, while the femur regained only 38% of the lost mineral mass. This research shows that mineral loss caused by immobilization can be reversed to some extent but that the recovery does not occur as rapidly as the loss of bone. Furthermore, the degree of recovery is related to the length of immobilization (Loitz-Ramage & Zernicke 1996). These potent immobilization and remobilization effects are likely fueling the strong interest in the use of fracture braces and early mobilization in the management of orthopedic injuries.

Articular Cartilage Biomechanics

Understanding the synergy among collagen fibers, proteoglycans, and fluid is essential for understanding the mechanical behavior of articular cartilage—the thin layer of hydrated soft tissue covering the ends

of the bones of diarthrodial joints. Normally, these components "perform their functions so well that we are often not even aware of their existence nor the functions they provide until injury strikes or arthritis develops" (Mow, Ratcliffe, & Poole 1992, 67).

Type II collagen is the principal fibrous protein in hyaline cartilage. Figure 4.5 schematically shows how collagen fibers are "recruited" as a tensile load is applied. Initially (toe region), the fibers are partially relaxed and wavy in appearance. As the tensile load continues to increase (linear region), the fibers straighten and become taut. If the load is increased even further, individual fibers begin to tear, and finally large groups of fibers fail in tension (failure).

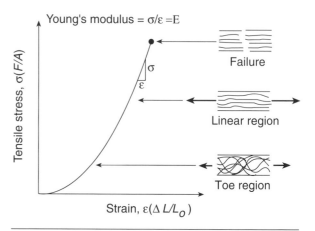

Figure 4.5 Recruitment of collagen fibers within articular cartilage as a tensile load is applied to the tissue.

From "Cartilage and diarthrodial joints as paradigms for hierarchical materials and structures" by V.C. Mow, A. Ratcliffe, & A.R. Poole, 1992, *Biomaterials, 13* (Fig. 20, p. 84). Copyright by IPC Science and Technology Press. Adapted by permission.

We generally think of a tensile load applied to tissue as tending to pull the tissue apart. With a straight tendon, a simple tensile load is easy to envision. With articular cartilage, however, recall that collagen changes its orientation throughout the depth of the cartilage (see figure 2.8b). The superficial tangential zone's fibers are generally oriented parallel to the surface of the joint, while in the middle region the fibers are more randomly arranged. In the deepest layer the radially directed fibers penetrate into the underlying bone.

So how is tension applied to these collagen fibers in the cartilage matrix? The answer is, in many ways. Shearing forces can be generated along the surface of the articular cartilage as the two bone ends move past each other. The surface collagen fibers can be deformed in this way. Also, recall that the negatively charged and hydrophilic proteoglycan aggregates (aggrecan) tend to repel each other and draw water into the extracellular matrix. The cartilage has a natural tendency to swell, and this tendency to expand is resisted by the matrix collagen. Thus, there is a homeostatic balance, or equilibrium, that develops because of the cartilage's swelling pressure and the tensile restraint of the collagen fibers.

Creep refers to the deformation of a tissue as a constant load is applied, and the creep response is a flow-dependent mechanical behavior of the cartilage. That is, a constant load causes extracellular fluid to exude from the matrix. After time, the cartilage reaches a stable compression deformation, or equilibrium strain. If the compressive load is released, the fluid is drawn into the matrix by the hydrophilic proteoglycans (Mow, Ratcliffe, & Poole 1992). Cartilage replete with water is easier to compress, and cartilage densely packed with charged glycosaminoglycan is more resistant to compression.

The cyclic loading and unloading of cartilage allows for a dynamic flow of fluid (with accompanying nutrients and waste products) into and out of the tissue. Thus, cyclic loading of cartilage can be beneficial for normal matrix and cell health. Excessive loading, however, can be destructive to the matrix.

Lubrication Mechanisms

Diarthrodial joint surfaces have remarkably low coefficients of friction. Articular cartilage contributes significantly to joint lubrication by means of cartilage's intrinsic properties and fluid flux. The coefficient of friction for articular cartilage in some human diarthrodial joints has been reported to range from 0.01 to 0.04. By comparison, the coefficient of friction for ice sliding on ice at $0°$ C ranges between 0.01 and 0.10, and the coefficient of friction for glass sliding on glass is 0.90. Diarthrodial joints have been called natural bearings that are nearly frictionless and nearly wear resistant throughout our lives (Mow, Ratcliffe, & Poole 1992).

How is this elegant system of lubrication achieved? Several hypotheses have been proposed, but the answer remains elusive. Two principal types of lubrication mechanisms have been proposed: boundary and fluid-film. *Boundary lubrication* happens when a layer of molecules adheres to each of the two surfaces that are gliding past each other. *Fluid-film lubrication* exists when two nonparallel surfaces move past each other on a thin layer of fluid. The fluid wedge is trapped between the two moving surfaces and maintains a distance between the two

surfaces. If the two moving surfaces are nondeformable, this produces a subtype of fluid-film lubrication called *hydrodynamic lubrication*. If one or both of the surfaces are deformable (usually considered as isotropic and linear elastic), this second subtype is called *elastohydrodynamic lubrication*. This latter type of lubrication commonly is used to model the lubrication in diarthrodial joints, because the articular cartilage is a deformable substance (Bray, Frank, & Miniaci 1991; Mow, Ratcliffe, & Poole 1992).

Additional theories of cartilage fluid-film lubrication have been proposed (Bray, Frank, & Miniaci 1991). One mechanism has been called *squeeze-film lubrication*. In this model the two surfaces move at right angles to each other, as might happen in your knee joint at the instant of heel strike in walking. The weight of your body tends to bring the distal femur and proximal tibia closer together, and fluid is forced out of the cartilage to produce a fluid interface between the two surfaces. This type of lubrication would be effective only for a short duration, and it works better with heavier loads.

Boosted lubrication is a potential mechanism that incorporates elastohydrodynamic and squeeze-film types of lubrication. Boosted lubrication may occur, for example, in the knee joint during the stance phase of walking or running. As the femoral and tibial articular surfaces assume load and slide past each other, the articular cartilage of both surfaces is deformed. As the deformation happens, matrix fluid is forced into the space between the surfaces, and this dynamic fluid flow increases the fluid's viscosity, which in turn boosts the effectiveness of the lubricating fluid film.

Articular Cartilage Adaptation

Articular cartilage generally is extremely well adapted for its purpose in synovial joints. As with many load-bearing connective tissues, articular cartilage has an amount of use that provides optimal function. If the cartilage is used too little (e.g., immobilization) or too much (e.g., excessive loading), a breakdown in the quality of cartilage can occur. The active loading and unloading of articular cartilage, it is believed, facilitates the diffusion of nutrients through the cartilage matrix, which is avascular in the adult. As we will later describe, cartilage does adapt, but in many cases the adaptation is degenerative, leading to osteoarthritic changes to the joint.

Development, Maturation, and Aging

Immature articular cartilage looks quite different from adult tissue. Immature cartilage appears blue-white and is comparatively thicker. The thickness appears to be a function of the substantially greater number of cells in young cartilage, which are found not only on the articular surface, but also in the epiphyseal plate.

Besides the morphological differences in young versus older articular cartilage, there appears to be a substantial difference in the biochemistry of articular cartilage as a function of age. The relative water content in immature articular cartilage is substantially greater than in the adult. Conversely, the collagen concentration increases with maturity, and proteoglycan content in articular cartilage is highest at birth and diminishes slowly throughout growth. The protein core and the glycosaminoglycan chains are longer in immature articular cartilage, and with advancing age, synthesis of proteoglycan decreases. The average length of the proteoglycan protein cores appears to decrease with aging (Mankin et al. 1994). Recall the analogy of the bottle brush (see chapter 2). As articular cartilage ages, there are fewer and shorter bristles on the brush. This change in proteoglycan may account for some of the changes in the mechanical properties and resilience of articular cartilage as an individual ages.

Use Versus Disuse

In both animals and humans, exercise produces a swelling of articular cartilage (Walker 1996). Prolonged exercise in animals may produce chondrocyte hypertrophy, an increase in the pericellular matrix, and an increase in the number of cells per unit of cartilage (Engelmark 1961). These effects are already evident after brief bursts of exercise, but long-term exercise produces a more lasting change in the cartilage. In some instances an exercise program has resulted in positive changes in components of articular cartilage, such as proteoglycans (Säämänen et al. 1986), but more typical findings are that "wear-and-tear" changes can accompany exercise (Vasan 1983). Particularly with excessive loading, synthesis can decrease and degradation increase within articular cartilage. These changes may lead to osteoarthritis, the most common joint disease in humans and the leading cause of chronic disability in the elderly. In describing the pathogenesis of osteoarthritis, Brandt (1992, 75-76) states that

> [osteoarthritis] develops in either of two settings: (1) the biomaterial properties of the articular bone and cartilage are normal but excessive loads applied to the joint cause the tissues to fail, or (2) the applied load is physiologically reasonable, but the biomaterial properties of the cartilage or bone are inferior. . . . In general, the earliest progressive degenerative changes in [osteoarthritis] occur at those sites within the joint that are subject to the greatest compressive loads.

Nevertheless, the exact cause of osteoarthritis is still unknown. It is likely that there is no single cause nor common final pathway, but rather a variety of factors may contribute to the end stage of osteoarthritis. Among the factors that may contribute are heredity; alterations in chondrocyte activity; changes in humeral-, synovial-, and cartilage-derived chemical mediators (e.g., interleukin-1); and altered joint mechanics—especially excessive joint laxity due to previous ligament injury (Mankin et al. 1994).

At the other end of the spectrum, if there is a substantial reduction in loading of articular cartilage, the cartilage can also significantly atrophy or degenerate. When a cartilage is left unloaded for substantial lengths of time, there can be a marked reduction in the synthesis and amount of proteoglycan in the cartilage, an increased fibrillation of the surface of the cartilage, and a decrease in the size and amount of the aggregated proteoglycan. Similarly, the mechanical properties of articular cartilage are degraded with prolonged immobilization. Cartilage that has been immobilized deforms much more rapidly when it is compressed, as the fluid rapidly exudes from the matrix. All of the biochemical and biomechanical changes that occur in articular cartilage as a consequence of immobilization are reversible, in part, after remobilization of the joint (Mankin et al. 1994).

Thus, articular cartilage can be compromised by both too little and too much loading. Figure 4.6 illustrates the hypothetical effects of intermittent loading on the biological properties of articular cartilage. The generally accepted notion is that either a lack of stress or excessive stress causes degeneration in the articular cartilage and that there is a normal physiological zone of cyclic loading that promotes optimal cartilage health.

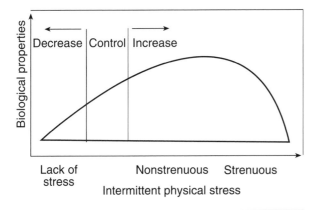

Figure 4.6 Hypothetical effect of cyclic physical stress on the biological properties of articular cartilage. Tammi and colleagues (1987) suggest that atrophy or injury occurs in articular cartilage because of hypophysiological or hyperphysiological physical stresses. When stresses occur within the physiological limits, the cartilage's biological properties may actually improve.

Adapted from Tammi et al. 1987.

Tendon and Ligament Biomechanics

The average ultimate tensile stress of tendons and ligaments ranges between 50 and 100 MPa. The *ultimate load* is related to the cross-sectional area of the specific tendon or ligament. Ultimate loads in tendons, for example, can be extremely large, particularly in tendons such as the Achilles tendon or the patellar tendon. As explained in chapter 6, the patellar tendon of a competitive weight lifter was able to withstand an estimated 14.5 kN (more than 17.5 times the body weight of the weight lifter) before rupturing (Zernicke, Garhammer, & Jobe 1977).

Like bone and articular cartilage, both tendon and ligament exhibit viscoelastic behaviors such as cyclic and static force-relaxation (figure 3.42), hysteresis (figure 3.40b), and creep (figure 3.41). By comparison, bone is much more sensitive to changes in strain rate; nonetheless, the mechanical responses of both tendons and ligaments exhibit moderate strain-rate sensitivity. For example, if a tendon is stretched at a fast strain rate, its stiffness will be greater than if it is stretched at a slower strain rate. This differential effect of strain rate on bone and ligament can have an influence on which structure is injured as a load is applied. If the tensile load is applied very quickly, it is more likely that the ligament will fail, whereas if the load is applied very slowly, it is more likely that a piece of bone at the

ligament attachment site will fail (avulsion fracture).

A classical stress-strain curve for a ligament loaded in tension is shown in figure 4.7. At low stresses (toe region), the crimp, or waviness, of the collagen fibers begins to disappear. As the collagen fibers straighten, the linearity develops, and it is in this relatively linear portion of the curve that the material stiffness (elastic or Young's modulus) can be measured. As noted earlier, the elastic modulus is the slope of the linear region of the stress-strain curve. Note that the strains in the toe and linear regions are relatively small (0% to 4% strain).

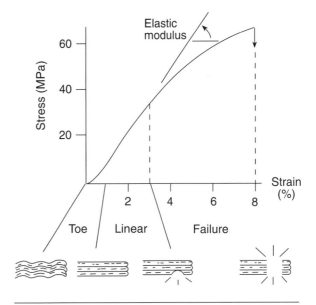

Figure 4.7 Example of a stress-strain curve for collagen fibers in a ligament. The stress-strain curve provides estimates of the material properties of the ligament independent of the size of the structure.

Reprinted from Butler et al. 1978.

Near the latter part of the linear loading region, some of the collagen fibers may exceed their load-bearing capacity and break. If the load or stress was removed at that point, there would be a partial failure of the tendon or ligament, but the remaining intact fibers of the structure might still be able to carry out the load-transmission function. The partial tear may induce an inflammation response, and subsequent healing eventually will form scar tissue (see chapter 5). If the tensile stress was increased even further, the remaining fibers of the tendon or ligament would fail (figure 4.7).

Like that of bone, the geometry of a ligament or tendon affects its structural mechanical behavior.

Figure 4.8, a and b, depicts two different situations to better highlight how ligament (or tendon) size could affect its mechanical function in the body. In figure 4.8a we show how two ligaments of equal fiber length but different cross-sectional areas can have different mechanical behaviors. The 2*A* ligament has twice the cross-sectional area (six collagen fibers in parallel) of the *A* ligament (three collagen fibers in parallel). As a tensile load is applied to each of the ligaments, the 2*A* ligament with twice the cross-sectional area will have double the tensile strength and stiffness of the *A* ligament. The elongation to failure, however, will be the same in both ligaments.

In figure 4.8b, contrast the responses of two other ligaments—*L* and 2*L*. Here, we show the mechanical response of a long ligament versus a short ligament. Ligament 2*L* is twice the original (resting) length of ligament *L*, but each of the ligaments has the same number of collagen fibers in parallel (same cross-sectional area). If a similar load is applied to each ligament, the 2*L* ligament will have one half the stiffness and twice the elongation at failure as the *L* ligament. But because each of the ligaments has the same cross-sectional area, the structural strength is the same for both ligaments.

Finally, in figure 4.8c we show that all four of these ligaments (even with their very different geometry) can have the same material properties, such as elastic modulus. Obviously, this is because the material properties of stress, strain, and elastic modulus are determined from values that are normalized to the differences in the geometry of the structures.

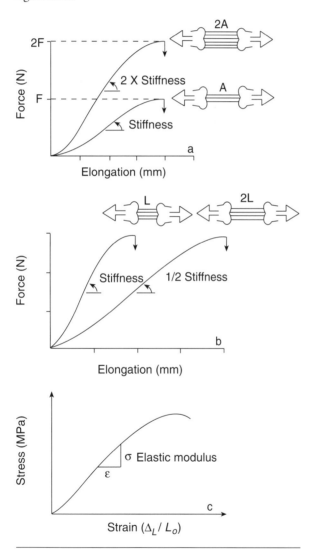

Figure 4.8 Effects of a ligament's (*a*) cross-sectional area and (*b*) original length on its structural properties. (*c*) The normalizing effect of stress and strain calculations to estimate the material properties of ligaments of different sizes.

Parts (*a, b*) reprinted from Butler et al. 1978.

Tendon and Ligament Adaptation

Several decades ago tendons and ligaments were frequently considered to be passive and inert cords for transmitting loads. Since then, much research has been done to reveal the marked adaptive abilities of these fibrous connective tissues.

Development, Maturation, and Aging

The mechanical properties and composition of tendons are greatly influenced by age. Prior to skeletal maturity, tendons and ligaments are slightly more viscous and are relatively more compliant (Frank 1996). With age, the stiffness and modulus of elasticity increase within the linear range up until the point of skeletal maturity, and then these properties remain relatively constant (Woo et al. 1994). In middle age, the insertional points of ligaments or tendons into bone begin to weaken, viscosity begins to decline, and the collagen becomes more highly cross-linked and less compliant (Frank 1996; Woo et al. 1994). With age, bones also become more fragile, and the insertion between a ligament or tendon to the bone becomes a weak link. Avulsion fractures (in which a piece of bone pulls away from its attachment site) become more common as aging progresses.

Use Versus Disuse

Dense, fibrous connective tissues, such as ligaments and tendon, are sensitive to both training and disuse (Booth & Gould 1975; Buckwalter, Maynard, & Vailas 1987). With exercise, normal tendons and ligaments generally adapt to the greater loads by becoming larger and hypertrophying or by changing their material properties to become stronger per unit area (Butler et al. 1978; Kiiskinen 1977; Tipton et al. 1975; Woo et al. 1980).

The primary effects of exercise on ligaments are increases in structural strength and stiffness. Normal, everyday activity (without training) is apparently sufficient to maintain about 80% to 90% of ligament's mechanical potential (Frank 1996). Exercise appears to have the potential to increase ligament strength and stiffness by up to an additional 10% to 20% (figure 4.9).

Compared to ligaments, fewer quantitative data are available about the exercise-related adaptations of tendon. Data suggest that exercise can increase the number and size of collagen fibrils and increase the cross-sectional area of tendons when compared with the tendons of sedentary controls (Michna 1984). Exercise can lead to increased collagen synthesis in growing tendons (Curwin, Vailas, & Wood 1988) and an increased number of fibroblasts in tendons (Zamora & Marini 1988).

Load deprivation or joint immobilization produces a rapid deterioration in ligament biochemical and mechanical properties, due in part to atrophy, which causes a net loss in ligament strength and stiffness (Frank 1996; Butler et al. 1978). Immobilization or disuse decreases ligaments' glycosaminoglycans and water content, increases the nonuniform orientation of the collagen fibrils, and increases collagen cross linking (Woo et al. 1975). Collagen synthesis and degradation rates increase with immobilization, so the ratio of new collagen to old increases in immobilized ligaments (Amiel et al. 1982). Furthermore, decreases occur in ligaments' total collagen mass (Amiel et al. 1982) and stiffness (Noyes et al. 1974). Tipton and colleagues (1975) concluded that the strength of the bone-ligament junction is related to the type of exercise regimen and not only the duration of the exercise—with endurance training being more effective. In general, exercise increases the strength of the bone-ligament junction (Tipton et al. 1975).

The general effects that exercise, immobilization, and remobilization have on ligaments and bone are shown in figure 4.9 (Woo et al. 1982). The effect of

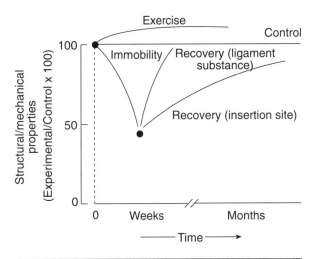

Figure 4.9   Schematic illustration of ligament responses to exercise, immobilization, and remobilization. Starting at the first black dot (0 Weeks), the "y" axis is in percent, with 100% being a constant "normal" (Control) level of structural and mechanical properties (e.g., stiffness or maximal tensile stress). The notation, "Experimental/Control x 100," on the "y" axis illustrates how the data for the curves were estimated. For example, if ligament strength in the experimental immobilization group was only one half the strength of non-immobilized normal controls, then the experimental ligaments would be 50% compared to control. The "x" axis is time, with early responses shown in "Weeks" and later responses extending to "Months." Exercise tends to moderately enhance the structural and mechanical properties of ligaments over time, whereas immobilization has a dramatic negative effect within 8-12 weeks (e.g., see second black dot). The two curves emanating from the second black dot show how moving (remobilizing) a joint after a period of immobilization is different for properties of the ligament substance (rapid recovery) versus ligament insertion site to bone (slower recovery).

Adapted from Woo et al. 1987.

immobilization or disuse is dramatic and rapid. With immobilization, major deterioration occurs within a few weeks as ligament cells produce inferior-quality ligament material, which in turn contributes to the structural weakening of the ligament complex (Frank 1996). At the same time, there is an osteoclast response at the bone-ligament junction that decreases the strength of the insertional bone.

Skeletal Muscle Biomechanics

The fundamental properties of muscle are linked to force, length, and velocity. In chapter 2 we reviewed muscle contractile dynamics (figures 2.13 and 2.14) and basic length-tension and force-velocity relationships (figure 2.17).

Muscle Force Production

The fundamental mechanical events of a muscle contraction relate to twitch properties, unfused tetanic contraction, and tetanus. A single twitch develops in a muscle when the muscle is stimulated once. If another stimulus arrives to depolarize the muscle before it completely relaxes, the stimuli have an additive effect, and the force produced in the muscle is greater than with a single twitch. As the volleys of stimuli (impulses) arrive faster and faster, the tension developed in the muscle will continue to rise, until at maximal stimulation the muscle is tetanized, and a steady maximum tension is achieved. If the stimulation rate is slightly less than maximum, then fluctuations in the tension are seen; this is called unfused tetanic contraction.

The total force developed in a skeletal muscle is proportional to the number of cross-bridges in parallel, while the rate at which force can be developed in a muscle is proportional to the number of sarcomeres in series. From a functional standpoint, it is *work output* (*power* as work done per unit time) that is important. That is, a muscle must be able to contract forcefully and with high velocity to have a high power output.

Muscle Strain Injuries

As seen in many different occupations, sports, and physical activities, skeletal muscles have the capacity to generate high forces (and power) without sustaining injury. But if too much force is transmitted through a muscle-tendon unit, which regions of the muscle-tendon unit are the most likely to be damaged?

Research has shown that when muscle-tendon-bone units are pulled to failure, the tears could happen at bone-tendon junctions, within the muscle belly, or at the myotendinous junctions (McMaster 1933). Later experimental studies also revealed tears in muscle-tendon units at the myotendinous junction (Garrett et al. 1988) or at sites within the muscle cell approximately 0.5 mm from the myotendinous junction (Tidball & Chan 1989).

Much of this work probed the failure characteristics of passive (unstimulated) muscle-tendon units, and certainly injuries can happen to noncontracting muscles. But two studies (Garrett et al. 1987; Tidball, Salem, & Zernicke 1993) provide interesting findings about the sites of muscle-tendon failure in stimulated versus quiescent muscle.

Garrett and coworkers (1987) compared the biomechanical properties of passive versus stimulated muscle (rabbit extensor digitorum longus) that was rapidly lengthened to failure. They found no significant difference in the amount of lengthening at which the failure happened, regardless of activation state. But when muscles were stimulated, they achieved 14% to 16% greater peak forces at failure than if the muscle was passive. Also, substantially more energy was absorbed to the point of failure in the stimulated than in the unstimulated muscle-tendon units. They reported that the site of failure was typically at the myotendinous junction.

Tidball, Salem, and Zernicke (1993) used an electron microscope to locate the specific sites of the muscle-tendon interface that failed in tetanically stimulated versus unstimulated bone-tendon-muscle-tendon-bone units, using a frog semitendinous muscle. The specimens were strained at physiological strain rates to failure, and all failures happened at or near the proximal (tendon of origin) myotendinous junction in both stimulated and unstimulated muscle.

Consistent with the earlier findings of Garrett and coworkers (1987), Tidball and colleagues (1993) found that the stimulated muscle-tendon units required about 30% more force and about 110% more energy to reach failure. Interestingly, the electron-microscopic analysis revealed systematic differences in the sites of failure, which varied with the state of activation of the muscle cells at the time of injury. Also, the breaking strength of the Z-disk when the muscle was stimulated was different from when it was unstimulated—suggesting that two load-bearing systems may be in parallel within the Z-disks.

Figures 4.10, 4.11, and 4.12 are extracted from Tidball, Salem, and Zernicke (1993), and these figures show more clearly the variation in failure site with activation state of the muscle. A transmission electron micrograph (figure 4.10a) illustrates a longitudinal section from an unstimulated muscle, and figure 4.10b illustrates a similar section from a stimulated muscle. In the unstimulated muscle, the site of failure was within the muscle, near the myotendinous junction. Failure happened in a single transverse plane of each cell within Z-disks, and other Z-disks in the area remained stretched—with residual strains of several hundred percent (figure 4.10a). In contrast, figure 4.10b

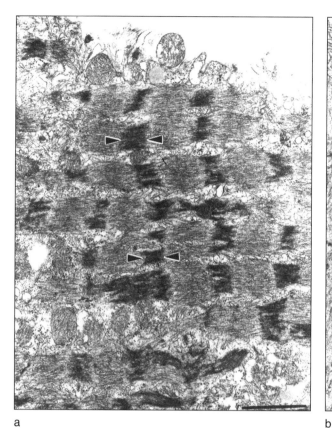 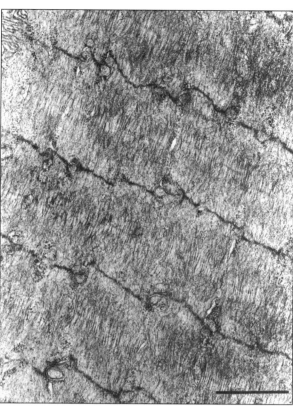

a
b

Figure 4.10 (*a*) Longitudinal section from an *unstimulated* muscle loaded to failure. This transmission electron micrograph shows an incomplete tear through a muscle fiber about 80 μm from the site of the complete tear. The Z-disks (between the arrowheads) show extensive residual strain. (*b*) Longitudinal section taken through a *stimulated* muscle that was strained to failure. The site in the photograph is about 100 μm from the failure site. The Z-disks are distinct and show no signs of persisting strain. The inset bar (1.5 μm) is the same in both photographs.

Reprinted from Tidball, Salem, & Zernicke 1993.

was taken from a stimulated muscle at a site about 100 μm from the failure site. Here you can see the relatively normal-looking Z-disks; they show no residual strains.

When the sites of failure were examined more closely in the unstimulated muscle, tears were found in the tendon near the myotendinous junction (outlined by the arrowheads in figure 4.11a). Identical-appearing tears were seen at the myotendinous junctions of both unstimulated and stimulated specimens. Large separations (denoted by S in figure 4.11b) were seen within the tendon near the myotendinous junction of an unstimulated muscle. In figure 4.12 (an electron micrograph taken through the myotendinous junction for a stimulated muscle), note that the site of failure (complete separation) is immediately external to the membrane of the myotendinous junction, and no connective tissue appears connected to the junction membrane (see arrowheads).

Skeletal Muscle Adaptation

Skeletal muscle is a tissue capable of enormous adaptation, as can be readily appreciated by contrasting the muscular development of an Olympic gymnast or weight lifter with the wasted muscles of an individual who has been bedridden for years. The type of training influences the type of muscle adaptation. Endurance training enhances a muscle's oxidative potential, whereas resistance training increases a muscle's myofibrillar diameter (Zernicke & Loitz 1990).

Development, Maturation, and Aging

As explained in chapter 2, skeletal muscle cells are derived from the mesoderm. The typical muscle

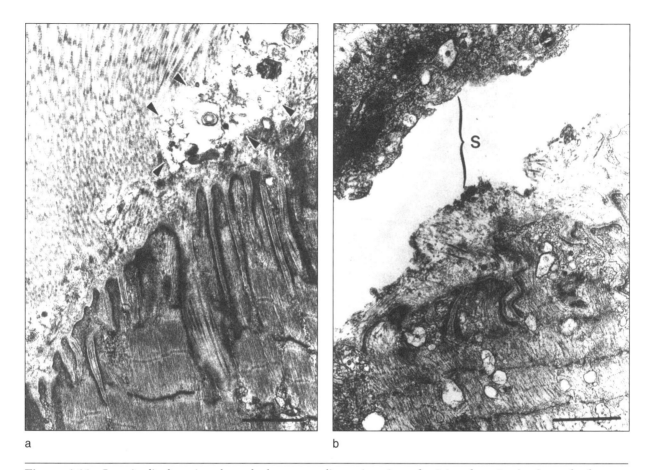

a   b

Figure 4.11 Longitudinal section through the myotendinous junction of origin of *unstimulated* muscle that was strained to failure. (*a*) Tears existed in the tendon, near the myotendinous junction (outlined by the arrowheads). Identical-looking tears were found at the myotendinous junctions of both unstimulated and stimulated fibers. The inset bar is 2.0 μm. (*b*) Large separations (S) within the tendon near the myotendinous junction were observed in some preparations, although complete tears were located in the fibers for these preparations. The inset bar is 2.5 μm.
Reprinted from Tidball, Salem, & Zernicke 1993.

fiber type in the early fetus is a primitive fast-twitch fiber (Bandy & Dunleavy 1996). As the neurological and muscular systems mature, histochemically identifiable fiber types begin to emerge (Vogler & Bove 1985). Williams and Goldspink (1981) indicate that while muscle development is not fully complete at birth, the number of muscle fibers in the body is probably set at birth, and continued muscle growth is a result of the increase in fiber size (both in width and in length). After the first year of life, an individual-specific distribution of fast-twitch and slow-twitch fibers begins to emerge in the musculoskeletal system. The developmental addition of sarcomeres and the hypertrophy of muscle fibers continue until growth ceases and adult fiber size is reached (approximately 15 years of age).

Although a bone has growth plates that allow it to extend in a longitudinal direction, the length associated with skeletal muscle growth is usually derived from the addition of sarcomeres to the muscle fibers, primarily in the region of the myotendinous junction. If a muscle-tendon unit is stretched, additional sarcomeres are typically added at the region of the myotendinous junction (Garrett & Best 1994).

Compared with the amount of information on muscle adaptation in adults, the data related to muscle adaptation in children are relatively sparse. Bandy and Dunleavy (1996) indicate that in prepubescent boys who are undergoing a program of progressive resistance training, for example, muscle strength increases occur without any appreciable change in cross-sectional area. The researchers suggest that the increased strength is a result of improved coordination of muscle groups responsible for the movements as opposed to changes in fiber size. Maximal strength in men and women is generally reached between the ages of 20 and 30 years, about the same time that the cross-sectional area of

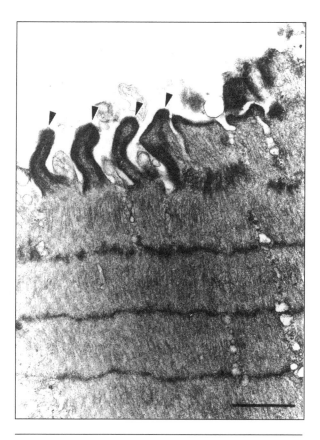

Figure 4.12 Longitudinal section through the myotendinous junction of origin of a *stimulated* muscle that was loaded to failure. The site of complete separation is immediately external to the junctional membrane so that no connective tissue is found associated with the junctional processes (see arrowheads). Inset bar is 2.0 μm.

Reprinted from Tidball, Salem, & Zernicke 1993.

muscle is the greatest. The strength level tends to plateau through the age of 50, followed by a decline in strength that accelerates by 65 years of age and beyond.

The loss of strength with aging may be related to the loss of muscle mass associated with a reduction in the number of muscle fibers. Typically, the fast-twitch muscle fibers are hit harder than slow-twitch muscle fibers as aging progresses. Skeletal muscle of elderly individuals responds to resistance training with increases not only in performance, but also in muscle mass and muscle fiber size, particularly in fast-twitch fiber areas. Individuals in their 60s, 70s, and older are able to respond to progressive resistance training by increasing strength through hypertrophy of skeletal muscle. Such increases in strength (or maintenance of strength) may have significant consequences for maintaining neuromotor coordination and reducing the likelihood of falls and injury (Bandy & Dunleavy 1996).

Gender-Related Effects

Before puberty, gender differences in athletic performance are not obvious. Girls do not experience a significant change in muscle mass during puberty, and before the onset of puberty the muscular strength of girls and boys is essentially equal. At ages 11 to 12 years, girls are approximately 90% as strong as boys, and at ages 13 to 14 years, the girls' percentage strength decreases to about 85% that of boys (Komi 1992). By the ages of 15 to 16, girls are typically only 75% as strong as boys. These diverging strength values are consistent with the differences that exist between men and women in the adult range. For example, the average percentage muscle mass (per total body mass) for a conditioned female athlete is about 23%, whereas in the conditioned male athlete it is 40%. The average percentage fat (per total body mass) for conditioned women is in the range of 10% to 15%, while in conditioned men it is less than 7%. For the unconditioned woman, the average percentage body fat is 25%, whereas for the unconditioned man it is closer to 15%. Similarly, there are differences in average heart size; in adult women the heart is 10.7 cm in diameter, while in adult men it is 12.1 cm in diameter. Also, average total lung capacity for adult women is 4,200 ml versus 6,000 ml for men; the average vital lung capacity for women is 3,200 ml, while in men the value is closer to 4,800 ml (Åstrand & Rodahl 1986).

The relative proportions of muscle fiber types are similar in men and women, but the total cross-sectional area of women's muscles is only about 75% that of men, which accounts for the differences in overall strength (Cureton et al. 1990). Strength differences between men and women are greater in the upper extremities than in the lower extremities (Wells 1991). Women are able to gain relative strength similarly to men (Cureton et al. 1990). Wilmore (1979) indicates that although men have greater upper-body muscle strength, elite female athletes are nearly equivalent to their male counterparts in strength per unit size and muscle fiber type. Ikai and Fukunaga (1968), who examined the strength of muscle elbow flexors in men and women in comparison to muscle size, found that there is little or no difference in the relative strength of men and women. The quality of a muscle fiber in exerting force is independent of gender (Bandy and Dunleavy 1996). There is some indication that men and women can increase strength to a similar degree following resistance training, but muscle hypertrophy seems to be less pronounced in women. One of the factors that may contribute to the greater hypertrophy in men is their 20- to 30-times-higher levels of testosterone, with its potent anabolic function in building muscle tissue (Hetrick & Wilmore 1979).

Use Versus Disuse

Hypertrophy is the dominant feature in muscle adaptation. Hypertrophy is an enlargement of the individual fibers within the muscle, which implies an increase in the amount of contractile proteins. There is also a strong neurological component to strength training, as it is likely that part of the gains in strength are associated with more-effective recruitment of motor units and greater synchronization of muscle activation.

Skeletal muscle adaptation is specific to imposed demands. Two modes of training include *strength training* (or *resistance training*) and *endurance training* (Garrett & Best 1994). Within a strength-training regime, a person progressively increases the resistance against which the muscle is active (either shortening or lengthening). Relatively high resistance coupled with a low number of repetitions leads to increases in the strength and size of the muscle. In contrast, muscle endurance is increased by training against a resistance that can be repeated many times. Recall that the greatest force a muscle can generate is closely linked to the cross-sectional area of the muscle; a larger muscle generates greater force than a smaller muscle. Many studies that have looked at increases in strength associated with training have concluded that the muscle hypertrophy produced by resistance training is a result of the enlargement of the muscle fiber and not an increased number of fibers (Bandy & Dunleavy 1996).

Training to increase muscle endurance involves a different challenge to the muscle, and different adaptations will occur. Endurance training involves the enhancement of the muscle's energy supply rather than its size. An important element is the increase in oxidative metabolism associated with the mitochondria, which increase in size, number, and density in endurance-trained skeletal muscles. With endurance training, the metabolic pathways adapt to a more effective use of fatty acids for fuel instead of glycogen. Different muscle fiber types respond differently to endurance training, although the oxidative capacity of all three fiber types can increase with endurance training.

Dietary intake can also affect the endurance capacity of muscle. Glycogen, which is stored in muscle fibers and the liver, is used extensively in exercises of moderate to high intensity. If high quantities of carbohydrates are eaten prior to competition, muscle and liver glycogen stores can be replete and provide the maximum energy availability for contractions.

The converse of hypertrophy is atrophy. *Muscular atrophy* is a decrease in the size of muscle tissue that can result from several causes, such as immobilization, bed rest, or a sedentary lifestyle after a period of high-intensity training. The clinical signs of atrophy include decreases in muscle circumference, strength, and endurance. The decreases in strength and endurance become the principal concerns during rehabilitation after injury or when resuming training. The changes in fiber size that occur with atrophy are most likely related to a decreased rate of protein synthesis and an increased rate of protein degradation (catabolism). With immobilization and disuse the atrophy that occurs in skeletal muscle is more likely to affect the more tonically recruited slow-twitch (type I) fibers than the fast-twitch (type II) fibers.

Finally, in terms of functional adaptation, a region in the muscle-tendon complex that is particularly important is the myotendinous junction. As noted earlier, this is a region where sarcomeres are added to increase the length of muscles. It is an active and very dynamic (and injury-prone) region. Surprisingly, very little is known about how the myotendinous junction adapts to training. With overload training, there is no change in the relative junctional angle between the myofibril and the collagen at the myotendinous junction, which may mean that its strength capacity is near optimal (Tidball 1983). Thus, adaptation at the myotendinous junction may be related to changes in the quality of the collagen and sarcolemmal membrane rather than to changes in the morphology of the junction.

Concluding Comments

For load-bearing connective tissues such as bone, cartilage, tendon, ligament, and muscle, it is clear that form and function are inextricably linked. All of these tissues are able to adapt to their environment to a greater or lesser extent. The mechanical, biochemical, hormonal, and molecular ability of these tissues to adapt favorably to environmental influences is a primary attribute of healthy tissues. On the other hand, the inability of these tissues to adapt to excesses (either high or low) is a leading factor associated with degradation and injury. In chapters 6, 7, and 8 we explore the types of injuries and damage that can occur to these tissues in major joints and regions of the body.

Suggested Readings

Bone

Currey, J.D. (1985). *The Mechanical Adaptations of Bones.* Princeton, NJ: Princeton University Press.

Kaplan, F.S., Hayes, W.C., Keaveny, T.M., Boskey, A., Einhorn, T.A., & Iannotti, J.P. (1994). Form and function of bone. In: Simon, S.R. (Ed.), *Orthopaedic Basic Science* (pp. 127-184). Park Ridge, IL: American Academy of Orthopaedic Surgeons.

Loitz-Ramage, B.J., & Zernicke, R.F. (1996). Bone biology and mechanics. In: Zachazewski, J.E., Magee, D.J., & Quillen, W.S. (Eds.), *Athletic Injuries and Rehabilitation* (pp. 99-119). Philadelphia: Saunders.

Martin, R.B., & Burr, D.B. (1989). *Structure, Function, and Adaptation of Compact Bone.* New York: Raven Press.

Articular Cartilage

Bray, R., Frank, C.B., & Miniaci, A. (1991). Structure and function of diarthrodial joints. In: McGinty, J.B. (Ed.), *Operative Arthroscopy* (pp. 79-123). New York: Raven Press.

Mankin, H.J., Mow, V.C., Buckwalter, J.A., Iannotti, J.P., & Ratcliffe, A. (1994). Form and function of articular cartilage. In: Simon, S.R. (Ed.), *Orthopaedic Basic Science* (pp. 1-44). Park Ridge, IL: American Academy of Orthopaedic Surgeons.

Mow, V.C., Ratcliffe, A., & Poole, A.R. (1992). Cartilage and diarthrodial joints as paradigms for hierarchical materials and structures. *Biomaterials, 13,* 67-97.

Walker, J.M. (1996). Cartilage of human joints and related structures. In: Zachazewski, J.E., Magee, D.J., & Quillen, W.S. (Eds.), *Athletic Injuries and Rehabilitation* (pp. 120-151). Philadelphia: Saunders.

Tendon and Ligament

Bray, R., Frank, C.B., & Miniaci, A. (1991). Structure and function of diarthrodial joints. In: McGinty, J.B. (Ed.), *Operative Arthroscopy* (pp. 79-123). New York: Raven Press.

Curwin, S.L. (1996). Tendon injuries: Pathophysiology and treatment. In: Zachazewski, J.E., Magee, D.J., & Quillen, W.S. (Eds.), *Athletic Injuries and Rehabilitation* (pp. 27-54). Philadelphia: Saunders.

Frank, C.B. (1996). Ligament injuries: Pathophysiology and healing. In: Zachazewski, J.E., Magee, D.J., & Quillen, W.S. (Eds.), *Athletic Injuries and Rehabilitation* (pp. 9-26). Philadelphia: Saunders.

Woo, S.L.-Y., An, K.-N., Arnoczky, S.P., Wayne, J.S., Fithian, D.C., & Myers, B.S. (1994). Anatomy, biology, and biomechanics of tendon, ligament, and meniscus. In: Simon, S.R. (Ed.), *Orthopaedic Basic Science* (pp. 45-87). Park Ridge, IL: American Academy of Orthopaedic Surgeons.

Skeletal Muscle

Alexander, R.M., & Goldspink, G. (1977). *Mechanics and Energetics of Animal Locomotion.* London: Chapman & Hall.

Bandy, W.D., & Dunleavy, K. (1996). Adaptability of skeletal muscle: Response to increased and decreased use. In: Zachazewski, J.E., Magee, D.J., & Quillen, W.S. (Eds.), *Athletic Injuries and Rehabilitation* (pp. 55-70). Philadelphia: Saunders.

Garrett, W.E., Jr., & Best, T.M. (1994). Anatomy, physiology, and mechanics of skeletal muscle. In: Simon, S.R. (Ed.), *Orthopaedic Basic Science* (pp. 89-126). Park Ridge, IL: American Academy of Orthopaedic Surgeons.

Hill, A.V. (1970). *First and Last Experiments in Muscle Mechanics.* Cambridge: Cambridge University Press.

McMahon, T.A. (1984). *Muscles, Reflexes, and Locomotion.* Princeton, NJ: Princeton University Press.

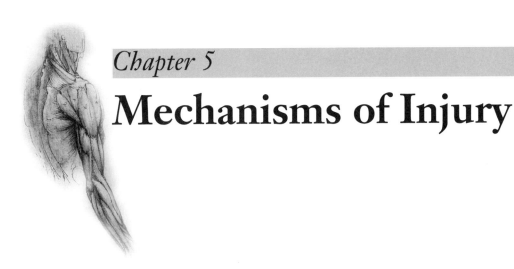

Chapter 5

Mechanisms of Injury

Kindnesses are easily forgotten;
but injuries!—what worthy man does not keep those in mind?
William Makepeace Thackeray (1811-1863)

The question typically first asked in assessing injury is "How did it happen?" Accurately answering this query may establish a cause-and-effect relation between the events surrounding the injury and the injury itself. In biomechanical terms, this is the mechanism of injury. Mechanism, in this context, can be defined as the fundamental physical process responsible for a given action, reaction, or result. Retrospective and accurate identification of injury mechanisms is essential for diagnosis, effective treatment, and prevention of future injuries.

Most everyone has experience in identifying injury mechanisms. Consider, for example, a basketball player who, in descending from a jump shot, lands on an opponent's foot and crumples to the floor in pain. Her coach rushes over and asks, "What happened?" The player grimaces and responds, "I twisted my ankle." In simple terms, the player specified the mechanism of her injury. Knowledge of the mechanism provides the coach, trainer, and physician with insights that can help determine the proper course of action.

Now imagine an elderly man found lying on a sidewalk one January night. Responding paramedics, after checking vital functions, determine that the man is in no immediate danger, though in considerable pain. The man indicates that he slipped on an icy patch of sidewalk and "landed on my tailbone and hands." Again, by describing the mechanism of the fall, the man gave paramedics valuable information to help them determine how to proceed. With further questioning, more details of the fall may emerge.

Trained professionals can translate the simple description of an injury, as illustrated in the two preceding examples, into more discipline-specific terms. A physician, for instance, may explain a "twisted ankle" as rapid loading of the lateral aspect of the ankle and foot, with possible injury to the anterior talofibular and calcaneofibular ligaments. A biomechanist might approach a "slip and fall" from a mechanistic perspective, focusing on the coefficient of friction at the foot-ground interface and the velocity of the body at the instant of ground contact. In both cases, the practitioner uses knowledge of the mechanism of injury in establishing a cause-and-effect relation.

The description of an injury mechanism depends in part on the perspective of the person involved. Physicians, athletic trainers, coaches, supervisors, physical therapists, and injury victims undoubtedly will describe the mechanism of a particular injury differently, each correct from his or her perspective.

While sometimes a single mechanism is responsible for a particular injury, mechanisms often act in combination. Accurate identification of the mechanisms involved is important for appropriate conditioning, treatment, and rehabilitation. Many of these mechanisms have been alluded to in our earlier discussions and will be explored further in the next section and in subsequent chapters.

Do not confuse mechanisms with the related but different concept of predisposing or contributory factors. Mechanisms establish a cause-and-effect relation. Contributory factors increase or decrease the likelihood of occurrence and the level of the effect; contributory factors are discussed in more detail later in this chapter.

Overview of Injury Mechanisms

The mechanisms responsible for injury are many and varied. Categorization of injury mechanisms is based on mechanical concepts, tissue responses, or a combination of the two. From a sports medicine perspective, for example, one useful classification system identifies seven basic mechanisms of injury: (1) contact or impact, (2) dynamic overload, (3) overuse, (4) structural vulnerability, (5) inflexibility, (6) muscle imbalance, and (7) rapid growth (Leadbetter 1994). Another source lists crushing deformation, impulsive impact, skeletal acceleration, energy absorption, and the extent and rate of tissue deformation as causal mechanisms (Committee on Trauma Research 1985).

The variability among types of injury suggests that there are many potential injury mechanisms.

Understanding these mechanisms is essential for proper diagnosis and treatment. Treatment of an injury's symptoms, without identification and consideration of its causal mechanisms, will result in ineffective treatment and the potential for injury recurrence.

Principles of Mechanical Loading

In chapter 3 we defined load as the application of an external force to a body and identified seven factors that characterize load: magnitude, location, direction, duration, frequency, variability, and rate. Body tissues continuously experience loads during normal activity with no obvious injury. Typical loads are said to be within a physiological range. The probability of injury increases when loads exceed the physiological range. In this case, the tissue experiences an overload.

Injury can result when a single overload exceeds a tissue's maximum tolerance. Use is normal functional loading, whereas repeated overload is overuse. Many injuries (e.g., tendinitis and carpal tunnel syndrome) are called overuse injuries because they result from repeated overloads with insufficient time for recovery. Some specific examples of overuse injuries are described in chapters 6 through 8.

Overuse injuries exemplify a broad class of conditions distinguished by an etiology of repeated force application. Such injuries are chronic injuries and may also be referred to as *cumulative trauma disorders* or *repetitive stress syndromes*. In contrast, injuries resulting from a single or a few loading episodes are called acute injuries. Chronic and acute injuries are usually distinguishable, but sometimes a relation exists between the two. For example, chronic loading (overuse) may weaken a tissue, lower its maximum strength, and increase the likelihood of an acute injury. A person with a chronic inflammation of the Achilles tendon has an increased likelihood of an acute rupture of that tendon.

Principles of Injury

In the context of musculoskeletal biomechanics we defined injury as damage caused by physical trauma sustained by tissues of the body. As you may expect, injury biomechanics has its own vocabulary that draws heavily from medicine and mechanics.

Varus, Valgus, Vexation!

In 1980, Houston and Swischuk published the paper "Varus and Valgus—No Wonder They Are Confused" in the *New England Journal of Medicine* that took issue with the use of the terms varus and valgus. Excerpts from their notes highlight the confusion caused by the use of these terms in the medical literature.

"In lecturing on pediatric bone disease to medical students, we have become painfully aware that the terms varus and valgus cause great confusion. Every year, when shown a radiograph of coxa valga and asked for the appropriate diagnosis, about a third of the students vote for coxa vara, a third for coxa valga, and a third admit that they do not know.

"Since radiologists, orthopedic surgeons, and pediatricians use varus and valgus regularly in their conversation and in their reports, we have attributed the ignorance of medical students to their inexperience, coupled with the unfortunate omission of high-school Latin as a prerequisite for entrance to medical school. This year one of us criticized the incorrect usage of the term varus in reviewing a book written by the other. This led to consultation with current and early dictionaries and to a survey of major orthopedic textbooks.

"To our surprise, we learned that the original Latin meaning of varus was knock-kneed, and of valgus bowlegged, exactly opposite to current pediatric and radiological usage.

"To show that current usage is consistently opposite to the derivation and the definitions of most dictionaries through the years, one of us checked 24 current orthopedic textbooks. . . . To our surprise, we could find a definition of the terms in only two of these texts. W.A. Crabbe's *Orthopedics for the Undergraduate* (1969) provided this definition of varus: 'Deviation of a limb towards the midline of the body.' Robert B. Salter's *Textbook of Disorders and Injuries of the Musculoskeletal System* (1970) gave detailed and helpful definitions and was the only one of the 24 to mention the historical discrepancy. Under the heading, 'Varus and Valgus,' Salter stated, 'This particular pair of terms has caused more confusion than any other pair, partly because the original Latin terms had the opposite meaning to that which is now universally accepted.' All 24 texts referred to bowlegs as genu varum, even though the knee in this condition is away from the midline of the body. Eleven of the texts somewhat paradoxically used tibia vara to describe other instances of the same directional deformity, where the distal tibia tilts towards the midline of the body. Thus, varus is now used to indicate a tilt toward the midline of the bone beyond the joint, regardless of whether the prefix is the name of the joint or the bone beyond it. This obviously is confusing.

"Since confusion is universal, since current usage is directly contrary to derivation, and since use of these terms in the directional sense is at the least misleading and at the most dangerous, we suggest that the simple English words bowlegged and knock-kneed are far superior to genu valgum and genu varum.

"In summary, it would seem best to avoid the terms varus and valgus altogether. Anyone who persists in using them should follow the lead of Crabbe and Salter and define them clearly. Furthermore, dictionaries should point out, in unambiguous fashion, not only the derivation of these terms, but the opposite way in which they are used in modern orthopedic literature."

Houston and Swischuk's recommendation that use of varus and valgus be avoided has apparently not found favor in the scientific and medical communities. Both terms are still widely used and continue to create confusion. We are tempted not to use these terms but feel that given their continued prevalence in the literature, you will be best served by our using the terms varus and valgus in the following chapters. In so doing, we will provide precise definitions for each term.

Although general agreement exists on most definitions, some exceptions lead to confusion and lack of clarity.

Confusion also arises when nonspecific, catch-all terms are used to describe an injury or group of injury conditions. "Tennis elbow," "shinsplints," "jumper's knee," "Little League elbow," and "whiplash" are nebulous terms and have minimal clinical or biomechanical utility. We sometimes use these vague but all-too-common descriptors; nevertheless, we discourage their general use and encourage more specific and appropriate terminology.

The mechanical how and why of injury are the keystones of our approach, and this section presents general principles of injury important to the later discussions of specific injury mechanisms.

Level of Dysfunction

Some injuries are simply annoyances and relatively trivial. These injuries do not limit function appreciably and heal quickly. Increasing injury severity, however, produces greater dysfunction. At the extreme are catastrophic injuries that result in permanent disability or death.

Progression of Injury

Relatively minor injuries that are ignored may, with repeated loading or insult, progress to more severe injuries. Delayed, improper, or inadequate treatment may also contribute to the progression to a more serious injury. Athletes or workers may try to do too much too soon. A minor injury, given inadequate time to heal, may progress to a more debilitating level.

Assessment of Injury Severity

Every injury is unique, and though it may be similar to other injuries, it is never exactly the same. This presents challenges in the assessment of injuries and classification of their severity. All categorization systems create discrete groupings and assign similar characteristics to all injuries in that group. Thus, while two different head injuries categorized as "mild concussions" may share similar characteristics, they are not identical injuries. Diagnosis and treatment must remain specific to each injury based on its own characteristics.

Clinical classification schemes are useful, though, in assigning general or common characteristics to similar injuries. Many such schemes exist (and differ), based on the tissues (e.g., bone vs. ligament) and body regions (e.g., head vs. leg) involved. A typical, three-level classification system for ligament injury, for example, specifies the structural involvement, physical signs, and level of dysfunction (mild, moderate, and severe) (table 5.1). Similarly, a five-level system for classification of concussions has been proposed (table 5.2).

Injury severity is linked to the amount of damage experienced by the tissue. In mild and moderate injuries, there is typically a partial disruption of the tissue structure. The damaged tissue is still able to accept load, though of smaller magnitudes than preinjury levels. In cases of complete failure the tissue's continuity is totally disrupted, and load transmission is not possible. In some cases appearances can be deceptive; a tissue may appear to be intact and capable of load acceptance, but in reality the fibers are disrupted and possess little or no ability to transmit loads.

Table 5.1 Classification of Ligament Injury Severity

Grade	Severity	Degree	Structural involvement	Exam	Performance deficit
1	Mild	First	Negligible	No visible injury, locally tender only, joint stable	Minimal to a few days
2	Moderate	Second	Partial	Visible swelling, marked tenderness, +/– stability	Up to 6 wk (may be modified by protective bracing)
3	Severe	Third	Complete	Gross swelling, marked tenderness, antalgic posture, unstable	Indefinite, minimum of 6-8 wk

Reprinted from Leadbetter 1994.

Table 5.2   Classification of Concussions

| Grade | Amnesia | | Loss of consciousness |
	Post traumatic	Retrograde	
I	No	No	No
II	Yes	No	No
III	Yes	Yes	No, or seconds
IV	Yes	Yes	Yes, 5-10 min
V	Yes	Yes	Yes, prolonged

Reprinted from Marion 1994.

Chronic Versus Acute Injury

Injuries can result from a single insult (acute injury) or from long-term, repeated loading (chronic injury). Continuing chronic insults to tissues may lead progressively to degenerative conditions that set the stage for an acute injury.

Microtrauma Versus Macrotrauma

Chronic injury can begin as microscopic damage to a tissue's structure. For example, the damage could be microscopic tendon fiber tears or bone microcracks. Repeated loading can exacerbate the injury, and eventually the injury becomes macroscopic. If left untreated, tendon microtears presage eventual tendon rupture. Similarly, X-ray findings of a patient complaining of a dull ache in the foot may be negative because of the microscopic nature of the bone cracks, but continued reloading may generate a stress fracture.

Primary Versus Secondary Injury

Primary injury means that the injury is a direct, immediate consequence of trauma. A skull fracture from blunt trauma or a torn medial collateral knee ligament from a violent lateral impact are two examples of primary injuries.

A *secondary injury* can happen in one of two ways. A secondary injury can surface some time after the initial trauma. In cases of traumatic head impact, primary brain injury can occur as a direct and immediate result of the impact. Delayed (or secondary) brain injuries, such as diffuse axonal injury and local or regional ischemia (localized decrease in blood flow to a tissue), may not appear until days after the initial trauma. Effects of these secondary injuries are often potentially reversible.

Alternatively, a secondary injury can develop as an accommodation to the primary injury. When an injured person alters his or her movement patterns in response to the pain or dysfunction of a primary injury, the altered movements redistribute loads through other joints in the body. These changes in loading can generate injuries remote from the primary injury. A woman with a sprained ankle, for example, may alter her gait and place unaccustomed loads on both ipsilateral and contralateral joints and tissues. These sites, not accustomed to these redistributed forces, may be injured.

One notable example of this type of secondary injury happened to Dizzy Dean, a Hall of Fame baseball pitcher. In the 1937 All-Star Game, the right-handed Dean's left big toe was struck by a line-drive hit. The toe was broken. Rather than wait until the toe healed completely, Dean returned to action too soon. He altered his pitching mechanics to accommodate the pain caused by the toe injury. In doing so, Dean suffered a career-ending injury to his pitching shoulder. Dean was the unfortunate victim of a secondary injury, now sometimes referred to as a "Dizzy Dean syndrome."

Tissue Structure

The mechanical response of biological tissue depends largely on its noncellular structural makeup, including its constituent material, orientation, density, and connecting substances. Bone, for example, with its mineral latticework and collagen fibers, is designed to transmit compressive, shearing, and tensile loads of high magnitude. Any change in the relation between structure and load, as might occur in an osteoporotic bone or in a bone experiencing abnormal and unaccustomed loading, increases the likelihood of bone injury.

Similarly, the collagen fibers of tendon and ligament afford them exceptional load-bearing capacity parallel to the fiber orientation. Off-angle forces, because of the anisotropic nature of these tissues, may expose the tissue to a greater risk of injury. The interaction between tissue structure and loading behavior creates a complex synergistic relationship that has important consequences for proper function and potential injury.

When different tissues form a functional unit, the weakest-link phenomenon typically occurs during an injury. This means that when a combined structure is mechanically loaded, it will likely fail first at the weakest link in the structural chain. In the human body the factors that contribute to making the weakest link are many, interrelated, and often not easily identified or well understood.

Contributory Factors

Simply stated, injury happens when an imposed load exceeds the tolerance (load-carrying ability) of a tissue. Many contributory factors, however, make this anything but a simple relation between load and injury. The following are examples of contributory factors.

Age

In general, during our formative years, perhaps into our 20s, our tissues are growing and developing. Later, tissues may begin to degenerate and lose strength, compliance, density, and energy-carrying capacity. Acute injuries are more common in younger people. As we age, chronic injuries happen more often, as do unintentional injuries from slips and falls.

It is important to recognize, however, the difference between chronological age and physiological age. The former is based on calendar years, while the latter is based on the physiological quality of the tissues. A 60-year-old person may potentially have tissues with better physiological and mechanical properties than those of a 45-year-old. Remember, while generalities are routinely used to describe aging responses, each person's response is unique and may be quite different from another person's.

Gender

Gender-specific differences in structure, hormones, sociology, activity patterns, and many other measures dictate that one gender may be at greater or lesser risk of injury than the other in some circumstances. For example, the number of fatalities from unintentional injury is higher for men in all categories except for strangulation, ignited clothing, falls from the same level, and certain types of poisoning. The male-to-female fatality ratios due to falls from ladders and scaffoldings are 29:1, injuries from machinery 23:1, electric current 19:1, boat-related drownings 14:1, and motorcycling 11:1 (Baker et al. 1992). Similar ratios exist for nonfatal injuries as well.

Women do not hold an advantage in all areas, however. For example, they are more likely than men to suffer the consequences of osteoporosis. Osteoporotic bone has decreased density, diminished strength, and is more susceptible to fracture. Men can also suffer from osteoporosis, but women are more likely to experience its effects, especially in the postmenopausal epoch. Estrogen deficiency is not the only factor involved in osteoporosis, making this condition a useful example of how complex the analysis of injury-contributing factors can become. Other contributory factors in osteoporosis include disuse due to sedentary lifestyle, paralysis, or immobilization; chronic liver disease; rheumatoid arthritis; alcoholism; diabetes; malignancy; stress; poor diet; and smoking (Sanders & Albright 1987).

Genetics

Genetic factors influence tissue matrix composition and are implicated in the predisposition toward certain injuries, including intervertebral disk and rotator cuff degeneration, carpal tunnel syndrome, and tendon ruptures.

Physiological Status and Physical Condition

A person's physical condition is a primary factor in his or her chances of suffering from an injury. The fitter the person is, the less likely he or she will be injured. If injury does occur, a better-conditioned person generally will have a less severe injury and will recover more quickly.

Nutrition

Diet provides the raw materials to build, sustain, and repair the body's tissues and therefore plays an indirect yet essential role in injury biomechanics. Tissue homeostasis depends on remediating nutritional deficiencies, excesses, or imbalances.

Psychological Status

Psychological parameters can influence the incidence of injury. These factors include stress levels, inattention, distraction, fatigue, depression, excitation, human error, risk evaluation, personality factors, and coping resources.

Fatigue

Physical and mental fatigue increase the likelihood of injury because of compromised muscle strength, coordination, mental attentiveness, and concentration. Fatigue-related injuries tend to happen later in an activity period; for example, truck drivers were found to have twice the risk of crash involvement after six hours of driving compared with the first two hours and to be asleep at the wheel or inattentive in 38% of commercial vehicle accidents (Harris & Mackie 1972). Athletes also tend to show greater risk of injury during the latter stages of a practice session or game. For example, ski injuries are more likely to happen after multiple runs down the mountain.

Environment

Numerous environmental factors contribute to injury, including location (e.g., indoors vs. outdoors, urban vs. rural), weather conditions (e.g., temperature, humidity, visibility), time of day or night, terrain (e.g., flat vs. inclined, smooth vs. rough, slippery vs. sticky), altitude, and activity (e.g., work vs. recreation).

Equipment

Equipment often plays a central role in injury, either in prevention, causation, or both. Equipment can include clothing and other worn items (e.g., pads or protective devices) and implements, such as tools, machinery, or computers. Apparel can be protective, especially in environments likely to produce injury. Implements such as bullet-proof vests, helmets, and shields also aid in injury prevention. Equipment can also be associated with acute injuries (e.g., finger severed in machinery) or chronic injuries (e.g., carpal tunnel syndrome caused by long-term, repetitive typing by a computer operator).

The same piece of equipment can protect a person from or contribute to injury. A football player's helmet and pads, for example, protect the head and body from direct impact. However, the helmet and pads may also contribute to heat stress (by decreasing thermoregulatory capacity and increasing heat production and retention) or to cervical injury if the helmet fits improperly.

Ergonomics and Injury

The economic and personal costs of work-related injuries are staggering. For example, the National Safety Council (1996) estimates that the monetary cost of work-related injury was $119.4 billion in 1995 and that total time lost due to injury was 120 million days. These figures indicate that each of the 124.4 million workers in the United States must produce goods and services valued at nearly $960 each year to offset the costs of injury (National Safety Council 1996).

Efforts to reduce these costs fall under the province of *ergonomics,* or *human factors,* which is the field of study that "discovers and applies information about human behavior, abilities, limitations, and other characteristics to the design of tools, machines, systems, tasks, jobs, and environments for productive, safe, comfortable, and effective human use" (Sanders & McCormick 1993, 5). In simple terms, ergonomics seeks to improve the things that people use and the environments in which they work and live. In many ways the problems associated with workplace injuries are more complex than sports-related injuries.

Sanders & McCormick (1993, 5) identified several characteristics that uniquely define the human factors, or ergonomics, profession:

- Commitment to the idea that things, machines, and so on are built to serve humans and must be designed always with the user in mind

(continued)

(continued)

- Recognition of individual differences in human capabilities and limitations and an appreciation for their design implications
- Conviction that the design of things, procedures, and so on influences human behavior and well-being
- Emphasis on empirical data and evaluation in the design process
- Reliance on the scientific method and the use of objective data to test hypotheses and generate basic data about human behavior
- Commitment to a systems orientation and a recognition that things, procedures, environments, and people do not exist in isolation

Despite the considerable progress that has been made in many areas of injury prevention, complex challenges remain for human factors professionals and others responsible for promoting society's health and well-being.

Human Interaction

Interactions among people can be social, occupational, or competitive, as seen in sports. Whenever people interact, the potential for injury exists. The possibility may be remote at a dinner party, for example, but it becomes a prime factor in a rugby match.

Previous Injury

Following any serious injury, elements of the injury can persist, whether physically or psychologically. The repaired tissues are often not equal to their preinjury condition and for many reasons may be more susceptible to a subsequent injury. A person's psychological status following injury can be different, as the prior injury can stay in mind.

Disease

Many diseases increase the risk of injury. For example, an osteosarcoma (malignant bone tumor) weakens bone, atherosclerosis damages arterial walls, and diabetes predisposes one to skin ulcers, particularly on the plantar surface of the foot.

Drugs

The wide variety of drugs available for either volitional or medical purposes can produce positive or negative effects on the body's tissues and alter human performance so that risk of injury is changed. These agents include alcohol, caffeine, anabolic steroids, pain medications (e.g., aspirin, ibuprofen, acetaminophen), nonsteroidal anti-inflammatory drugs (NSAID), and many other prescription drugs that may be prescribed for an injury or for another unrelated condition. In addition, drugs and other chemical agents may also indirectly contribute to an injury because of their systemic effects.

The use of drugs or ergogenic aids has become more and more insidious and widespread, perhaps most noticeably in competitive sports. Ergogenic refers to the work-generating or power-generating potential of these aids, which can include a host of substances or treatments that purportedly improve a person's physiological performance or remove the psychological barriers associated with more intense activity (Haupt 1991). Many of the pharmacological aids have been banned by official sports bodies because of the unfair advantage some substances give athletes during competition and because of the negative side effects that can occur, including a greater risk of injury in some instances. For example, since their infiltration into sport in the 1950s, anabolic steroids (e.g., oral or injectable forms of synthetic testosterone) have permeated many sports, from the high school level to the Olympic and professional levels. Anabolic steroids may have little or no effect on anaerobic performance. They may increase body size and muscular strength, although these increases are rapidly lost after discontinuing their use. Besides the potential of overuse or acute muscle-tendon injuries associated with the heightened training that may accompany anabolic steroid use, individuals who take anabolic steroids may experience increased acne on the face and upper body, testicular atrophy, changes in sex drive, irritability, aggression, and possible liver damage.

Rehabilitation

The success in returning a person to preinjury status depends on the nature of the injury, the person's motivation, the expertise of the rehabilitation therapist, and the sophistication of the available rehabilitation methods. Sometimes even the best rehabilitation methods are unable to return a person to her or his preinjury capacity. In cases of severe injury, even the most dedicated rehabilitation may not be sufficient, and the injury may be permanently disabling and career threatening. On the other hand, rehabilitation has the potential for returning a person not only to preinjury condition, but potentially to an even higher level of function.

Inflammation is a prime result of an injury to a joint or tissue of the musculoskeletal system, as described more fully in the upcoming section. Inflammation can lead to joint pain, with its potential for tissue atrophy as a consequence of inactivity and lack of motion. Many effective modalities are used to counteract the inflammatory process, including cryotherapy (e.g., ice, cold compresses, cooling sprays) and thermotherapy (e.g., moist hot packs, whirlpool baths, heating pads, ultrasound).

Anthropometric Variability

People come in many shapes and sizes. Differences in body dimensions often play a critical role in injury. Analysis of our structural variability is the province of anthropometry, the study of comparative measurements of the human body. Anthropometric measures such as height, weight, body composition, muscle mass, and shape (somatotype) can all play a central role in assessing injury. Obese individuals, for example, are three times more likely to suffer a fatal heat stroke in comparison to nonobese people. Anthropometric measures are also involved in determining body posture and flexibility (joint range of motion), both of which—either alone or in concert—can affect the risk of injury.

Skill Level

The adeptness with which a person performs a task influences the risk of injury. Especially in high-risk activities (e.g., auto racing) the skill level of the performer may be the most important determinant of injury. Novice or less-skilled performers are more likely to be injured. The converse may prove true, however, when a person's skill level permits the attempt (sometimes ill-advised) of particularly dangerous tasks with a high risk of injury.

Experience

Closely related to skill level is the experience of the individual. While related, these two factors (skill and experience) are not synonymous. An individual may be experienced, having performed a task many times, but be unskilled. Another person may be naturally gifted with a skill but have little experience at the task. Usually, however, the two factors are closely linked. Experienced performers typically exhibit efficiency of movement, along with sound judgment and decision-making abilities. These all combine to lower the risk of injury.

Pain

Sensation of pain is fundamental to any discussion of injury. Pain, the body's message of distress, accompanies most injuries of consequence and often serves as the limiting factor in continued participation in an activity. Pain derives from various biomechanical and inflammatory sources. Pain is one factor used in determining an injury's severity and in prescribing and monitoring the rehabilitation during postinjury therapy. Pain also influences movement patterns (recall the Dizzy Dean syndrome). It may be a hindrance to further activity or preclude participation altogether.

Tissue Injury

The physical damage resulting from injury is unique to each injury. The human body, however, does have a generalized response to injury that occurs in all cases regardless of the specific body region or tissues affected. This immediate reaction to injury is termed the inflammatory response.

Inflammation

The inflammatory response, or *inflammation*, is a generalized pathological process affecting blood vessels and adjacent tissue. It happens in response to a variety of stimuli, especially injury. The cardinal signs of inflammation were identified long ago by Aulus Cornelius Celsus (30 B.C.-A.D. 38). Celsus described the inflammatory response as having "*rubor et tumor cum calore et dolore*," or redness and swelling with heat and pain. A fifth sign, *functio laesa*, or functional loss, was added by Galen (A.D. 129-199) and is often present in inflammation as well.

Inflammation (indicated by the suffix *-itis*) can develop in response to an acute injury or may develop from chronic irritation, as seen in arthritis, bursitis, or tendinitis. The redness and heat of inflammation are due to a vascular response characterized by blood vessel dilation and increased flow. Increases in intracapillary hydrostatic pressure and enhanced capillary permeability combine to cause inflammatory swelling. Pain develops from the swelling-related increase in pressure on nerve endings and is most pronounced when a confined space (e.g., synovial joint) is inflamed. Swelling can restrict function, and the tendency to swell may persist as the damaged tissues (e.g., torn ligament or tendon, or fractured bone) heal.

An injury produces a vasoconstrictive response known as the coagulation phase. This is followed within minutes by a vasodilatory phase, during which an increase in vascular permeability permits the flow of materials from the vessels into the surrounding tissues. These moving substances are termed *exudate* and consist of fluid and plasma proteins, including fibrinogen (a precursor to fibrin, a protein instrumental in the coagulation process). Though the edema (swelling) caused by the exudate may contribute to pain, the exudate has a number of positive functions: It dilutes and inactivates toxins; provides nutrients for inflammatory cells; and contains antibodies, complement proteins, and fibrinogen.

The inflammatory process is controlled by substances known as chemical mediators. This includes the immediately available histamine, as well as other mediators—such as serotonin, bradykinin, prostaglandins, leukotrienes, and plasmin—produced at the site of inflammation or by leukocytes (white blood cells) drawn to the injury site through chemotaxis (cellular attraction due to chemical action).

The chemical mediators of the inflammatory response are joined by cells that perform specific functions. Among these are a general class of cells known as phagocytes (which degrade bacteria and necrotic tissue), the most predominant of which are polymorphonuclear neutrophils (PMNs), responsible for phagocytosis (the engulfing and destruction of particulate matter by phagocytes) and defense against fungal and bacterial infections. Several immune system cells—for example, accessory cells and lymphocytes (B cells, T cells, and NK cells)—also assist in defending against foreign substances (collectively known as antigens).

The essential purpose of inflammation is to serve as the body's first line of defense against insult such as that imposed by injury. The details of the process are complex and in some cases unknown. But for all the apparent complexity of the inflammatory process, "it seems . . . that the more we learn about inflammation, the simpler its message becomes: Our cells and humors defend the self against invisible armies of the other. We call our losses 'infection' and our victories 'immunity'" (Weissmann 1988).

Our comments on injury thus far have applied to most biological tissues and structures. In addition to these general principles, each tissue possesses unique characteristics determined by its own structure and function. The following sections examine these characteristics of the major tissues involved in musculoskeletal injury.

Bone

The viability of bone as a tissue depends on the proper function of the bone's cellular component and the ability of these cells to produce extracellular matrix and perform other important physiological processes. Any disease or injury that compromises osteocyte performance jeopardizes the structural integrity of both the affected bone and the skeletal system in general. Three general conditions that affect bone tissue are described briefly in the following paragraphs. Specific injuries involving these conditions will be examined in detail in chapters 6, 7, and 8.

Osteonecrosis refers to the death of bone cells resulting from a cessation of the blood flow necessary for normal cellular function. In describing the general condition of bone cell death, the term *osteonecrosis* is preferred to the commonly used terms *avascular necrosis* (i.e., cell death due to an absent or deficient blood supply) and *aseptic necrosis* (i.e., cell death in the absence of infection) since osteonecrosis best describes the histopathological processes involved and does not implicate any specific etiology (Ostrum et al. 1994).

The mechanisms of compromised circulation that may lead to osteonecrosis are mechanical disruption of vessels, occlusion of the arterial vessels, injury to or pressure on arterial walls, and occlusion of venous outflow. These conditions may result from bone fracture, joint dislocation, infection, arterial thrombosis, or a number of conditions that affect circulatory integrity. While the bone's noncellular structures (e.g., organic and inorganic matrix) may not be immediately affected, over time they may suffer deleterious effects from the absence of cellular production. A decrease in extracellular matrix production, for example, may result in decreased bone strength and increased likelihood of fracture.

Osteoporosis literally refers to a condition in which bone experiences an increase in porosity (more and/or larger holes). Based on the types of osteoporosis seen clinically, osteoporosis may be more accurately described as a condition "in which a progressive diminution of skeletal mass renders bone increasingly vulnerable to fracture" (Sanders & Albright 1987). Osteoporosis was identified as a prominent public health issue more than 50 years ago and has been the subject of extensive research and scientific debate ever since. Histological, radio-

logical, and clinical evidence has clearly demonstrated that progressive bone loss begins in the fourth decade of life, and the rate of loss increases with advancing age (figure 5.1).

Osteoporosis most affects trabecular bone and the endosteal surface of cortical bone. It occurs earlier (in a person's 20s) in bones of the axial skeleton than in the appendicular skeleton (beginning about age 40). Osteoporosis is a multifactorial problem that continues to frustrate researchers in their attempts to identify the precise etiological factors and pathogenic mechanisms involved in both the onset and progression of the condition.

Among the factors most often included in discussions of osteoporosis are dietary status, physical activity patterns, hormone dynamics, calcium absorption, and physical stress. Some of the clinical conditions associated with osteoporosis are listed in table 5.3. With the average age of the population increasing, osteoporosis will undoubtedly continue to be a major public health concern and will provide fertile ground for research in the coming decades.

The injury most commonly associated with bone is fracture, derived from the Latin *fractura*, meaning to break. While the term *fracture* is also used to describe disruption to cartilage and the epiphyseal plate, it is most closely associated with breaks in the structural continuity of bony tissue. In a simple sense, fracture occurs when an applied load exceeds the bone's ability to withstand the force. The many factors involved in specifying the loading conditions and the response characteristics of the loaded bone, however, make the study of fracture mechanics anything but a simple task.

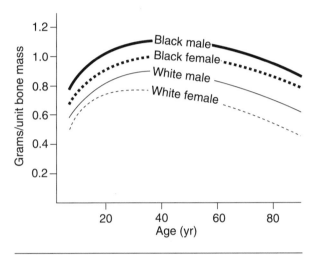

Figure 5.1   Bone mass as a function of age, gender, and race.

From "Effects of aging on bone structure and metabolism" (Fig. 1-3, p. 3) by R. Pacifici & L.V. Avioli, 1993. In: *The Osteoporotic Syndrome: Detection, Prevention, and Treatment* (3rd ed.), New York: Wiley-Liss. Copyright 1993 by Wiley-Liss, Inc. Reprinted by permission of Wiley-Liss, Inc., a subsidiary of John Wiley & Sons, Inc.

Table 5.3   Clinical Conditions Associated With Osteoporosis

Menopause or aging	Acromegaly
Disuse; immobilization, paralysis, weightlessness	Scurvy
Corticosteroid treatment	Alcoholism
Cushing's syndrome	Diabetes
Osteogenesis imperfecta	Lactase deficiency
Partial gastrectomy	Malignancy
Malabsorption syndromes	Mastocytosis
Chronic liver disease	Acid-rich diet
Heparin treatment	Decreased physical stress
Hyperparathyroidism	Amenorrhea in runners
Hyperthyroidism	Smoking
Rheumatoid arthritis	

From "Bone: Age-related changes and osteoporosis" (Table 9-2, p. 277) by M. Sanders & J.A. Albright, 1987. In: J.A. Albright & R.A. Brand (Eds.), *The Scientific Basis of Orthopaedics* (2nd ed.), Norwalk, CT: Appleton-Lange. Copyright 1987 by Appleton-Lange. Reprinted by permission.

The fracture resistance of bone is determined by both the material properties of bone as a tissue and the structural properties of bone as an organ. It is influenced by the complex interaction of viscoelastic characteristics (e.g., strain rate), bone geometry (e.g., cross-sectional dimensions), anisotropic effects (e.g., microstructural orientation with respect to the loading direction), and bone porosity (Hipp, Cheal, & Hayes 1992).

The nature of bone loading determines in large part the potential for injury and the type of fracture produced. Fracture may occur in response to a single, large-magnitude loading, as occurs in a violent collision (acute loading). Alternately, fractures may result from repeated application of lower-magnitude forces (chronic loading), as is characteristic of a metatarsal fatigue fracture (stress fracture) resulting from excessive running or jumping.

A fracture at the specific site of force application is termed a direct injury. When the fracture is remote from the location of force application, it is an indirect injury. Indirect injuries result from force transmission through other tissues. An example of indirect injury is when a force applied to a tendon or ligament is transferred to its bony attachment site and causes an *avulsion fracture* at that location (a piece of bone is pulled out at the insertion site).

The risk of fracture also depends on the type of bone being loaded. Cortical (compact) bone, because of its relatively low porosity (i.e., high density), is generally more fracture resistant than less-dense trabecular (cancellous) bone. In general, factors that contribute to an increase in bone density serve to increase bone strength and thus decrease fracture risk. Conversely, factors that contribute to decreased bone density increase the risk of bone injury.

A diagnosed fracture can be classified in various ways, but the following factors are commonly considered (Salter 1983):

- Injury site—Fractures may be classified according to their location, such as diaphyseal, epiphyseal, or metaphyseal fractures.

- Extent of injury—Fractures may be either complete or incomplete, depending on whether the damage completely traverses the entire bone or only partially encompasses the bone structure.

- Configuration—In cases where there is only a single fracture line, the shape of the line may be either transverse, oblique, or spiral. When there is more than one fracture line, the fracture may be classified as a comminuted or butterfly fracture.

- Fragment relations—Bone fragments may be either undisplaced or displaced. In the latter case, the fragment displacement may occur in many ways, including angulation, rotation, distraction, overriding, impaction, or sideways shifting.

- Environmental relations—Fractures, even if displaced, that remain within the body's internal environment are termed closed fractures. Those penetrating the skin and resulting in exposure of bone to the external environment are open fractures. For obvious reasons, open fractures pose a much greater risk of infection than do closed fractures. Historically, closed and open fractures sometimes have been called simple and compound fractures, respectively. This terminology somewhat misrepresents the nature of the fractures and can be misleading. Many clinicians and other professionals, therefore, discourage the use of simple and compound as fracture descriptors, preferring the closed and open designations.

- Complications—Some fractures are accompanied by few, if any, complications. Many, however, have complications that may be immediate (e.g., skin, vascular, neurological, muscular, or visceral injury), early (e.g., tissue necrosis, infection, tetanus, pneumonia), or late (e.g., osteoarthritis, growth disturbances, post traumatic osteoporosis, refracture) (Salter 1983).

- Etiological factors—In some cases, fracture is preceded by conditions that predispose a bone to injury. Examples of predisposing etiological factors are repetitive-use microfractures that precede stress fractures and inflammatory disorders, bone disease, congenital abnormalities, and neoplasms that contribute to pathological fractures.

- Combination injuries—Bone fracture may be associated with or caused by other tissues. Multiple fractures and fracture-dislocation injuries are examples of such combined injury conditions. Another combination condition results from the "connectedness" of tissues. Forces applied to an osteotendinous junction, for example, can produce a tendon injury, bone fracture, or both. The weakest-link argument predicts that if the bone is stronger, the tendon will be strained. Conversely, if the tendon is relatively stronger, the bone will experience an avulsion fracture. Here, the viscoelastic properties of bone and tendon may come into play. If the injury load is applied slowly, the bone is more likely to be fractured (avulsion fracture), whereas the tendon is more likely to tear if the load is applied rapidly. An avulsion fracture and various other frac-

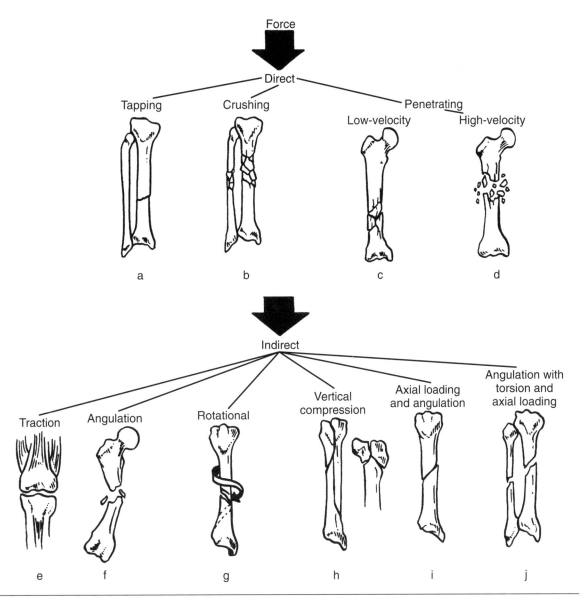

Figure 5.2 Classification of fractures according to the mechanism of injury. Direct force: (*a*) Tapping mechanism from relatively small forces over a small area causes transverse fracture. (*b*) Crushing from large forces over a large area results in extensive comminuted fracture. Large force over a small area at either (*c*) low velocity or (*d*) high velocity results in penetrating, comminuted fracture. Indirect force: (*e*) Traction mechanism from tensile loading results in either transverse fracture or avulsion fracture. (*f*) Angulation (bending) mechanism results in angulated, or butterfly, fracture. (*g*) Rotational mechanism from torsional loading results in spiral fracture. (*h*) Vertical, or axial compressive, loading causes oblique fracture. (*i*) Combination of axial compression and angulation produces a combination of transverse fracture (on the convex side) and oblique fracture. (*j*) Combination of angulation (bending) with torsion and axial loading results in complex fracture pattern.

From *Rockwood and Green's Fractures in Adults* (4th ed.) (Fig. 1-15, p. 11) by C.A. Rockwood, D.P. Green, R.W. Bucholz, & J.D. Heckman (Eds.), 1996, Philadelphia: Lippincott-Raven Publishers. Copyright 1996 by Lippincott-Raven. Adapted by permission.

ture types and their commonly associated injury mechanisms are shown in figure 5.2.

Fracture healing can be divided into three phases: inflammation, initial union of the bony ends, and remodeling of the callus. Immediately following injury, a hematoma (pool of blood) develops around

the fracture site. Within three days, mesenchymal cells arrive in the area and produce a fibrous tissue that envelopes the fractured bone ends. The outer layer of the fibrous material begins to form the new periosteum. Until this point, stable and unstable fractures react similarly, but between 3 to 5 days after the fracture the degree of stability influences subsequent healing steps. Microscopic examination of the fibrous tissue reveals that in a stable fracture the tissue is well vascularized, but in an unstable fracture the fibrous tissue contains no vessels.

Where the fibrous tissue meets the original bony cortex—in both stable and unstable fractures—new trabeculae are formed by osteoblasts lying on the old bone surface. In a stable fracture, new bone forms along the periosteal surface of the fibrous layer and spans the fracture site. In an unstable fracture, new bone also forms along the periosteal surface of the fibrous material but does not span the fracture line. In humans, minimal periosteal bone formation occurs at this point in healing, and periosteal union is further delayed. As bony trabeculae continue to form, the bony collar becomes more compact, and the periosteum increases in thickness.

In the gap between the bony ends (rather than along the periosteal surface), the first cells to invade after injury (approximately day 9) are macrophages, followed by fibroblasts and capillaries. Macrophages remove cell and matrix debris, while the fibroblasts generate the structural matrix for cells and vessels. Osteoblasts begin bone deposition by 2 wk postfracture, and bony union across the fractured ends is established (optimally) by 3 wk. If the bone adjacent to the fracture site dies secondary to disruption of its blood supply at the time of fracture, osteoclasts may be present to resorb the dead tissue. Otherwise, osteoclasts are not routinely present in all fractures.

In small gaps (< 10 mm) or where fracture ends contact, healing is via direct Haversian remodeling: Osteoclasts resorb a cone of bone, osteoblasts deposit new Haversian bone, and osteocytes maintain the new bone after mineralization. In 10- to 30-mm gaps (too large for Haversian remodeling but too small for cells to move) osteoclasts may resorb the bone to increase the gap width. Osteoblasts later arrive to lay down disorganized lamellae across the gap. The disorganized bone is then remodeled.

In an unstable fracture, periosteal bone formation continues from the old bone ends toward the fracture line, but across the fracture line (where the fibrous material is avascular) chondrocytes proliferate and lay down a cartilage matrix. In a sequence identical to that which happens during endochondral ossification of long bones, the cartilage bridging the fracture ends is gradually replaced by bone. In humans, good stability is generally achieved by 6 wk. With the improved stability, blood vessels and fibroblasts proliferate in the fracture gap.

Remodeling of the fracture callus begins as soon as the fracture site regains stability. The dynamics of this remodeling are similar to those of Haversian remodeling: Old bone is resorbed by osteoclasts, and new bone is deposited by osteoblasts. The process is vigorous in the area where the periosteal callus meets the surface of the old bone. Prior to remodeling, this line is clearly visible, but after remodeling, the junction is indistinguishable between the old bone and the callus.

Articular Cartilage

The articular surfaces of bones in synovial joints are, with few exceptions, covered with a thin (1 to 5 mm) layer of hyaline articular cartilage. This layer serves several important functions, including load distribution and minimization of friction and wear. Injury to articular cartilage can severely compromise normal joint function and, in advanced cases, may necessitate joint replacement.

Experimental data suggest that excessive joint loading leads to three types of articular damage: (1) loss of cartilage matrix macromolecules, alteration of the macromolecular matrix, or chondrocyte injury (any or all of these can occur with no detectable disruption of the tissue), (2) isolated damage to the articular cartilage itself in the form of chondral fracture or flap tears, and (3) injury to the cartilage and its underlying bone, a condition known as an osteochondral fracture.

When significant damage happens to articular cartilage, repair with new hyaline cartilage rarely occurs. The inability of articular cartilage to repair defects of any significant size is attributed to its lack of blood vessels and the relative lack of cells in cartilage. This inability of articular cartilage to effect substantial self-repair is a contributory factor to degenerative joint disease.

Degenerative joint disease, commonly referred to as *osteoarthritis*, is a noninflammatory disorder of synovial joints, particularly those with load-bearing involvement, that is characterized by deterioration of the hyaline articular cartilage and bone formation on joint surfaces and at the joint margins (figure 5.3). Osteoarthritis is often accompanied by the formation of bony outgrowths of ossified cartilage (osteophytes), typically at the joint margin. Osteoarthritis results in a degradation of articular cartilage and may be initiated by mechanical trauma and attendant chemical process alterations.

Advances in Joint Replacement

The debilitating pain of advanced osteoarthritis of the hip and knee severely limits a person's mobility. Joint replacement surgery (arthroplasty), in which the damaged structures are replaced by artificial materials, provides remarkable pain relief and restores function in most cases. Because of the load-bearing responsibilities of the lower extremities, it is not surprising that the hip and knee are the leading arthroplastic sites, accounting for 38.4% and 35.8%, respectively, of all arthroplasty procedures (Praemer, Furner, & Rice 1992).

The most common procedure involves replacement of the hip. More than 120,000 hip replacements are performed each year in the United States (National Institutes of Health 1994). In light of continued advances in biomaterials and surgical technique, computer-assisted design and manufacture (Crowninshield 1990), and an aging population, the number of arthroplasties will continue to rise.

Total hip replacement (THR) involves excision of the femoral head and part of the neck and enlargement of the acetabulum. A metallic femoral prosthesis (figure 5B.1) is inserted into the medullary canal of the femur. The prosthesis may be cemented into the canal using methyl methacrylate. An alternative, cementless technique uses a prosthesis with porous structure that encourages bony ingrowth. The success of cemented versus cementless prostheses remains a subject of debate.

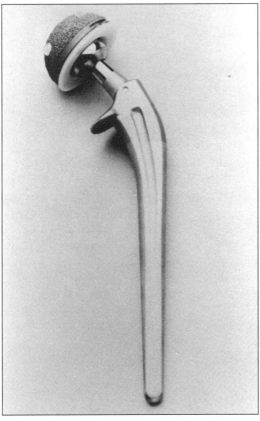

a

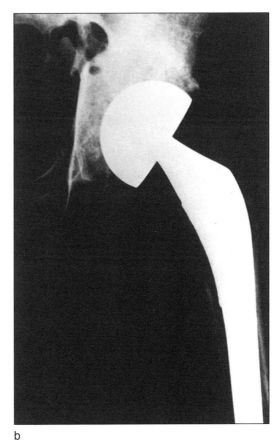

b

Figure 5B.1   Hip prosthesis used in arthroplasty. (*a*) Femoral and acetabular components. (*b*) Implanted prosthesis.

Reprinted from Stillwell 1987.

(continued)

(continued)

The prosthetic femoral head fits into an acetabular prosthetic component that is inserted into the enlarged acetabulum. The acetabular component consists of a high-density polyethylene articulating surface backed by a metallic foundational base.

Arthroplasty procedures are not without potential complications. Prosthetic component loosening and infection are the most common problems after the surgical procedure. Nonetheless, the relief provided to the arthritic patient far outweighs any potential difficulties. This has led Coombs and colleagues (1990, p. xxi) to conclude boldly, "No operation has done more to alleviate human suffering than hip replacement."

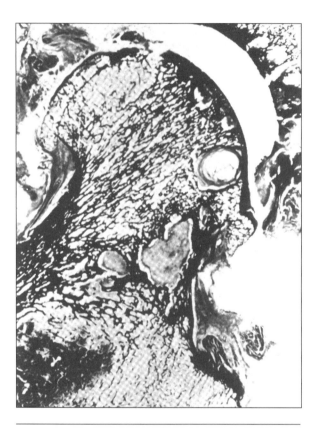

Figure 5.3 Histological section of the upper end of the femur showing principal features of osteoarthritis, including joint space narrowing, sclerosis of the bony end plates, cysts, and osteophytes at the medial and lateral joint margins.

From "Articular cartilage, cartilage injury, and osteoarthritis" (Fig. 2-13, p. 29) by H.J. Mankin, 1993. In: J.M. Fox & W. Del Pizzo (Ed.), *The Patellofemoral Joint*, New York: McGraw-Hill. Copyright 1993 by McGraw-Hill. Reproduced with permission of The McGraw-Hill Companies.

The degenerative process is characterized by cartilage fibrillation, cell loss, *chondromalacia* (cartilage softening), loss of elastic support, and disruption of the collagen framework (Fulkerson, Edwards, & Chrisman 1987). These structural alterations increase the susceptibility of the articular cartilage to shearing loads and thereby predispose it to injury.

Among the factors implicated in the pathogenesis of osteoarthritis are obesity, genetics, endocrine and metabolic disorders, joint trauma, and activity patterns determined by a person's occupation or choice of recreation. Epidemiological evidence suggests that up to 90% of the population shows some degree of osteoarthritic involvement by the age of 40, though in many cases with no clinical symptoms.

Fibrocartilage

Fibrocartilage serves as a transitional tissue at osteotendinous and osteoligamentous junctions, facilitating the distribution of forces at attachment sites and lowering the risk of injury. Fibrocartilage is also found in certain joints as *menisci*, interposed fibrocartilage pads that act as shock absorbers and as wedges at the joint periphery that improve the structural fit of the joint. Menisci are found in the joints of the tibiofemoral, acromioclavicular, sternoclavicular, and temporomandibular joints. Meniscal injuries at several of these joints are discussed in later chapters.

Fibrocartilage is also found in the outer covering (*annulus fibrosus*) of the intervertebral disks. Injury to the fibrocartilage of the annulus fibrosus plays a central role in the mechanisms of low-back pain caused by so-called slipped disks.

Tendon

As the agents responsible for force transfer from skeletal muscle to bone, tendons provide a critical link in the musculoskeletal system. Injury to tendinous structures can restrict or even prevent normal movement and function. The connective structure of tendon creates three structural zones: the body of the tendon itself (tendon substance), the connec-

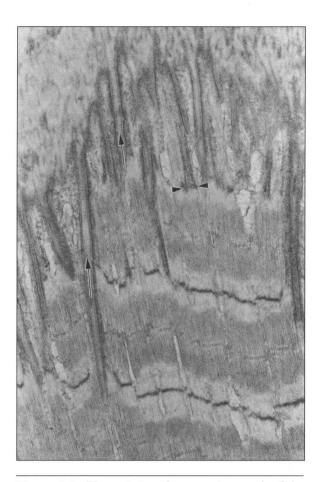

Figure 5.4 Transmission electron micrograph of the myotendinous junction. Collagen fibers (arrows) extend into the folded cell membrane. Densely bundled filaments meet at the terminal Z-disk (arrowheads).
Reprinted from Tidball 1991.

tions of tendon with bone (osteotendinous junction), and the connections with its accompanying muscle (myotendinous junction; figure 5.4).

Tendon injury may result from a direct insult, as is commonly seen in tendons of the hand and fingers that are lacerated by sharp implements such as knives, saws, and other bladed tools. Tendinous injury may also be indirect, resulting from excessive tensile loads applied to the tendon structure. Attempted transmission of loads exceeding the ultimate strength of fibers (or the whole tendon) leads to tendon injury.

Injuries to musculotendinous units are termed *strains*. Like skeletal muscle injuries, tendon injuries are categorized according to their severity. Mild strain is characterized by negligible structural disruption, local tenderness, and minimal functional deficit. Moderate strain exhibits partial structural defect, visible swelling, marked tenderness, and some loss of stability. Severe strains have complete

structural disruption, marked tenderness, and functional deficits that typically necessitate corrective surgical intervention.

Severe tendon strain (complete rupture of the tendon's structure) is often preceded by undetected tissue damage that existed before the specific incident of rupture. Such cases have been termed spontaneous tendon rupture and are typically seen in middle-aged individuals engaged in strenuous activities. The injured often have no history of injury or any prior recognized distress. These spontaneous tendon ruptures are accompanied by a popping sensation and occur unexpectedly. Postinjury investigation during surgery often identifies preexisting pathology, suggesting that previous, undetected tendon degeneration may facilitate the spontaneous failure (Woo et al. 1994). Examples of spontaneous ruptures in the Achilles and patellar tendons are described in chapter 6.

Repetitive overloading of a tendon may lead to an inflammatory response, or tendinitis. The reaction may be acute (in response to a limited session or event) or chronic (a result of repeated overuse). In addition to inflammation of the tendon substance itself, related structures that facilitate tendon sliding may also become inflamed and subsequently injured (e.g., peritenon, tendon sheath, and accompanying bursa).

At the risk of creating confusion, it is important to note that some variability exists in the terminology used to describe tendon and tendon-related conditions. The terms *tendinitis* (also spelled *tendonitis*), *tenosynovitis*, *tendinosis*, and others may be used by clinicians and researchers in different contexts to describe different conditions, as indicated in table 5.4. Caution is warranted in using these terms, and specification of the injured tissue should be exact.

A great deal is known about the healing of severed tendons that have been surgically repaired. After an initial inflammatory response, synthesis of glycosaminoglycans and collagen, which are used in restoring the matrix integrity of the tendon, is triggered. Rest, ice, and immobilization are recommended to avoid additional tissue damage for the first week after a tendon is acutely injured. Then in the second and third weeks, cyclic low loads applied to the healing tendons may help to align the new fibers and strengthen the repairing tendon. In addition, stretching and activation of the muscle-tendon unit may prevent excessive muscle atrophy and joint stiffness. After the third week, progressively increasing the stress on the tendon optimizes the tissue's healing.

Table 5.4   Tendon Injury Terminology

New	Old	Definition
Peritenonitis	Tenosynovitis Tenovaginitis Peritendinitis	An inflammation of only the peritenon, either lined by synovium or not
Peritenonitis with tendinosis	Tendinitis	Peritenon inflammation associated with intratendinous degeneration
Tendinosis	Tendinitis	Intratendinous degeneration due to atrophy (aging, microtrauma, vascular compromise, etc.)
Tendinitis	Tendon strain or tear	Symptomatic degeneration of the tendon with vascular disruption and inflammatory repair response

Reprinted from Leadbetter 1994.

Much less is known about the processes and healing responses associated with chronic tendinitis.

In addition to injuries of the tendon substance, damage can also occur at the myotendinous and osteotendinous junctions. The myotendinous junction has been implicated as the site of many injuries. The structure of the junction shows an interdigitation of skeletal muscle fibers with tendinous collagen fibers in a characteristic membrane-folding pattern. This folding pattern serves to reduce stress at the myotendinous junction during muscular contraction, thus lessening the likelihood of injury.

Injury also occurs at the osteotendinous junction, where the tendon attaches to the cortical bone surface. The structure of this attachment exhibits four zones of increasing mechanical stiffness as the material transitions from tendon, to fibrocartilage, to mineralized fibrocartilage, and finally to bone, as shown in figure 5.5a. These transition zones serve to distribute the tensile forces and lessen the chance of injury. Figure 5.5b is an electron micrograph showing an intact osteotendinous junction, and figure 5.5c shows a disrupted osteotendinous junction in which the applied force exceeded the maximum tolerance of the tissues.

Ligament

Injury to a ligament, termed a ligamentous *sprain*, may compromise a ligament's stabilizing ability and impair its ability to control joint movements. The severity of the sprain is clinically specified with a three-level scheme as shown in table 5.1. Mild and moderate sprains are most common. Complete ligament tearing (severe sprain) happens in a minority of cases.

Recall that ligaments can be intracapsular (located within the joint capsule), capsular (appearing as a thickening of the capsule structure), or extracapsular (extrinsic to the capsule). The location and attachments of these different ligament types help determine their function, their response to mechanical loading, and their susceptibility to injury. Examples in chapters 6 and 7 illustrate these ligament-specific responses in lower- and upper-extremity joints.

The attachment of ligament to bone follows a structure similar to that at the osteotendinous junction. The osteoligamentous junction can also exhibit transitional zones of fibrocartilage and mineralized fibrocartilage intervening between the ligament and the cortical bone to which it attaches. This zonal structure facilitates load distribution at the ligament attachment sites. Additionally, fibers of the ligament can travel relatively parallel to the surface of the bone and gradually blend with the periosteum.

Frank (1996) outlines the three major phases of ligament healing: (1) bleeding and inflammation, (2) proliferation of bridging material, and (3) matrix remodeling. The first step, the inflammatory response, parallels the description in the preceding section on inflammation. The platelets from the blood promote clotting, a fibrin clot is deposited, growth factors are released to promote the inflammatory cascade, local vessels dilate, acute inflammatory cells infiltrate, and the fibroblastic scar cells arrive on the scene. The second phase of ligament

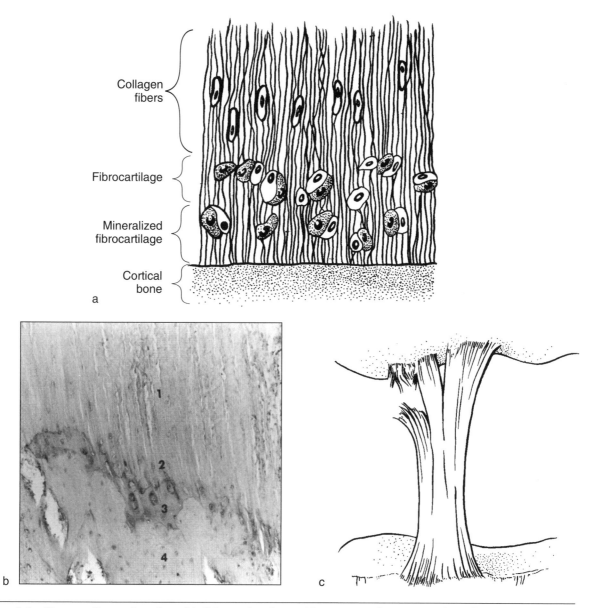

Figure 5.5 Osteotendinous junction. (*a*) Schematic of transition zones of progressively stiffer tissues (tendon, fibrocartilage, mineralized fibrocartilage, cortical bone). (*b*) Electron micrograph of patellar insertion from a dog with zones of (1) tendon, (2) fibrocartilage, (3) mineralized fibrocartilage, and (4) cortical bone. (*c*) Drawing of a disrupted osteotendinous junction.

Part (*b*) reprinted from Cooper & Misol 1970.

healing comprises the generation of a scar matrix. The scar that is produced and eventually remodeled in phase three, however, is not normal ligament. The collagen fibers in the scar are typically smaller in diameter than in normal ligament, and the alignment of the collagen fibers in the scar is generally more haphazard than in normal ligament. Matrix remodeling constitutes the third phase of ligament healing. Once bridging happens, the scar matrix diminishes in size and becomes less viscous and

more dense and organized. The scar, with time, may start to look and function more like an uninjured ligament, but it never becomes the same as a normal, uninjured ligament.

Skeletal Muscle

Injury to skeletal muscle is common. It can take several forms and involve various mechanisms. A strain injury (not to be confused with mechanical strain, discussed in chapters 3 and 4) occurs when damage is inflicted to a musculotendinous unit. The specifics of tendon injury were discussed previously; here we concentrate on three forms of skeletal muscle injury: (1) acute muscular strain, (2) contusions, and (3) exercise-induced muscle injury (Leadbetter 1994).

Acute muscular strain typically results from overstretching a passive muscle or from dynamically overloading an active muscle, either concentrically or eccentrically. The severity of tissue damage depends on the magnitude of the force, the rate of force application, and the strength of the musculotendinous structures. Mild strains are characterized by minimal structural disruption and rapid return to normal function. Moderate strains are accompanied by a partial tear in the muscle tissue (often at or near the myotendinous junction), pain, and some loss of function. Severe muscle strains are defined by complete or near-complete tissue disruption and functional loss, as well as marked hemorrhage and swelling.

Muscle injury may also happen as a result of a direct compressive impact. Such contact may cause a muscle bruise (contusion), which is distinguished by intramuscular hemorrhage. Muscular contusion commonly occurs in contact sports (e.g., basketball, football, soccer) when an athlete's thigh has a violent impact with another participant's knee. Such a thigh injury is often termed a "Charley horse," but we again caution against the use of such catch-all designations as they are nonspecific and inconsistently applied. Repeated mechanical insult to a damaged muscle prior to healing may worsen the injury and lead to serious secondary conditions, such as myositis ossificans (deposition of an ossified mass within the muscle).

A third condition, known as exercise-induced muscle injury, results from connective and contractile tissue disruption following exercise. It is characterized by local tenderness, stiffness, and restricted range of motion. This type of injury, also referred to as delayed-onset muscle soreness (DOMS), typically happens 24 to 72 h after participation in vigorous exercise, especially following eccentric muscle action in contractile tissue unaccustomed to the activity's demands. While the underlying mechanism of DOMS remains elusive, its symptoms and metabolic events (e.g., pain, swelling, presence of cellular infiltrates, increased lysosomal activity, and increased levels of some circulating acute-phase proteins) are similar to that of acute inflammation and suggest a relation between the two (Smith 1991).

While not particularly injurious itself, the common muscle cramp may be indicative of conditions predisposing to injury. Excessive demands placed on such a sustained and often painful muscular spasm may result in muscle strain. The mechanisms of muscle cramps, despite the frequency of their occurrence, are not fully understood. Most cramps occur in a shortened muscle and are characterized by abnormal electrical activity. Many factors have been implicated in the etiology of muscle cramps, including dehydration, electrolyte imbalances, direct impact, fatigue, and lowered levels of serum calcium and magnesium. Cramps happen in many muscles, especially the gastrocnemius, semimembranosus, semitendinosus, biceps femoris, and abdominals, and can be relieved by antagonistic muscle activity or manual stretching of the afflicted muscle. Stretching warrants care since excessive force applied to a muscle in spasm may result in muscle strain.

Skin

Injury to the skin can take various forms and may involve many causal mechanisms, some of which are mechanical in nature. Sufficient friction between the skin and an opposing surface may result in superficial injury such as an abrasion (scraping away of the superficial skin layer, usually by mechanical action) or deeper injury such as a blister (a fluid-filled structure under or within the epidermis, caused by heat, chemical, or mechanical means).

Nonpenetrating skin injury is termed a contusion, or bruise, which usually results from a direct, violent impact. Internal hemorrhage typically accompanies contusion injury and, in severe cases, can be quite debilitating.

Sharp implements that penetrate the skin create puncture wounds, which not only damage the dermal and epidermal layers, but may, with sufficient penetration depth, result in injury to intervening internal structures as well. The mechanics of puncture injury often result in a wound that appears on the skin surface to be much less severe than it may actually be, since the skin often closes on implement removal to obscure deeper damage. The wound often appears to be "clean," leaving little visible external evidence of the damage created internally. Jagged tearing of the skin (laceration) is characteristic of cut wounds by a knife or other sharp implements, because the mechanism of injury is tearing rather than puncture. The external appearance of a laceration is usually more obvious than that of a puncture wound.

Any injury that penetrates the skin, to any depth, carries with it the risk of infection. Caution is warranted in treating any penetrating injury, however slight, since the damaging effects of infection resulting from an improperly treated injury may far exceed the deleterious effects of the original injury itself.

Given the proximity of venous vasculature to the dermis, skin injuries are often characterized by considerable bleeding (hemorrhage). Facial lacerations, for example, commonly produce effusive bleeding, especially in the areas immediately above (supraorbital) and below (infraorbital) the eye and on the chin.

Nervous Tissue

Nervous tissue is not classified as a musculoskeletal tissue, but since injury to nervous tissue can affect, either directly or indirectly, the function of musculoskeletal tissues, we present a brief outline of nervous tissue injury. Injury to nervous tissue has the potential to produce the most debilitating types of dysfunction. Damage to the brain and other supraspinal structures, spinal cord, spinal nerves, or peripheral nerves can impair the most essential of the body's communication systems, reducing or even eliminating sensory and motor processes. Injury to specific neural structures and the causal mechanisms of these injuries are considered in each of the three succeeding chapters. Injuries to structures of the peripheral nervous system are considered in chapters 6 and 7. Examples of injuries to the central nervous system (e.g., cerebral concussion) are presented in chapter 8. As a prelude, a brief review of nervous tissue injury is presented here.

Nerves are cord-like organs that serve as the communication conduits in the peripheral nervous system. Each nerve consists of many nerve fibers (axons) that are arranged in parallel bundles. These bundles are enclosed by layers of connective tissue. Each axon is covered by a delicate endoneurial sheath. Axons are grouped into nerve bundles (fascicles) that are surrounded by perineurium. Finally, the fascicles collectively form the whole nerve (nerve trunk) that is surrounded by a tough covering of epineurial tissue (epineurium).

Nervous tissue can be injured through chemical, thermal, ischemic, or mechanical means. We will focus on only the last of these. Mechanical influences on nervous structures can take one of two basic forms, namely, entrapment or trauma. In the former, nervous tissue becomes entrapped in a confined anatomical space or between other anatomical structures. The resulting forces impinge on the nervous tissue and can produce damage and compromise function.

The second form of nerve injury, trauma, results from a direct mechanical insult to the tissue or from indirect forces applied to surrounding structures being transmitted to the nervous tissue. Each of the three principal loading types may be present, either alone or in combination. Compressive loads result in pressure on nervous tissue. Tensile loading creates tissue elongation, which may result in stretch injury. Shear loading may lead to friction-related injury. In entrapment and traumatic situations the nature of any resulting dysfunction depends on the exact characteristics of the mechanical environment at the time of injury.

Traumatic peripheral nerve injury may produce a temporary block of nerve signal conduction in the absence of axonal discontinuity or in actual severance (partial or full) of the axon. In the latter case, injury to the axon typically leads to axonal degeneration, in which the axon and its myelin sheath disintegrate (Wallerian degeneration). This degenerative process results in a separation (denervation) between the axon's neuron (nerve cell) and its target organ. The cell's response depends on the location and severity of injury and may enable a regenerative response or may result in cell death.

The severity of injury, based on nerve histopathology, is commonly assessed with a qualitative five-level classification system (Sunderland 1978). Only the basic elements of these levels are presented in the following paragraphs.

The least severe level is termed a first-degree injury and is characterized by the presence of a conduction block. This interruption of nerve signal transmission may be brief, mild, or severe. First-degree nerve injuries do not involve any denervation effects and result in full recovery, though this recovery may take several months to occur. First-degree injury can happen after a prolonged, low-pressure compression (e.g., carpal tunnel syndrome) or an acute, high-compression event that results in a conduction block without axonal discontinuity, or neurapraxia.

Second-degree injury involves axonotmesis, an interruption of axonal structure with accompanying Wallerian degeneration but without severance of the nerve's supporting structure. These lesions may result from pinching or crushing mechanisms or from prolonged pressure. Recovery and regeneration of second-degree nerve injury normally occurs. Third-degree injury involves a loss of fiber continuity (neurotmesis), with damage to both the axon and the endoneurial sheath. Fascicular disorganization and intrafascicular hemorrhage, edema, and ischemia result. A third-degree injury results in complete loss of sensory and motor function. Recovery may be complete but typically is quite protracted.

Fourth-degree nerve injury involves a loss of axonal, endoneurial, and fascicular continuity, leaving only epineurial tissue to provide structural continuity. Successful recovery seldom occurs spontaneously, and surgical repair is indicated in most cases. The most severe (fifth-degree) injury results in complete severance of the nerve trunk. Regeneration, if it occurs at all, is usually incomplete and disrupted. This most severe category of nerve injury usually requires surgical repair.

Any level of compromised sensory or motor function can hasten or exacerbate musculoskeletal injury. Impaired sensory function, for example, may alter pain sensation, thus retarding the body's warning system and permitting a more severe injury than might occur with normal sensation.

Axonal damage that results in motor impairment can alter muscle recruitment patterns and produce uncoordinated and potentially dangerous movements. A runner, for example, with impaired motor control due to nervous tissue injury may experience selective muscle weakness that results in altered gait mechanics and eventual musculoskeletal injury.

Compartment and Entrapment Conditions

The fundamental mechanical relation between mass and volume plays a central role in various injury conditions that are broadly termed compartment, entrapment, or impingement syndromes. The common element of all such conditions is the ratio of mass and volume, or density, and its mechanical consequences on biological tissues. Increasing the density of material within a confined space increases the pressure exerted on the boundaries of the space and on the material within the space. Increasing density, either by increasing the mass or decreasing the volume (or both), will result in a pressure increase. This increase in pressure is transmitted to all structures within the enclosed space. In the case of biological systems, the structures affected are often

nerves and circulatory vessels. Pressure on nerves is felt as tingling, numbness, or pain. Pressure on circulatory vessels results in decreased arterial or capillary perfusion or restricted venous return. The tissues reliant upon proper neural and circulatory supply will be deleteriously affected.

Such situations are often either caused or worsened by inflammation—in particular the swelling that accompanies the inflammatory response. In many cases, the affected system becomes involved in a positive feedback loop, with increases in pressure causing restricted outflow, which in turn further increases pressure.

This fundamental pressure-density relation and its physiological effects can be seen in many instances of musculoskeletal injury, some of which are detailed in the following chapters. Included in the wide array of compartment-entrapment are conditions such as carpal tunnel syndrome, glenohumeral impingement syndrome, skeletal muscle compartment syndromes, synovial joint swelling, and cerebral edema. All are either caused or aggravated by the mechanical relation between mass, volume, and pressure.

Joint Injury

Skeletal articulations (joints), by virtue of their often intricate structure, are susceptible to injury and involve complex mechanical loading of multiple tissues. While not well understood in many cases, the dynamics of joint mechanical loading determine the actual injury or injuries that occur. Since numerous joint injuries are examined in detail in subsequent chapters, we limit our discussion here to basic concepts and terminology of joint injury.

When sufficient force is applied to a joint, the articulating bones may become displaced with respect to their normal structural relationship. This results in a complete dislocation (*luxation*) or a partial dislocation (*subluxation*) (figure 5.6). Dislocations, whether partial or complete, often are accompanied by additional injuries, including ligamentous sprain and tears of the fibrous joint capsule.

The inner surface of the joint capsule is lined by the *synovial membrane*, a thin layer of tissue that has negligible biomechanical function but plays an important role in the physiology of both normal and injured joints. Irritation or trauma to the synovium may lead to *synovitis*, a condition with inflammatory symptoms that may in turn limit joint function.

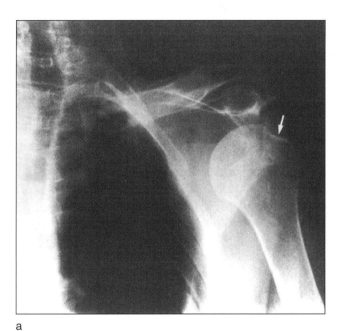

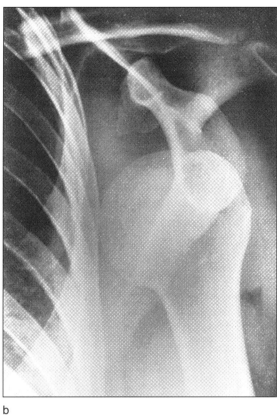

a   b

Figure 5.6   X ray of (*a*) partial dislocation (*subluxation*) and (*b*) complete dislocation (*luxation*).
Part (a) from Julin & Mathews 1990. Part (*b*) from Gusmer & Potter 1995.

Arthritis refers to inflammation of a joint or a state characterized by joint inflammation. It comprises many conditions that have either primary or secondary inflammatory involvement. Among the major types are those resulting from chronic and excessive mechanical loading (e.g., osteoarthritis), systemic disease (e.g., rheumatoid arthritis), or biochemical imbalances (e.g., gouty arthritis). Arthritis may be a primary condition or may develop secondarily in response to a noninflammatory insult, as is the case in osteoarthritis. In any case, arthritis and its sequelae have the potential to inflict debilitating pain and loss of function to joints of the musculoskeletal system.

Concluding Comments

We have briefly described general concepts of injury mechanics, basic terminology, and fundamental mechanisms of musculoskeletal injury, setting the stage for discussions in the next three chapters of specific injuries and their causal mechanisms. The tenets and principles of mechanical load and overload, use and overuse, level and progression of injury, and the many contributory factors involved in injury combine to form a complex and fascinating backdrop for viewing specific musculoskeletal injuries. Since it would be impossible to examine all injuries, the injuries discussed in succeeding chapters were selected because of their epidemiological pervasiveness and their value in illustrating the principles of injury biomechanics.

Suggested Readings

Adams, J.C., & Hamblen, D.L. (1992). *Outline of Fractures* (10th ed.). Edinburgh: Churchill Livingstone.

Albright, J.A., & Brand, R.A. (1987). *The Scientific Basis of Orthopaedics* (2nd ed.). Norwalk, CT: Appleton & Lange.

Curwin, S., & Stanish, W.D. (1984). *Tendinitis: Its Etiology and Treatment*. Lexington, MA: Collamore Press.

Finerman, G.A.M., & Noyes, F.R. (Eds.). (1992). *Biology and Biomechanics of the Traumatized Synovial Joint: The Knee as a Model.* Rosemont, IL: American Academy of Orthopaedic Surgeons.

Fu, F.H., & Stone, D.A. (1994). *Sports Injuries: Mechanisms, Prevention, Treatment.* Baltimore: Williams & Wilkins.

Garrett, W.E., Jr., & Duncan, P.W. (1988). *Muscle Injury and Rehabilitation.* Baltimore: Williams & Wilkins.

Rockwood, C.A., Green, D.P., Bucholz, R.W., & Heckman, J.D. (Eds.). (1996). *Rockwood and Green's Fractures in Adults.* Philadelphia: Lippincott-Raven.

Tencer, A.F., & Johnson, K.D. (1994). *Biomechanics in Orthopedic Trauma: Bone Fracture and Fixation.* Philadelphia: Lippincott.

Tidball, J.G. (1991). Myotendinous junction injury in relation to junction structure and molecular composition. In: Holloszy, J.O. (Ed.), *Exercise and Sport Sciences Reviews* (pp. 419-445). Baltimore: Williams & Wilkins.

Woo, S. L.-Y., & Buckwalter, J.A. (1988). *Injury and Repair of the Musculoskeletal Soft Tissues.* Park Ridge, IL: American Academy of Orthopaedic Surgeons.

Zachazewski, J.E., Magee, D.J., & Quillen, W.S. (Eds.). (1996). *Athletic Injuries and Rehabilitation.* Philadelphia: Saunders.

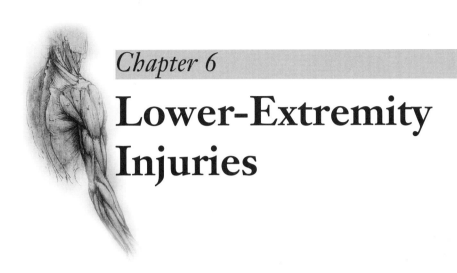

Chapter 6

Lower-Extremity Injuries

Fractured, hell! The damn thing's broken!

Dizzy Dean, Hall of Fame baseball pitcher, commenting on his injured toe

---

Injuries to lower-extremity joints, in particular the knee and ankle, are among the most common of all musculoskeletal disorders. Given the importance of the lower extremities in everyday activities such as walking, running, and postural maintenance, injury to these joints assumes a practical urgency. The circumstances of lower-extremity injury can vary, ranging from the acute, high-energy trauma of a sprained ankle to the more gradual onset of a metatarsal stress fracture. The lower-extremity injuries presented in this chapter were selected based on their prevalence and their value in illustrating specific injury mechanisms. Representative injuries are presented for the major lower-extremity joints (hip, knee, ankle) and the regions spanning these joints (thigh, lower leg, foot).

Hip Injuries

The hip joint is formed by articulation of the femur with the pelvic girdle (coxal bone), specifically by the articulating surfaces of the femoral head and the acetabulum (figure 6.1). The bony fit is improved by the acetabular labrum, a fibrocartilage pad attached to the bony rim of the acetabulum. The hip joint is reinforced anteriorly by the iliofemoral ligament, posteriorly by the ischiofemoral ligament, and anteroinferiorly by the pubofemoral ligament. The ligament of the head of the femur provides limited structural support, serving primarily to contain the vasculature supplying the femoral head. Additional support is provided by the articular joint capsule, whose fibers form a fibrous collar around the femoral neck and help secure the femoral head in the acetabulum.

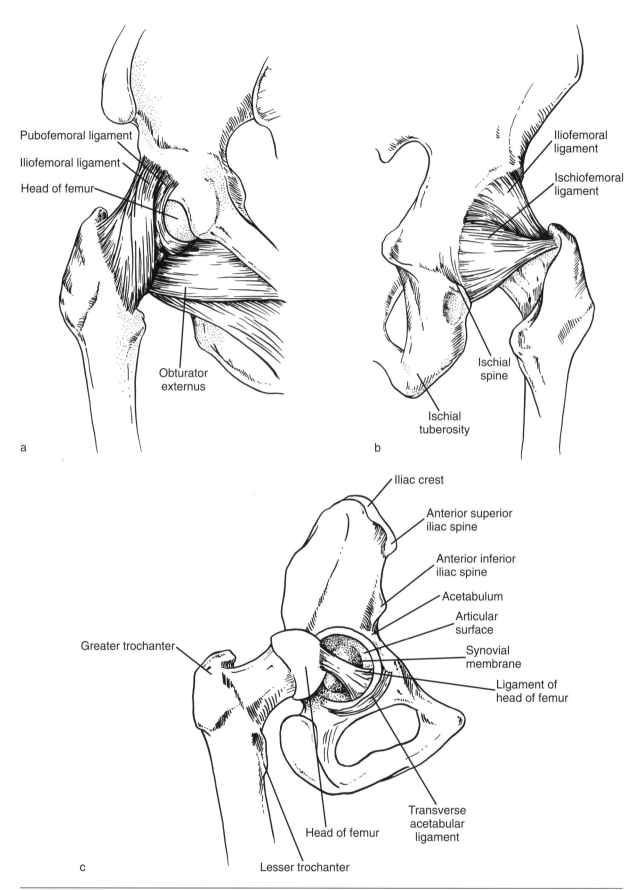

Figure 6.1　Ligaments of the hip joint: (*a*) anterior view, (*b*) posterior view, and (*c*) lateral view.

Table 6.1   Muscles of the Hip

Muscle	Action

Adductor group
    Adductor brevis
    Adductor longus
    Adductor magnus
	Adducts and laterally rotates the thigh

Biceps femoris (long head)	Extends the thigh
Gluteus maximus	Extends and laterally rotates the thigh
Gluteus medius	Abducts and medially rotates the thigh
Gluteus minimus	Abducts and medially rotates the thigh
Gracilis	Adducts the thigh
Iliopsoas (psoas major & iliacus)	Flexes the thigh; flexes the trunk when femur is fixed
Pectineus	Adducts, flexes, and laterally rotates the thigh
Piriformis	Laterally rotates the thigh; assists in extending and abducting the thigh
Rectus femoris	Flexes the thigh
Sartorius	Flexes the thigh
Semimembranosus	Extends the thigh
Semitendinosus	Extends the thigh
Tensor fasciae latae	Assists in flexion, abduction, and medial rotation of the thigh

The hip joint's ball-and-socket configuration permits movements in the three primary planes defined as flexion/extension (sagittal plane), abduction/adduction (frontal plane), and internal/external rotation (transverse plane). The muscles responsible for controlling movements about the hip joint are shown in figures 6.2 and 6.6; their actions are summarized in table 6.1. This considerable musculature further stabilizes the hip joint.

Hip Fracture

Bone fractures in the hip region typically result from high-energy forces such as those in falls from heights and automobile crashes. Pelvic fractures, while not as prevalent as femoral fractures, nonetheless present a significant problem. For example, it is estimated that in a single year, 15,300 pelvic fractures occurred in motor vehicle crashes (Moffatt, Mitter, & Martinez 1990). In motor vehicle accidents the direction of force largely determines the pattern of injury. Pelvic fractures resulting from severe motor vehicle accidents are significantly more frequent in side-impact collisions, occur at much lower speeds in side impacts than in frontal collisions, and have high mortality rates from associated injuries (Gokcen et al. 1994).

Proximal femoral (hip) fractures are a major health concern, with an estimated 250,000 fractures occurring each year in the United States (Praemer, Furner, & Rice 1992). While relatively rare in younger individuals, the likelihood of fracture increases markedly with advancing age. Hip fractures are common in older populations, with a prevalence of 4.5 per 100 people 70 years and older; women are three times more likely to suffer a fractured hip than men (Cummings et al. 1985).

Hip fractures in the young usually result from high-energy impacts, most commonly a result of motor vehicle accidents. These injuries are often associated with hip luxation. Two potential mechanisms for femoral neck fracture are direct impact to the greater trochanter, as might be seen in a fall, and a lateral rotation of the leg while the body falls backwards (figure 6.3). On rare occasions, young people experience a stress fracture of the proximal femur as a result of repeated loading during strenuous activity.

Hip fractures in the elderly are associated with falls, often caused by tripping or unsteady gait (table 6.2). This association raises an intriguing "chicken and egg" question: Does hip fracture cause the fall, or does the impact of landing from a fall cause the bone to break? In most cases, it seems that the force

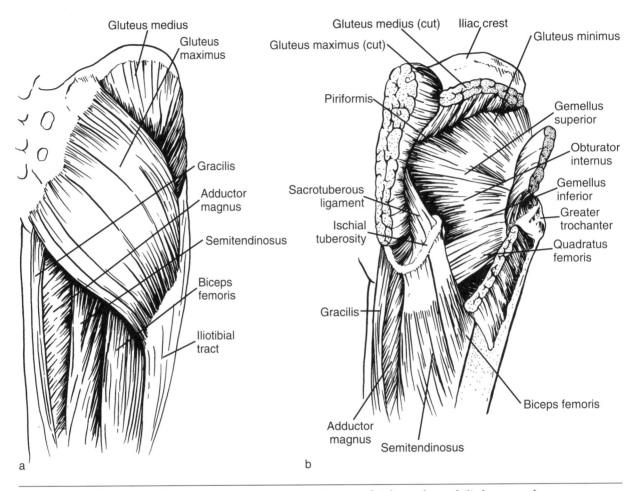

Figure 6.2 Musculature of the hip joint (posterior view): (*a*) superficial muscles and (*b*) deep muscles.

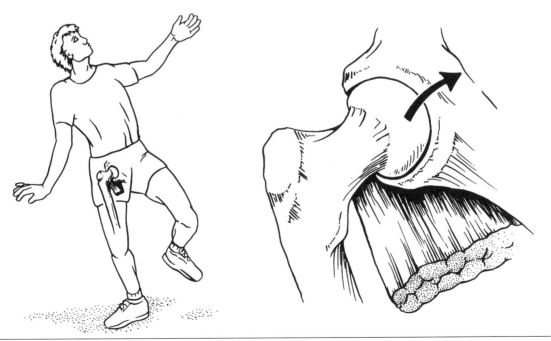

Figure 6.3 Mechanism of femoral neck fracture in which the subject falls backward with the right foot planted on the ground. The iliofemoral ligament secures the neck while the stiffened iliopsoas tendon provides a solid structure against which the femoral neck fractures.

Table 6.2   Predisposing Factors to Falls by Older People

Host factors	Environmental factors
Neurological disorders (e.g., seizures)	Home factors (e.g., wires, loose rugs, poor lighting, unstable furniture)
Cerebrovascular disorders (e.g., CVA)	
Cardiovascular disorders (e.g., cardiac arrhythmias)	Slippery or uneven walking surfaces
Cumulative effect of chronic illness and aging on gait; balance, sensory perception, muscle strength, coordination, reflexes	Stairs
	Other obstacles to routine daily activities
Previous history of falls	
Dizziness	
Postural hypotension	
Syncope	
Senile dementia	
Other cognitive disorders	
Drugs and alcohol	

Summarizes discussion in "Epidemiology of osteoporosis and osteoporotic fractures" by S.R. Cummings, J.L. Kelsey, M.C. Nevitt, & K.J. O'Dowd, 1985, *Epidemiologic Reviews, 7* (p. 178-208). Baltimore: John Hopkins University Press. Copyright 1985 by permission of Johns Hopkins University Press.

of impact precipitates the fracture, with only rare instances of a spontaneous fracture causing a fall. The energy created by a fall is much greater than that necessary to fracture a bone. Since hip fractures occur in fewer than 5% of falls, other tissues obviously are absorbing considerable energy. This observation is substantiated by the fact that risk of hip fracture is lower in people with an increased body mass index (weight/height^2). A recent study concluded that while the thicker trochanteric soft tissues in obese individuals do cushion the fall, this force attenuation is insufficient by itself to prevent hip fracture. Additional absorptive mechanisms (e.g., breaking the fall with outstretched arm or eccentric action of the quadriceps during descent) are probably involved in falls without fracture (Robinovitch, McMahon, & Hayes 1995).

Current research suggests that even though osteoporotic bone exhibits diminished strength and certainly increases the likelihood of fracture, the dynamics of the fall may be the dominant component in the incidence of fracture. Dynamic models of sideways falls predict peak trochanteric impact forces ranging from 2.90 to 9.99 kN. These forces are more than sufficient to cause fracture (van den Kroonenberg, Hayes, & McMahon 1995). Further research is needed to define the exact location, direction, and magnitude of forces experienced during actual falls. Osteoporosis appears to be but one piece in the hip fracture puzzle and must be considered in conjunction with bone quality, muscular strength, soft tissue character-

istics, and neuromuscular coordination in a comprehensive understanding of hip fractures.

Hip Luxation

Hip luxation (dislocation) occurs rarely, due in large part to the joint's strong ligamentous support and its substantial surrounding muscle mass. In most cases, hip luxation requires tremendous forces, so it should come as no surprise that motor vehicle accidents, falls from heights, and skiing accidents are among the most common causes. While isolated luxations have been documented, the large forces involved often produce accompanying fracture of the acetabulum, proximal femur, or both.

Force application causing hip dislocation can arise in several ways. Force may be applied to the greater trochanter, flexed knee, foot with ipsilateral knee extended, and, rarely, to the posterior pelvis (Levin & Browner 1991). Depending on their location and direction, the applied forces tend to translate and rotate the femur. In most cases these forces cause posterior dislocation of the femur relative to the acetabulum.

Automobile crashes have long been the leading cause of hip luxation. Six decades ago, Funsten and co-workers coined the term "dashboard dislocation" in describing 20 cases of traumatic dislocation (Funsten, Kinser, & Frankel 1938). The mechanism of injury, with few exceptions, is a violent collision of the occupant's knee against the dashboard (figure

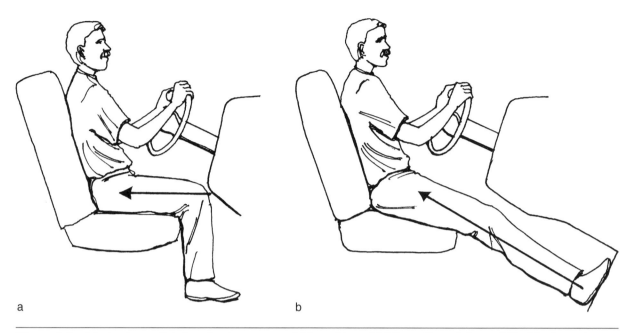

a   b

Figure 6.4   Mechanisms of hip luxation in a motor vehicle accident. (*a*) Hip and knee joints at 90° of flexion at impact with dashboard. (*b*) Knee fully extended to brace for axially directed impact force that drives femoral head out of the acetabulum posteriorly.

6.4), resulting in posterior hip dislocation and often accompanied by acetabular or, less commonly, femoral fracture. Not surprisingly, the victims of vehicle-related hip luxation invariably are not wearing seat belts.

Anterior hip luxations occur infrequently (10%-20% of all hip dislocations) and usually result in anteroinferior dislocation. Forcible abduction, the primary factor in anterior dislocation, presses the femoral neck or trochanter against the rim of the acetabulum and leverages the head of the femur out of its socket. Abduction combined with simultaneous hip flexion and external rotation result in obturator-type anterior dislocation. When combined with extension, abduction causes pubic- or iliac-type luxation.

Interestingly, there appears to be a relation between femoral structure and the likelihood of hip dislocation. It has been noted that patients suffering dislocations have significantly less anteversion than a control group. Thus, it seems that patients exhibiting relative retroversion may be predisposed to hip dislocations (Upadhyay, Moulton, & Burwell 1985). Given the anatomic stability of the normal hip and the rare occurrence of hip dislocation, these observations suggest that people who experience recurrent hip dislocations have a structural abnormality (Levin & Browner 1991).

While most hip luxations result from trauma, there is a class of injury occurring in young infants,

known as congenital dislocation, in which the hip spontaneously dislocates. These occurrences depend on joint position: Hamstrings acting on a flexed hip and extended knee are associated with posterior dislocation, and iliopsoas acting on an extended hip is associated with anterior dislocation.

Osteoarthritis

Osteoarthritis (OA), also referred to as osteoarthrosis and degenerative joint disease (DJD), is the most common joint disorder. Strictly speaking, OA is not an arthritis, since it does not initially manifest as an inflammatory condition. Inflammation may be secondary to the underlying tissue degeneration. Technically, DJD may be a more appropriate designation. However, because the condition is almost universally labeled OA, we will use that term in our discussion.

OA is a progressive condition, initially characterized by softening of articular cartilage due to a decrease in matrix proteoglycan content. Subsequently, the cartilage thins, and its surface becomes rougher with characteristic pitting, fissuring, and ulceration. The cartilage damage results in enzyme release that results in further breakdown. Advanced cartilage degeneration is accompanied by subchondral bone necrosis and osteophyte formation at the joint margin. Normal and OA-damaged cartilage are shown in figure 6.5. The severity of OA is

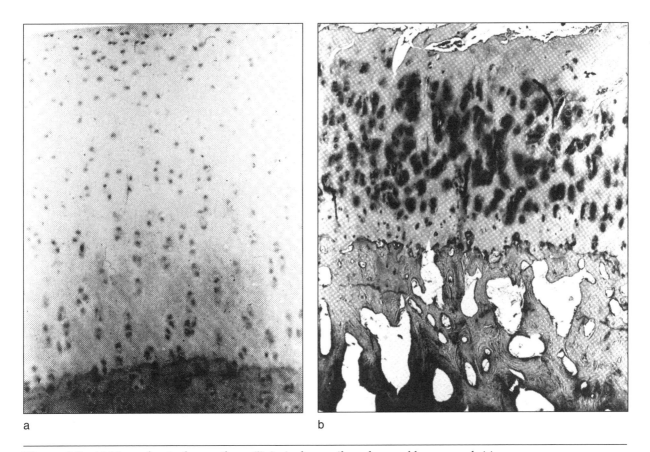

a   b

Figure 6.5 (*a*) Normal articular cartilage. (*b*) Articular cartilage damaged by osteoarthritis.

Part (*a*) from "Biphasic and quasilinear viscoelastic theories for hydrated soft tissues" (Fig. 3A, p. 219) by V.C. Mow, J.S. Hou, J.M. Owens, & A. Ratcliffe, 1990. In: *Biomechanics of Diarthroid Joints,1*, New York: Springer-Verlag. Copyright 1990 by Springer-Verlag. Reprinted by permission.

Part (*b*) from "Articular cartilage" (Fig. 14, p. 330) by C.C. Edwards & O.D. Chrisman, 1979. In: *The Scientific Basis of Orthopaedics*, New York: Appleton-Century-Crofts. Copyright 1979 Appleton-Century-Crofts. Reprinted by permission.

typically graded according to the degree of joint space narrowing, osteophyte formation, sclerosis, and joint deformity.

OA is strongly associated with advancing age. Radiological evidence of OA is rare in persons under age 25, but by age 75 almost all persons exhibit evidence of OA in their hands and about half of these people show some degree of OA in the feet (Lawrence et al. 1989). The onset of OA at specific joints varies, occurring earliest at the metatarsophalangeal joints, next at the wrist and spine, later in the interphalangeals and first carpometacarpal, next in the tibiofemoral, and last in the hip. The reasons for this sequential appearance are unclear, but anatomic ultrastructural, biophysical, and biomechanical changes are likely involved. The development of OA in body joints is determined by an individual's predisposition to OA, abnormalities in the joint, and patterns of mechanical loading and use. The precise relation between these biological and mechanical factors largely remains a mys-

tery; identification of the specific mechanisms remains a challenge.

OA has been etiologically described as being either (1) primary, or idiopathic (i.e., of unknown origin), or (2) secondary, resulting from identifiable conditions such as trauma, metabolic disorders (e.g., calcium pyrophosphate dihydrate deposition disease [CPDD] and diffuse idiopathic skeletal hyperostosis [DISH]), existing inflammatory conditions, or crystalline diseases.

The causes of primary OA remain elusive. Postulated mechanisms include biomechanical, biochemical, inflammatory, and immunological factors. Classifying OA at the hip as "idiopathic" may be an overstatement. In summarizing the evidence from a number of studies, Harris (1986) concluded that in the large majority of cases reported as primary OA of the hip, mild and unrecognized developmental abnormalities (e.g., acetabular dysplasia, pistol-grip deformity) were the likely causal factors. Thus, a large proportion of OA is misclassified as primary OA.

Consensus allows that in cases of OA with known etiology, mechanical overuse plays a prominent role. This overuse can be acute (e.g., traumatic injury) or chronic (e.g., repeated heavy lifting). The mechanism of injury in chronic conditions often is occupationally related. For example, the incidence of OA among farmers has been linked to heavy lifting, walking on rough ground, and prolonged tractor driving. As expected, occupation-related OA has also been reported in the knees and spines of coal miners and the hands of cotton mill workers.

Somewhat surprisingly, obesity is not strongly associated with the onset of OA at the hip, but rather may be more involved in the progression of already established OA (Croft et al. 1992). This contrasts with the knee joint, where obesity, along with repeated use and previous injury, are strong risk factors for the occurrence of OA (Felson et al. 1988).

Thigh Injuries

The thigh region spans the hip and knee joints and consists of the longitudinally aligned femur surrounded by three muscular compartments (anterior, medial, posterior), which are defined by their location and muscular actions (figure 6.6). The anterior compartment includes the iliopsoas (psoas major and iliacus), tensor fasciae latae, pectineus, sartorius, and quadriceps group (vastus lateralis, vastus medialis, vastus intermedius, rectus femoris). Included in the medial compartment are the three adductor muscles (a. longus, a. brevis, a. magnus) and the gracilis. The posterior compartment contains three muscles (semitendinosus, semimembranosus, biceps femoris) collectively termed the hamstrings.

Quadriceps Contusion

Contusions are among the most common injuries, especially in contact sports such as soccer, football,

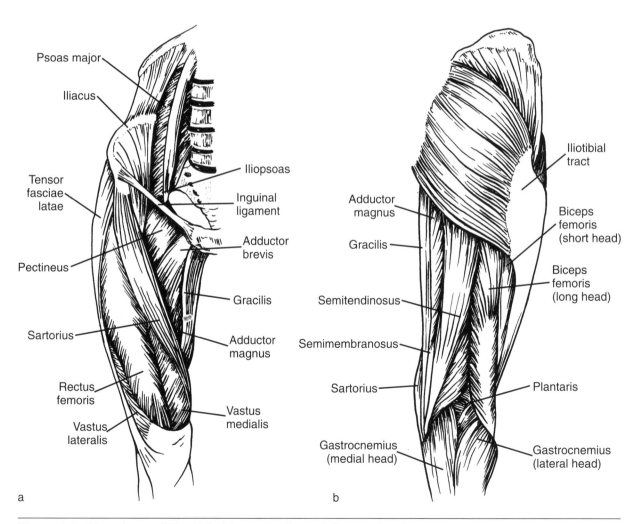

Figure 6.6 Musculature of the thigh: (*a*) anterior view and (*b*) posterior view.

and rugby. The anterolateral aspect of the thigh is frequently involved with resultant injury to the quadriceps muscle group. Compression from a nonpenetrating blunt force trauma is the predominant injury mechanism, most commonly in the form of an impactor's knee, helmet, or shoulder. The resulting capillary rupture, edema, inflammation, infiltrative bleeding, and muscle crush leads to pain, swelling, and decreased knee range of motion.

Despite extensive description of the symptoms, treatment, and sequelae of quadriceps contusion, little is known about the underlying pathophysiological mechanisms of tissue injury. One recent study examined selected biomechanical, physiological, and histological aspects of contusion injuries using a reproducible, single-impact model on the gastrocnemius muscle complex of anesthetized rats. In spite of some limitations and the speculative nature of extrapolating the results of animal studies to human clinical observations, the results prove enlightening. Gross observation of the muscle surface within 2 h after injury showed muscle disruption at the center of the impact site with extensive surrounding intramuscular-interstitial hematoma, but no damage at either the proximal or distal myotendinous junction. An observed increase of 11% in muscle weight was attributed to hemorrhage and edema. Acute injury also resulted in a 38% decrease in maximum tetanic tension compared to uninjured contralateral controls.

The course of acute injury, degeneration, regeneration, and normalization also were examined microscopically. At day 0, injury to the gastrocnemius was localized near the site of impact and extended deep into the muscle complex. Intracellular vacuolation of intact myofibers was present, along with gross disruption of myofibers. Two days postinjury, the muscle exhibited a marked inflammatory response, with evidence of macrophage, polymorphonucleocytes, and degenerating contractile proteins. By day 7, extensive cellular proliferation of myoblasts and fibroblasts was evident. Within 24 days the injured specimens were essentially indistinguishable from control muscles (Crisco et al. 1994).

This study also provides the following instructive observations with respect to impact mechanics and tissue responses: (1) Impact pressures on the skin produce stress to the underlying muscle tissue. When these stresses exceed some critical value, damage results. It is hypothesized that this is the mechanism of contusion injury. (2) Mass and velocity [see eq. (3.19)] of the impacting object alone are not sufficient to describe the event; the size and shape of the impacting object needs to be considered as well. (3) Assuming that passive failure (i.e., inactive muscle loaded to failure) is indicative of tissue strength, contusion injuries may be more susceptible to subsequent strain injuries at the site of injury.

Myositis Ossificans

Severe acute or repeated trauma to an injured muscle may lead to myositis ossificans, a condition characterized by calcified mass formation within the muscle, typically several weeks after the injury. One study found calcification in 17% of patients with quadriceps contusion (Rothwell 1982). This pathogenic bone may form contiguously with normal bone (periosteal) or free of any connection with bone (heterotopic) within the muscle belly. The precise mechanism of myositis ossificans remains unknown, but it has been theorized that the condition results from ossification of proliferating fascial connective tissue (Hait, Boswick, & Stone 1970).

Femoral Fracture

While femoral neck fractures present one of the most urgent health concerns of older people, fracture to other regions of the femur account for more than 58,000 hospital admissions annually (Praemer, Furner, & Rice 1992). Most fractures of the femoral diaphysis (shaft) result from high-energy trauma and can thus be both life threatening and a source of severe disability. One study of 520 femoral fractures reported that nearly 78% resulted from automobile, motorcycle, or automobile-pedestrian accidents (Winquist, Hansen, & Clawson 1984).

Fracture patterns typically are classified by the fracture's location, configuration (e.g., spiral, oblique, transverse), and level of comminution. One system for classifying femoral fractures uses the categories of segmental and comminuted (grades I-IV; figure 6.7). Grade I comminuted fractures have a very small piece of bone broken off. Grade II fractures are characterized by a larger fragment than grade I, but with at least 50% contact between adjacent bone surfaces. Grade III comminuted fractures exhibit less than 50% cortical contact that may allow further rotation, translation, and shortening of the fracture. The most severe (grade IV) comminuted fractures have lost contact between the proximal and distal fragments (Winquist & Hansen 1980).

Femoral fractures in adolescents (figure 6.8) require special consideration, especially when the fracture occurs near joints or through the epiphyses. There is a potential for long-term problems

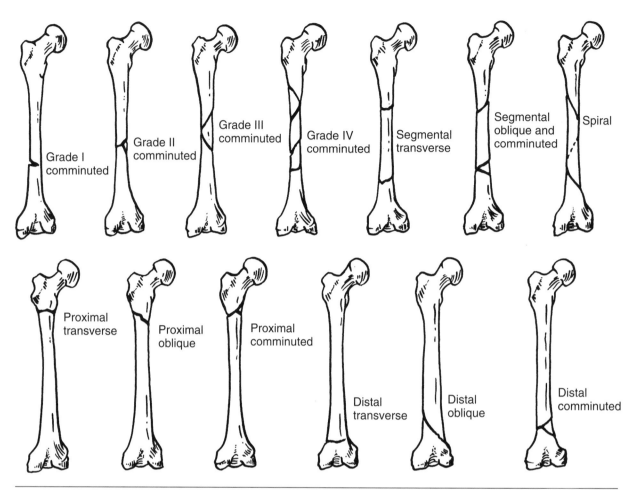

Figure 6.7 Types of femoral fractures. The upper left illustrates grades I to IV comminuted fractures (see text for description). The others show fractures based on location (e.g., proximal, distal) and configuration (e.g., transverse, oblique, spiral; see chapter 5).

associated with abnormal growth and development following injury and the possibility of subsequent osteoarthritis.

Gunshot, or ballistic, wounds provide a unique example of injury mechanisms. Obviously bullets can strike anywhere in the body, but we will restrict our attention here to those that happen to strike the femur. Gunshot fracture patterns depend on numerous factors, including bullet diameter (caliber), velocity, weight, shape, and tumbling characteristics (Brien et al. 1995). Low-velocity bullets ($< 600 \, \text{m·s}^{-1}$), typical of small-caliber handguns, tend to cause splintering of the femoral diaphysis. In one study the vast majority (93%) of low-velocity gunshot–related fractures were classified as grade III or IV (Wiss, Brien, & Becker 1991). In addition to causing severe bone fracture, high-velocity bullets ($> 600 \, \text{m·s}^{-1}$) from rifles and close-range shotgun blasts cause more extensive soft tissue damage and considerable cavitation.

A final example of femoral fracture mechanisms is provided by skiing. Femoral fractures, as in other skiing injuries, depend on skier ability, snow conditions, level of physical conditioning, age, and the mechanism of injury. Sterett and Krissoff (1994) examined 85 cases of femoral fractures in alpine skiing, focusing on the mechanisms of injury as a function of skier age. They reported that in the youngest age group (3-18 years), femoral fracture tended to result from torsional loading of the femoral shaft, usually while skiing fast and catching the ski in wet or heavy snow. In older skiers, such torsional loading would more likely result in soft tissue injury at the knee. Fractures in young adults (18-45 years) occurred mostly from high-energy, direct-impact collisions with an object (e.g., rock or tree) and not surprisingly resulted in high-grade comminuted fractures. In older skiers (> 45 years), the majority of fractures were localized in the hip area (femoral neck and peritrochanteric) and were caused by low-energy impact falls on firm snow. In general, expert skiers are much less likely to sustain injuries than novices. Femoral fracture, however, is one of the few

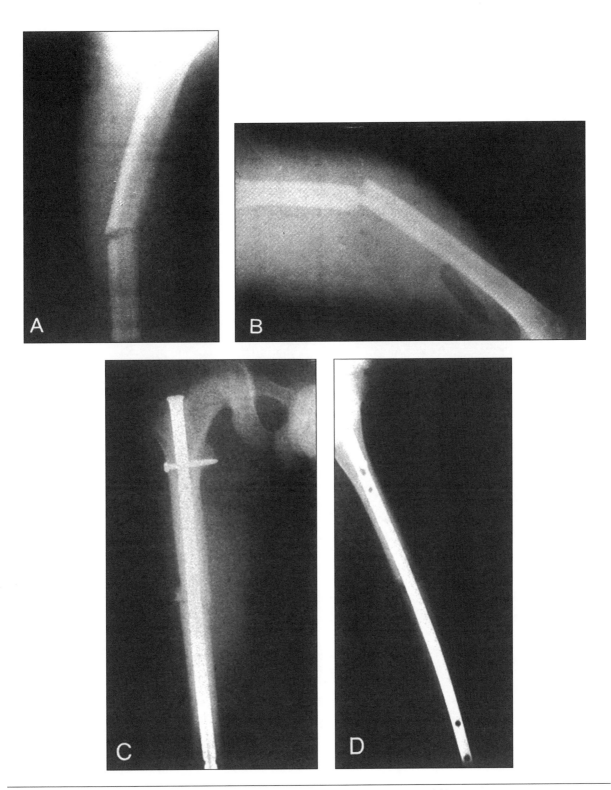

Figure 6.8 Radiographs of a fracture of the right, midshaft femur of a 15-year-old boy. Reprinted from Moreland 1994.

injuries more prevalent in advanced skiers than in beginners. This is due largely to the high energy levels required for femoral fracture. Advanced skiers typically ski at higher speeds and over more difficult terrain than novices. The greater speeds result in higher kinetic energy [see eq. (3.17)], which upon impact (e.g., with a rock or tree) is transferred to the musculoskeletal tissues, including the femur.

Hamstring Strain

Muscle strain (compare with mechanical strain in chapter 3) involves injury to the musculotendinous complex. It is classified as an indirect injury because it results from excessive tension loads and not from direct trauma. Injury typically occurs during forced lengthening or eccentric muscle action employed to control or decelerate high-velocity movements (e.g., sprinting, throwing). The significance of an active muscle to muscle strain has been well documented. For example, it has been observed that force generated at failure was only 15% higher in stimulated rabbit extensor digitorum longus muscles compared to unstimulated ones, while the energy absorbed was approximately 100% higher at failure in the activated muscles (Garrett et al. 1987). This suggests that any compromise in a muscle's contractile capacity (e.g., fatigue) may reduce its ability to absorb energy and increase the risk of injury. Muscle fatigue, along with other predisposing factors (e.g., muscle imbalance, lack of flexibility, insufficient warm-up) are implicated in muscle strain injuries (Worrell 1994).

Certain muscles seem more prone to strain injury than others. The hamstrings, in particular, are especially susceptible to muscle strain. Why is this the case? The muscles of the hamstring group, with the exception of the short head of the biceps femoris, have biarticular function. This structural arrangement dictates that muscle length is determined by the conjoint action of the hip and knee joints. Hip flexion and knee extension each serve to lengthen the semitendinosus, semimembranosus, and biceps femoris (long head). Simultaneous hip flexion and knee extension places the hamstrings in a lengthened state that contributes to the muscles' susceptibility to injury (figure 6.9).

The circumstances of hamstring strain in sprinters illustrate a common injury mechanism. Strain injury usually occurs late in the swing phase or early in the stance phase. During late swing the hamstrings work eccentrically to decelerate both the thigh and lower leg in preparation for ground contact. Early in stance the hamstrings act concentrically to extend the hip. Kinetic analyses have shown that peak torques at the hip and knee occur during these phases. An additional contributing factor may

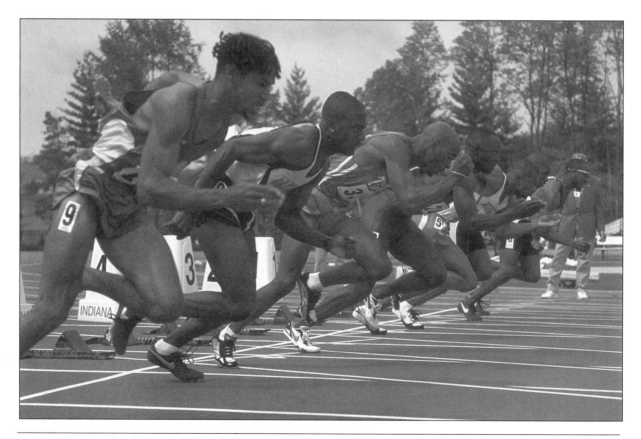

Figure 6.9 Simultaneous hip flexion and knee extension places the hamstring muscle group in an elongated position and increases the risk of strain injury.

be the relatively high proportion of fast-twitch muscle fibers found in hamstring muscles, which allows for higher levels of intrinsic force production. This combination of factors places the hamstrings at elevated risk of injury in high-velocity movements.

Locating the precise injury site often proves difficult. Which of the hamstring muscles, for example, is most likely to sustain injury? Computed tomography (CT) used to localize hamstring muscle strain showed that injuries tended to be proximal and lateral within the hamstring group, most often in the long head of the biceps femoris (Garrett et al. 1989).

Where in the muscle-tendon unit is injury likely to occur? Strain injury occurs most often at the myotendinous junction (MTJ). The MTJ's microscopic structure makes it a likely site for focused mechanical loading. Several factors contribute to

the MTJ's susceptibility to injury. First, the structural folding of the junctional membrane (figure 6.10) increases the surface area (by 10-20 times or more) and thus reduces stress. Second, the folding configuration aligns the membrane so that it experiences primarily shear forces rather than tensile forces. Third, the folding may increase the adhesive strength of the muscle cell to the tendon. Fourth, the sarcomeres near the junction are stiffer than those distant from the junction and thus have limited extensibility (Noonan & Garrett 1992).

In summary, the hamstrings' gross and microscopic anatomical structure, biarticular arrangement, and involvement in controlling high-velocity movement all contribute to making this muscle group at particular risk for muscle strain injury.

Knee Injuries

The knee joint comprises three articulations: those between the medial and lateral condyles of the femur and tibia (*tibiofemoral joint*) and between the patella and the femur (*patellofemoral joint*) (figure 6.11a). While often classified as a hinge joint (which implies uniplanar movement), the knee is more correctly classified as double condyloid, since it has movement potential both in flexion/extension and rotation (when the knee is flexed). The muscles acting about the knee joint are depicted in figures 6.6 and 6.11b and functionally summarized in table 6.3.

As a synovial joint, the knee has a strong fibrous capsule that attaches superiorly to the femur and

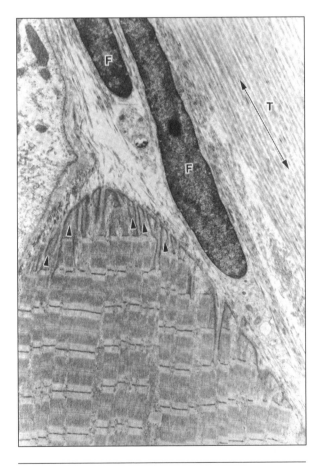

Figure 6.10 Electron micrograph of myotendinous junction. The muscle cell appears to interdigitate with the tendon (arrowheads). The tendon contains fibroblasts (F) and dense collagen fibers (T). (Inset bar = 3.0 µm.)

Reprinted from Tidball 1991.

Table 6.3 Muscles of the Knee

Muscle	Action
Gracilis	Flexes the leg
Sartorius	Flexes the leg

Quadriceps femoris group
  Rectus femoris
  Vastus intermedius
  Vastus lateralis
  Vastus medialis
	Extends the leg

Hamstring group
  Biceps femoris
  Semimembranosus
  Semitendinosus
	Flexes the leg

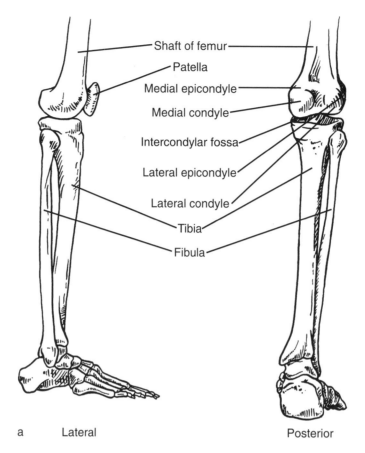

Shaft of femur

Patella

Medial epicondyle

Medial condyle

Intercondylar fossa

Lateral epicondyle

Lateral condyle

Tibia

Fibula

a   Lateral

Posterior

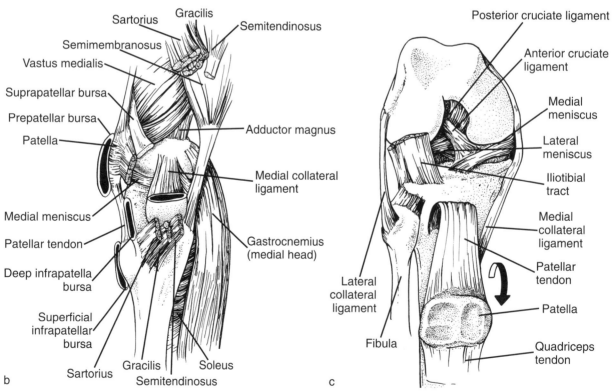

Sartorius

Gracilis

Semimembranosus

Semitendinosus

Vastus medialis

Suprapatellar bursa

Prepatellar bursa

Patella

Adductor magnus

Medial collateral ligament

Medial meniscus

Patellar tendon

Deep infrapatella bursa

Gastrocnemius (medial head)

Superficial infrapatellar bursa

Sartorius

Gracilis

Semitendinosus

Soleus

b

Posterior cruciate ligament

Anterior cruciate ligament

Medial meniscus

Lateral meniscus

Iliotibial tract

Medial collateral ligament

Patellar tendon

Patella

Lateral collateral ligament

Fibula

Quadriceps tendon

c

Figure 6.11   Anatomy of the knee. (*a*) Skeletal structures. (*b*) Muscle structures. (*c*) Knee ligaments (anterior view).

inferiorly to the articular margin of the tibia. Given its relatively poor bony fit, the knee relies on ligaments for much of its structural strength and integrity. Among the most important, and most often injured, are the collateral ligaments and the cruciate ligaments (figure 6.11c). The collateral ligaments span the medial and lateral aspects of the knee and serve to resist valgus and varus loading. Valgus loading at the knee results in an inward curvature of the leg at the knee (i.e., knock-kneed). Varus loading results in an outward curvature of the leg at the knee (i.e., bowlegged). The *lateral (fibular) collateral ligament* (LCL) is extracapsular and extends from the lateral epicondyle of the femur to the lateral surface of the fibular head. The *medial (tibial) collateral ligament* (MCL) spans from the medial femoral epicondyle to the superomedial surface of the tibia. Unlike the LCL, which is extracapsular, the MCL is a capsular ligament that connects directly to the capsule and the medial meniscus. This structural arrangement, as will be seen, has important implications for the MCL's susceptibility to injury. Reference to the MCL as a singular ligament understates its anatomical complexity. It is usually described as having superficial and deep components that act synergistically to restrict knee joint movements.

The two cruciate ligaments, named for their oblique, or X-shaped orientation to one another, extend between the femur and tibia. The weaker of the two, the anterior cruciate ligament (ACL) attaches proximally on the posteromedial aspect of the lateral condyle of the femur and distally on the anterior portion of the intercondylar surface of the tibia. The ACL is composed of two major bundles, the anteromedial bundle, which is tight in flexion and relatively lax in extension, and the posterolateral bundle, which is tight in extension and lax in flexion. The likelihood of injury to a bundle obviously depends on the degree of knee flexion at the time of injury. The ACL's primary function is to restrict anterior movement of the tibia relative to the femur (or conversely to limit posterior movement of the femur relative to the tibia) and secondarily to provide resistance to valgus, varus, and tibial rotation.

The stronger posterior cruciate ligament (PCL) attaches proximally on the anteromedial aspect of the medial condyle of the femur, passes medial to the ACL, and secures distally to the posterior portion of the intercondylar area of the tibia. The PCL also consists of two bundles. The larger anterolateral bundle tightens in flexion and is relatively lax in extension. The smaller posteromedial bundle is tightest in extension and relatively lax in flexion. The PCL serves to limit posterior movement of the tibia relative to the femur (or conversely to restrict

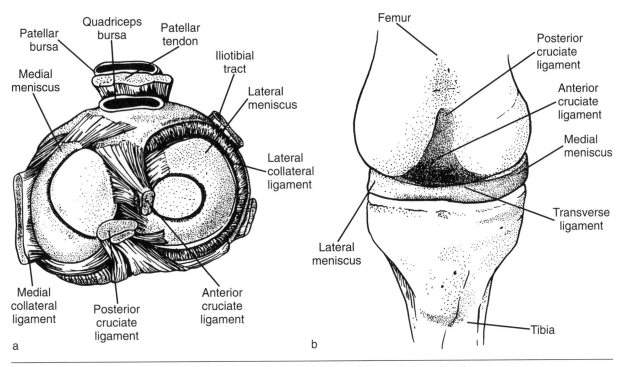

Figure 6.12 Menisci of the knee. (*a*) Superior view of the tibial plateau. (*b*) Anterior view.

anterior movement of the femur relative to the tibia). In addition, the PCL limits hyperflexion of the knee and assists in stabilizing the femur in situations of weight bearing on a flexed knee.

In addition to its capsular and ligamentous support, the knee contains two *menisci*. Each meniscus is a wedge-shaped fibrocartilage pad with peripheral attachment to the joint capsule. They project centrally and are freely moving in non-weight-bearing flexion. Both menisci have a characteristic crescent shape (figure 6.12).

The medial meniscus has a larger radius of curvature than the lateral meniscus and a semilunar shape. It averages about 10 mm in width in the posterior horn and is narrower in the middle and anterior zones. Several structural characteristics of the medial meniscus increase its risk of injury. These include its tight connection with the joint capsule and MCL and its frequent connection with the ACL.

The lateral meniscus exhibits a tighter curvature and forms a nearly closed curve. Its posterior horn is wider than the corresponding region of the medial meniscus. The lateral meniscus attaches posteriorly to the femoral intercondylar fossa and has only loose attachment to the joint capsule and no direct connection with the LCL. The nature of these attachments allows more mobility for the lateral meniscus than for the medial meniscus in both unloaded (figure 6.13) and loaded conditions.

The *patella*, located between the quadriceps tendon and its attachment on the tibial tuberosity, increases the mechanical advantage of the knee

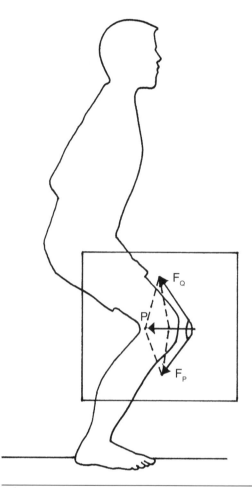

Figure 6.14   Patellofemoral joint reaction force (*P*). Vector *P* is formed by the vector sum of the force vector of the quadriceps tendon (F_Q) and the force vector of the patellar tendon (F_p).

extensor mechanism. The articulation of the patella with the femur forms the patellofemoral joint (PFJ). The PFJ experiences large loads when the knee is in a flexed position (figure 6.14) and thus is predisposed to certain injuries.

Cruciate Ligament Sprain

Considerable literature on cruciate ligament injury has accumulated since the first description of ACL rupture in the mid-19th century and initial attempts at surgical reconstruction early in the 20th century. Growing participation in exercise and sports in recent years has presaged an increased incidence of cruciate injuries. ACL injury is much more common than PCL injury. ACL injury occurs most often in response to valgus loading in combination with external tibial rotation or to hyperextension with internal tibial rotation. The first mechanism

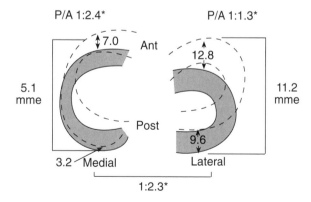

Figure 6.13   Diagram of mean meniscal excursion (mme) along the tibial plateau. Ant, anterior; Post, posterior; mme, mean meniscal excursion (millimeters); P/A, ratio of posterior to anterior meniscal translation during flexion. * $p < .05$ by Student's *t* test analysis.

Adapted from Thompson et al. 1991.

typically occurs when attempting a rapid cutting maneuver with the foot in contact with the ground and the knee flexed. The situation is exacerbated if, while the foot is in contact with the ground, a force is applied to the knee. This is common in contact sports such as football and rugby when another player contacts the lateral aspect of the knee, accentuating the valgus loading and rotation. The knee valgus, combined with external tibial rotation, severely stresses the ACL.

The second mechanism involves knee hyperextension with internal tibial rotation. While a less-common mechanism overall, hyperextension may be the predominant mechanism in certain populations such as basketball players or gymnasts, whose injuries often occur as they land following a jump (figure 6.15).

One recent approach to determine mechanisms of ACL injury uses magnetic resonance imaging (MRI) to assess the bone lesions associated with these injuries. Valgus loading, as previously described, results in compressive forces between the lateral femoral condyle and the lateral tibial plateau. Speer and co-workers (1992) have identified an injury pattern they term the "MRI triad" (ACL rupture, terminal sulcus osseous lesion, and bone or soft tissue injury [or both] at the posterolateral corner) and proposed several mechanisms consistent with this pattern of lesions. These mechanisms include valgus with subsequent lateral joint compression and hyperextension. The authors are prudent in their conclusions by making a statement that holds true for many injuries: "The great difficulty in resolving the injury into a single mechanism may be that the issue is not resolvable; that is, both mechanisms may come into play depending on the nature of applied extrinsic and intrinsic forces" (Speer et al. 1992, 387).

A similar approach has been taken to investigate the hypothesis that for downhill skiers, different mechanisms may be involved in ACL injury. Bone bruise patterns suggest there is less valgus loading in skiers, as evidenced by greater variety of presentation of injury across the posterior tibial rim (Speer et al. 1995). These data are consistent with observations that ACL injury in skiers is often associated with a backward fall (figure 6.16a). In a fall, the skis and boots accelerate forward relative to the body, and because of modern boot design, take the tibia along. This creates an "anterior drawer" mechanism that is consistent with ACL failure in what is termed a boot-induced ACL injury.

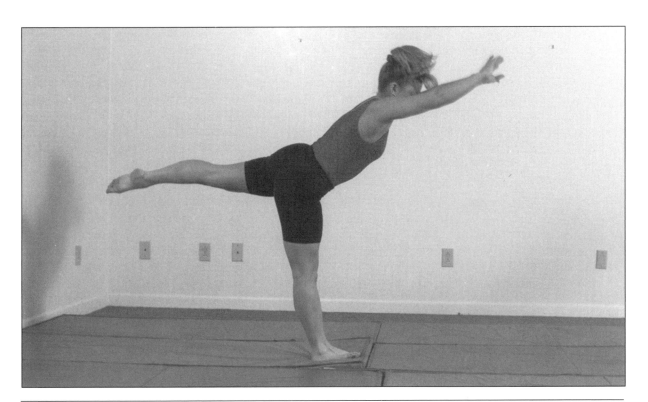

Figure 6.15 Mechanism of anterior cruciate ligament injury. Hyperextension of the right knee joint when landing a gymnastics skill.

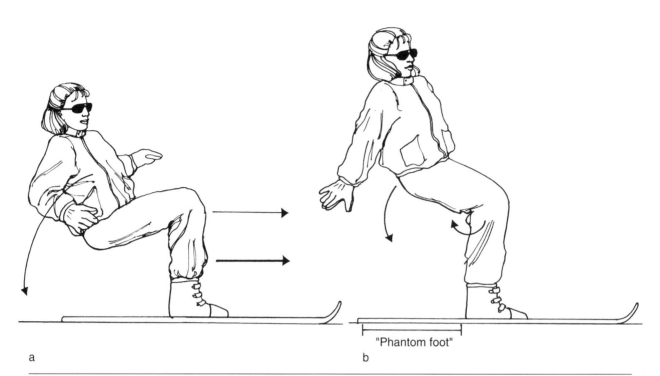

a   b

Figure 6.16 (*a*) Anterior cruciate ligament (ACL) injury caused by a backward fall. This mechanism forcibly pushes the tibia anteriorly relative to the femur and stresses the ACL. (*b*) Anterior cruciate ligament injury caused by the "phantom foot" provided by the section of ski posterior to the boot.

A second mechanism of ACL injury unique to skiing has been described as the "phantom foot," referring to the lever formed by the rear section of the ski that effectively forms another "foot" in the posterior direction. In a backward fall, this phantom foot levers the flexed knee into internal rotation and amplifies stress in the ACL (figure 6.16b).

Numerous studies have noted an alarming increase in the incidence of ACL injuries in female athletes. These injuries are disproportionate to those seen in men. Female intercollegiate soccer players, for example, are 2.6 times more likely to sustain ACL lesions than their male counterparts in the same sport. In basketball the difference jumps to 5.75 times. The reasons for these differences in ACL injury rates are unclear. Among the suggested predisposing factors are a woman's wider pelvis, greater flexibility, less-developed musculature, hypoplastic vastus medialis obliquus, narrow femoral notch, genu valgum, and external tibial torsion. Body movement in sport, muscular strength and coordination, shoe-surface characteristics, level of conditioning, joint laxity, limb alignment, and ligament size must also be taken into account (Arendt & Dick 1995; Ireland 1994). The exact combination of factors responsible for the gender discrepancies in ACL injury remains

elusive and is the subject of intensive clinical debate.

The posterior cruciate ligament (PCL) was once thought to be rarely injured. Improved diagnostic techniques have allowed better identification of PCL injury, but its prevalence is still much lower than that of ACL injury. The causes of PCL injury vary but about half of the cases are due to trauma resulting from vehicular crashes. Most of the remaining cases are caused during sporting activities. There are many mechanisms of PCL failure. Some are quite common; others are relatively rare. Five of these mechanisms are illustrated in figure 6.17. (1) Most commonly, PCL injury occurs in vehicular crashes when an unrestrained occupant is thrown into the dashboard. With the knee flexed 90°, the PCL is taut, and the posterior capsule is lax. The impact force drives the tibia posteriorly and causes PCL rupture. (2) In a fall onto a flexed knee with plantar-flexed foot, the impact occurs on the tibial tuberosity. The proximal femur is again driven posteriorly. (3) Forced knee flexion with the foot either plantar-flexed or dorsiflexed can result in PCL injury. (4) Sudden and violent hyperextension of the knee can cause PCL rupture, and it is not unusual for this mechanism to have accompanying ACL damage. (5) Rapidly shift-

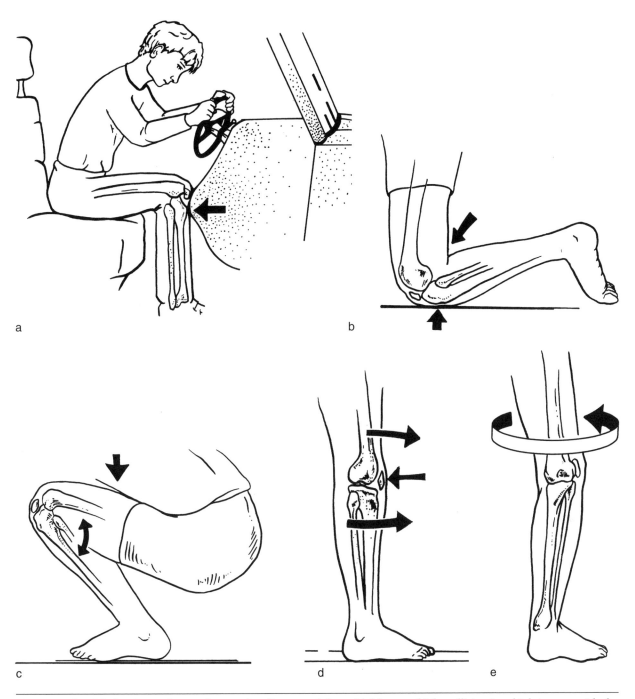

Figure 6.17 Mechanisms of posterior cruciate ligament injury. (*a*) Motor vehicle collision in which impact with the dashboard forces the tibia posteriorly relative to the femur. (*b*) Fall on a flexed knee pushing tibia posteriorly. (*c*) Forced knee flexion. (*d*) Forced knee hyperextension. (*e*) Cutting (changing direction) on a minimally flexed knee.

ing weight from one foot to another, rotating the body quickly on a minimally flexed knee, causes internal rotation and anterior translation of the femur and resulting PCL damage (Andrews, Edwards, & Satterwhite 1994).

Injury to either cruciate ligament may be an isolated injury or may occur in concert with damage to other structures. An example combination injury is one known variously as O'Donoghue's triad (or triangle), or the "unhappy" triad, in which the ACL, medial collateral ligament (MCL), and medial meniscus sustain damage. This injury typically involves the valgus–external rotation mechanism described earlier.

Meniscus Injury

The menisci once were believed to be useless remnants of intraarticular attachments. We now know that they serve an essential role in maintaining normal knee function. Physiologically, compression of the menisci facilitates the distribution of nutrients to adjacent structures. Of greater interest to us in our discussion of injury mechanisms are the mechanical functions of the menisci, specifically weight bearing, shock absorption, stabilization, and rotational facilitation.

The menisci transmit varying percentages of forces across the knee joint depending on knee position. In full extension the menisci accommodate 45% to 50% of the load, while in 90° of flexion, they accept 85% of the load (Ahmed & Burke 1983; Ahmed, Burke, & Yu 1983). The load distribution between the medial and lateral menisci differs. Medially, the meniscus and articular cartilage share the load equally. Laterally, the meniscus assumes 70% of the load transmission (Seedhom & Wright 1974; Walker & Erkman 1975). The tibiofemoral joint experiences a combination of compressive, tensile, and shearing forces that vary according to both the individual and the task. Most obvious is the compressive force created by the ground reaction forces of contact (e.g., at foot strike in walking or running). These compressive loads are typically accommodated through a *hoop effect* in which the forces are directed peripherally along the lines of greatest collagen fiber stiffness. Tensile forces are seen in the structures resisting distraction between the tibia and femur. Shear forces arise from the rotational loads in movements involving rapid change of direction.

Since meniscal injury often is caused by high rates of force application, the meniscus's biphasic (i.e., solid and fluid) character plays a fundamental role in determining the mechanical response. Even though circumferential stresses dominate the tissue's response (due to the hoop effect), circumferential strains are relatively small, and the fluid phase carries a significant part of the applied load (Spilker, Donzelli, & Mow 1992).

Knee joint movement is among the most complex of all joints in the human body. While its primary movement is flexion/extension, the joint's structure dictates a nonhingelike motion character-ized by a variable instantaneous axis of rotation and combined rotational, rolling, and gliding movements (figures 3.22 and 3.23). In addition to the predominant flexion and extension, the tibiofemoral joint also has rotational capability when the joint is flexed, as well as limited varus/valgus movement.

One unique motion feature of the tibiofemoral joint is the so-called *screw-home mechanism*. During the final few degrees of knee extension, there is a relative rotation between the tibia and femur that "locks" the joint in place at full extension by rotationally screwing the bones together. If the tibia is fixed, the femur rotates medially at extension. Conversely, if the femur is fixed, the tibia experiences a relative lateral rotation into place. At the initiation of flexion, the tibiofemoral joint unscrews, reversing the relative tibial and femoral rotations.

The combination of complex joint movement and continuously varying loading patterns creates a formidable puzzle in terms of identifying meniscal injury mechanisms. Nonetheless, certain mechanisms are implicated. Damage usually occurs when the meniscus is subjected to a combination of flexion-rotation or extension-rotation during weight bearing. For example, when an athlete, with foot planted on the ground, attempts a rapid change of direction, internal femoral rotation on a fixed tibia causes posterior displacement of the medial meniscus. The meniscal attachment to the joint capsule and MCL resists this movement and places the meniscus under tensile loading. Rapid extension of the knee results in forces sufficient to cause a longitudinal tear of the medial meniscus. On occasion the loading is large enough to cause a longitudinal tear that extends into the anterior horn, an injury termed a bucket-handle tear. The bucket-handle pattern more typically arises from repeated insult to a partial tear that then progresses to span a large portion of the meniscus (figure 6.18).

Predisposition to meniscal injury is activity dependent. Certain sports are associated with high incidence of meniscus injury. Leading the list is soccer, in which players experience frequent collisions with opponents and often change direction and body position while their cleats are embedded in the turf. Meniscal injury is also common in track and field (e.g., knee torsion in the shot put or discus) and skiing (e.g., ski slippage or catching that imparts a sudden twist to the knee). Occupations involving sustained or repeated squatting (e.g., mining, carpet laying, gardening) are also implicated in meniscus

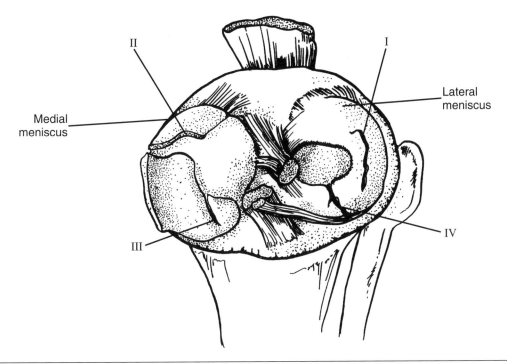

Figure 6.18 Meniscal injury. Four basic types of meniscal tears: I, longitudinal (bucket-handle); II, horizontal; III, oblique; IV, radial.

injury, often due to the degenerative processes that accompany prolonged knee flexion and its attendant structural loads.

Collateral Ligament Sprain

Injury to the medial collateral ligament (MCL) complex is quite common, with involvement of the lateral collateral ligament (LCL) much less frequent. Both injuries result from sudden and violent varus or valgus loading. LCL injury results from impact to the knee's medial aspect while the foot is planted on the ground. The resulting varus loading creates tensile forces in the lateral structures. Conversely, impact on the lateral side of the knee causes tensile loading of the medial aspect and produces MCL injury. The MCL is most effective in resisting valgus loading when the knee is flexed 25° to 30° (Swenson & Harner 1995). At full knee extension other structures play a relatively greater role than when the knee is partially flexed.

The role of the MCL in resisting valgus loading has been demonstrated experimentally (Grood et al. 1981; Piziali et al. 1980; Seering et al. 1980). The conclusion from the research is that the MCL is the primary valgus restraint, with only secondary involvement provided by the cruciate ligaments. In cases of isolated MCL failure, however, residual structures, particularly the ACL, are able to resist varus-valgus moments (Inoue et al. 1987). While most MCL injuries are acute and traumatic, overuse syndromes also have been implicated, specifically associated with the whip-kick technique used by swimmers performing the breaststroke.

Knee Extensor Disorders

The knee joint complex forms the critical middle link in the kinetic chain of the lower extremity. In this role, its loading and motion characteristics dictate effective limb function. Aberrations in any of its many functional components increase the risk of injury. Arguably the most important component is the so-called knee extensor mechanism (KEM) that consists of the quadriceps muscle group, the patellofemoral joint, and the tendon group connecting these elements.

The patella serves as the central structure in the knee extensor mechanism. In that role it acts as a fulcrum, or pivot, to enhance the mechanical advantage of the quadriceps during knee flexion and extension. The patella effectively moves the tendon line of action away from the instantaneous joint center (axis) and thus increases the moment arm (figure 6.19). A given force then produces a greater moment of force or torque.

Force created by the quadriceps is transmitted through the quadriceps tendon and patellar tendon (also patellar ligament) to the tibial tuberosity. Some researchers erroneously have assumed that the force in the quadriceps tendon (F_Q) is the same as that in the patellar tendon (F_P). However, this has been disproved by research that has shown that F_Q and F_P generally are not equal. The actual forces in each tendon depend on the knee joint angle (figure 6.20). Tendofemoral contact in positions of extreme flexion (e.g., in a deep squat) carries a significant portion of the contact force, thus reducing the load on the patella.

As forces are transmitted through the knee extensor mechanism, a component of the force is directed through the patella toward the joint center and pushes the patella against the femur. Near full extension, the patella rides high on the femur. As the knee flexes, the patella slides into the intercondylar

groove. This simultaneously changes the location of the patellofemoral joint reaction force and the moment arm about the instantaneous knee joint

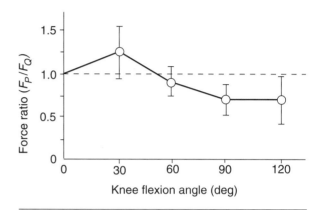

Figure 6.20 Ratio of patellar tendon force (F_P) to quadriceps tendon force (F_Q) as a function of flexion angle.

Adapted from Hayes, Stone, & Shybut 1984.

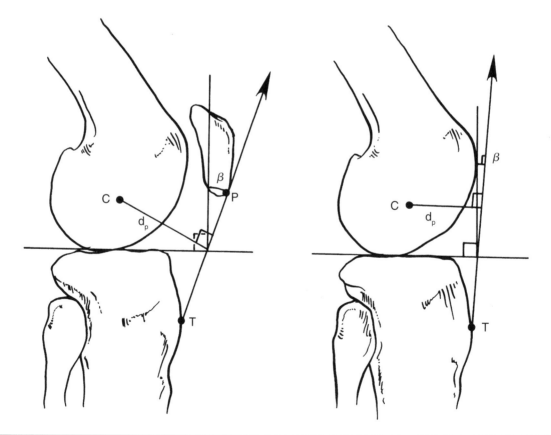

Figure 6.19 Effect of the patella in increasing the mechanical advantage of the knee extensor mechanism. The patella (*left*) effectively moves the tendon line of action away from the knee joint instantaneous center (axis of rotation, *C*), increasing the moment arm (d_p) of the quadriceps group and thus enhancing its mechanical advantage. Without a patella (*right*), the moment arm (d_p) is shorter and the mechanical advantage is reduced.

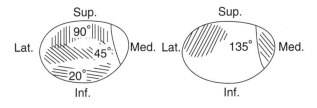

Figure 6.21 Patellofemoral contact areas as a function of change in degree of knee flexion. As the knee is flexed from full extension (0°) through 90°, the contact area migrates from the inferior retropatellar surface to the superior region. At 135° of flexion, the contact area is on both the superolateral surface and the medial odd facet.

From "Biomechanics of the patellofemoral joint" by D.S. Hungerford & M. Barry, 1979, *Clinical Orthopaedics and Related Research, 144* (Fig. 2, p. 11). Copyright 1979 by Lippincott-Raven. Adapted by permission.

axis. As the patella slides down within the groove, the retropatellar contact area changes (figure 6.21).

Movement of the patella along the femur is referred to as patellar tracking. Proper tracking depends on a complex interaction of muscle forces (i.e., vector sum of the individual force vectors of the vastus medialis, vastus lateralis, vastus intermedius, and rectus femoris) and structural considerations (e.g., Q-angle [angle formed by a line drawn from the anterior superior iliac spine to the mid-patella and a line drawn from the mid-patella to the tibial tuberosity], patella alta [patella positioned abnormally high on the femur], geometry of intercondylar groove). As the patella moves, contact pressures develop between the patella and femur. These pressures vary with the amount of knee flexion (figure 6.22).

Effective tracking depends on congruence between the patella and femur. This congruence is typically measured by congruence angle, lateral patellofemoral angle, and patellar tilt angle (figure 6.23). In summary, the integrity of patellofemoral movement is dictated by the neuromechanical synergy between patellofemoral tracking, patellofemoral contact pressures, and neuromotor control of patellofemoral agonists.

Disturbance of patellofemoral integrity often leads to injuries. Injuries to the knee extensor mechanism result from either direct trauma, indirect trauma, or chronic overuse. Whatever the cause, there is little doubt that the injuries are both myriad and prevalent.

In chapter 5, we cautioned against the use of nonspecific injury descriptors. Two such terms are used in referring to patellofemoral pathologies: jumper's knee and chondromalacia patella. The former term refers to tendon pain of the knee extensor mechanism developed through repeated jumping. We suggest the use of more clinically useful terms that identify the location and condition of the involved tissue (e.g., quadriceps tendinitis, patellar tendinitis, apophysitis of the tibial tuberosity, or Osgood-Schlatter disease).

The second term, chondromalacia patella, has evolved into an all-too-common descriptor for generalized patellar pain. The term chondromalacia patella is best reserved to describe specifically the degeneration of retropatellar articular cartilage. Once believed to be a primary condition of unknown etiology, chondromalacia patella is now thought to most often occur secondary to other mechanisms. These include both traumatic (e.g.,

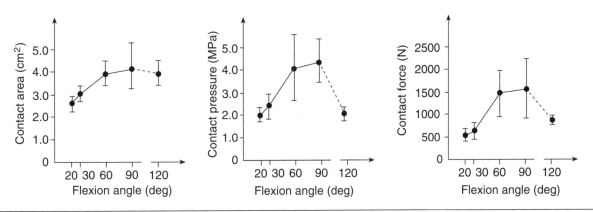

Figure 6.22 Patellofemoral contact area, pressure, and force vary with knee flexion angle.
Adapted from Huberti & Hayes 1984.

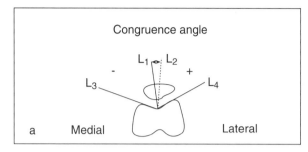

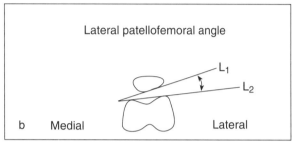

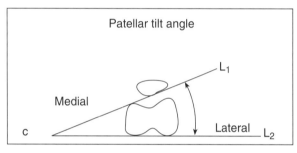

Figure 6.23 Patellofemoral angle measures. (*a*) Congruence angle (between lines L_1 and L_2). (*b*) Lateral patellofemoral angle. (*c*) Patellar tilt angle.

patellar fracture) and chronic (e.g., patellar malalignment, chronic subluxation, pathological patellar tracking) events.

Extreme forces or continued mechanical insult to an already weakened knee extensor mechanism may lead to tendon rupture. Quadriceps tendon rupture typically occurs in people over 40 years old and is localized at the osteotendinous junction of the superior patellar pole. Calcification at the rupture site suggests that quadriceps tendon rupture tends to occur in areas of previous microtrauma. In contrast, patellar tendon ruptures tend to afflict those under 40 years of age, most often tearing at the inferior patellar pole. The injury mechanism typically involves a violent quadriceps contraction against resistance at the knee and requires substantial loads to induce rupture. Instances of bilateral patellar tendon ruptures have also been reported in the literature. Some of these injuries have identifiable mechanisms, including jumping, tripping, or vari-

ous athletic tasks, while others appear as idiopathic events in otherwise healthy individuals.

Lower-Leg Injuries

The lower leg (also called leg or shank) spans the knee and ankle joints and contains two longitudinally aligned bones, the tibia (medial) and fibula (lateral). Four muscle compartments (anterior, lateral, superficial posterior, deep posterior) surround these bones, with tight fascia enclosing each compartment. The anterior compartment contains the tibialis anterior, extensor hallucis longus, extensor digitorum longus, and peroneus tertius. The lateral compartment comprises the peroneus longus and peroneus brevis. The largest compartment in terms of muscle mass is the superficial posterior compartment, which contains the gastrocnemius and soleus (together termed the triceps surae) and plantaris. The deep posterior compartment houses the popliteus, flexor hallucis longus, flexor digitorum longus, and tibialis posterior (figure 6.24). The actions of the foot and ankle muscles are summarized in table 6.4.

Compartment Syndrome

Acute injury or chronic exertion often increases fluid accumulation within muscle compartments of the arms, feet, and legs. The excess fluid may be due to hemorrhage, edema, or both. Given the relative inextensibility of the surrounding fascia, the fluid increase results in increased compartmental pressure. This creates a compartment syndrome, defined as "a pathologic condition of skeletal muscle characterized by increased interstitial pressure within an anatomically confined muscle compartment that interferes with the circulation and function of the muscle and neurovascular components of the compartment" (Garrett 1995, 48).

From a mechanical perspective, compartment syndromes are a consequence of the relation between mass, volume, and pressure (see chapter 5). Increasing the mass within a fixed volume increases the internal pressure. This is the essence of a compartment syndrome. Many conditions can lead to a compartment syndrome. These include soft tissue contusion, crush, bleeding disorders, venous obstruction, arterial occlusion, burn, prolonged compression after drug overdose, medical antishock trousers, and exercise.

Increased compartmental pressure compromises vascular and neural function and sets the stage for

Case Study: Patellar Tendon Rupture

Most musculoskeletal injuries do not happen under conditions that permit quantitative assessment of the injury dynamics. In most cases clinicians and researchers are limited to qualitative evaluation. On rare occasions, however, circumstances do allow for quantitative examination. One such case, in which a human patellar tendon ruptured during an actual sports competition, was reported by Zernicke, Garhammer, and Jobe (1977). A world-class light heavyweight lifter was attempting to complete the second phase of a clean-and-jerk movement using 175 kg when his right patellar tendon ruptured. The tendon was torn completely with evidence of damage at the distal pole of the patella and at the patellar-tendon insertion on the tibia.

The lift was attempted during a national weight-lifting competition and was being filmed for biomechanical analysis. Using a multilink, rigid-body model, Zernicke and co-workers were able to estimate the tensile force in the tendon at the instant of rupture. The force was approximately 14.5 kN, or more than 17.5 times the lifter's body weight!

This exceptional example highlights the complex dynamics of injury and provides evidence of the high stresses applied (and tolerated) to biological tissues and the importance of loading rate on tissue response to mechanical loading.

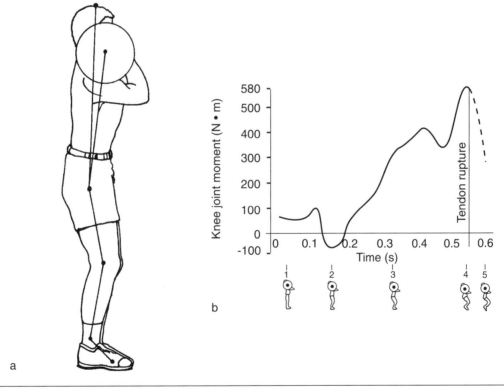

Figure 6B.1   Patellar tendon rupture. (*a*) Five-segment, rigid-body model of weight lifter. (*b*) Mean resultant knee joint moments from the beginning of the jerk movement until after tendon failure.
Adapted from Zernicke, Garhammer, & Jobe 1977.

ischemia and a self-perpetuating cycle of fluid accumulation and restricted flow. The situation is exacerbated by the mechanical properties of the fascia, which has been shown to increase in thickness and stiffness in response to *chronic compartment syndrome* (Hurschler et al. 1994). The situation is further

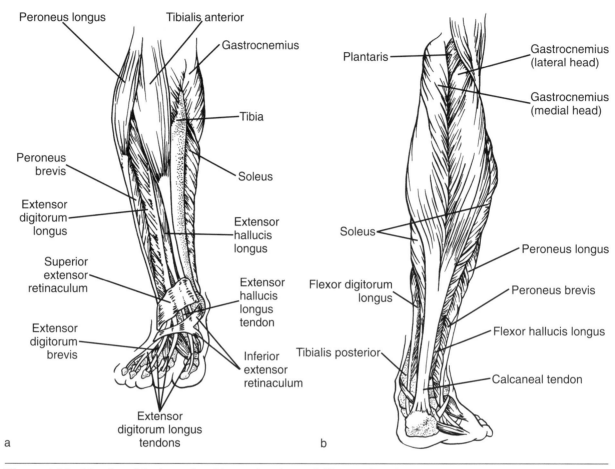

Figure 6.24 Muscles of the lower leg: (*a*) anterior view and (*b*) posterior view.

Table 6.4 Muscles of the Lower Leg and Ankle

Muscle	Action
Anterior compartment	
Tibialis anterior	Dorsiflexes the ankle and inverts the foot
Extensor hallucis longus	Dorsiflexes the ankle and inverts the foot
Extensor digitorum longus	Dorsiflexes the ankle and everts the foot
Peroneus tertius	Dorsiflexes the ankle and everts the foot
Lateral compartment	
Peroneus longus	Plantar-flexes the ankle and everts the foot
Peroneus brevis	Plantar-flexes the ankle and everts the foot
Superficial posterior compartment	
Gastrocnemius	Plantar-flexes the ankle and flexes the leg
Soleus	Plantar-flexes the ankle
Plantaris	Plantar-flexes the ankle and flexes the leg
Deep posterior compartment	
Popliteus	No action at ankle or foot; flexes and medially rotates the leg
Flexor hallucis longus	Plantar-flexes the ankle and inverts the foot
Flexor digitorum longus	Plantar-flexes the ankle and inverts the foot
Tibialis posterior	Plantar-flexes the ankle and inverts the foot

worsened by a decrease in compartment volume, as might be caused by compression wraps or tight clothing.

Sufficiently large compartment pressures result in vessel closure and potentially catastrophic physiological consequences. Venous collapse severely reduces blood return and leads to capillary congestion and decreased tissue perfusion. Local tissues then suffer the consequences of hypoperfusion (e.g., ischemia and eventual necrosis).

Transient increases in compartment pressures are normally seen in response to exertion. In people without *chronic compartment syndrome* (CCS), resting pressures vary, ranging from 0 to 20 mm Hg (Dayton & Bouche 1994). During exertion, pressures may exceed 60 to 70 mm Hg but quickly return to resting levels within minutes of exercise cessation. A person with CCS, in contrast, may exhibit resting pressures of 15 mm Hg that climb to more than 100 mm Hg during exercise, with prolonged postexercise decline (figure 6.25).

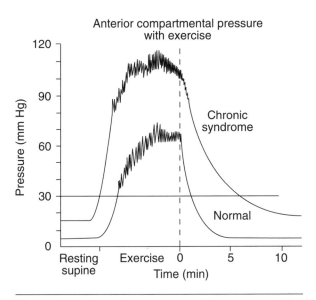

Figure 6.25 Anterior compartment pressures recorded in a patient with chronic anterior compartment syndrome and in a normal subject.

Reprinted from Mubarak 1981.

Relief from CCS is achieved surgically by fascial incision (fasciotomy) to "release" the compartment and effectively increase its volume and also reduce internal pressure. Some controversy exists over the threshold pressure above which fasciotomy is indicated. Suggested values range from 30 to 45 mm Hg. Using a single mechanical variable (i.e., compartment pressure) to determine surgical interven-

tion must be viewed with caution, as many other factors warrant consideration: (1) Intracompartmental pressures do not measure neuromuscular ischemia; (2) ischemic development depends on both the magnitude and duration of the elevated pressure; (3) patient tolerance to ischemia may vary; (4) injured muscle may be less tolerant of ischemia and elevated pressure than uninjured muscle (Gulli & Templeman 1994).

Tibial Stress Syndrome

Tibial stress syndrome (TSS) is an inflammatory reaction of the deep fascial tibial attachments in response to chronic loads. Pain is localized to the anterior or posteromedial crest of the tibia, or both, and results from excessive tension forces applied to the fascia by the eccentric action of musculotendinous units, most often the soleus, tibialis posterior, and flexor digitorum longus. The condition initially manifests as fasciitis and, with continued loading, progresses to periostitis and ultimately to endosteal activity.

Commonly seen in runners, TSS is a multifactorial overuse syndrome related to the runner's anatomical structure, training program, flexibility, muscle strength, footwear, and running mechanics. Changes in any of these parameters may lead to a TSS injury. Despite its prevalence, diagnosis of TSS remains problematic in light of differential diagnoses of stress reaction and stress fracture (see following section), tendinitis, musculotendinous strain, and chronic compartment syndromes.

Tibial Stress Reaction and Stress Fracture

Bone responds to repetitive loading by adapting its structure according to what is known as Wolff's law. This adaptation or remodeling process includes resorption of bone where the loading conditions deem it unnecessary and deposition in regions needed to sustain the new mechanical loads. If, however, the magnitude and frequency of loading exceed the bone's ability to adapt, injury occurs. The most recognizable form of injury is bone fracture. As discussed in the previous chapter, fracture may occur acutely (traumatic fracture) or in response to chronic loading (stress fracture). The term *stress fracture* itself suffers from overuse, or perhaps misuse, as it is used frequently to describe bone with no clear evidence of discontinuity or line of fracture. The term *stress reaction* describes bone with evidence of remodeling but with an absence of radiological evidence of fracture. Such stress reactions are quite common and are detectable using a combination of radiographs, bone scans, and magnetic resonance imaging scans (figure 6.26).

Actual fractures occur much less frequently than pure mechanical loading (i.e., material fatigue failure) alone would predict, suggesting that the process leading to stress reaction and subsequent stress fracture in fact involves physiological processes of bone adaptation to mechanical loading. This is not to discount completely the role of mechanical fa-

tigue, however, since microfractures have been detected at remodeling sites.

Verifiable stress fractures are most frequently found in the tibia, accounting for up to 50% of all stress fractures. From a mechanical perspective, it is interesting to note that the fracture location depends somewhat on activity. The mechanical demands of specific movements appear to play a prominent role in determining the fracture site. Runners, the most common victims of tibial stress fracture, exhibit fractures focused between the middle and

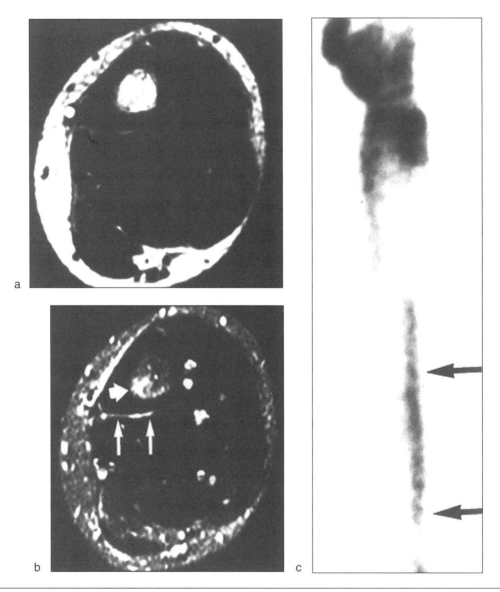

Figure 6.26 Stress reaction in the lower left leg of an 18-year-old female varsity runner. Axial T1-weighted magnetic resonance image (*a*) shows no detectable abnormality, but the T2-weighted image (*b*) shows moderate periosteal edema (long arrows) along the posterior and medial aspect of the tibia. There is also marrow edema (short arrow) in the adjacent part of the tibia. The bone scintigraphy (*c*) shows increased activity along the distal half of the tibial diaphysis (arrows).

Reprinted from Fredericson et al. 1995.

Shinsplints

Of the many catch-all terms used in the medical literature, perhaps none can match *shinsplints* when it comes to nonspecificity, lack of consensus on meaning, and being a continuing source of misunderstanding and confusion. As evidence, we present a few of the many and varied descriptions of shinsplints.

1. "Tenderness and pain with induration and swelling of pretibial muscles, following athletic overexertion by the untrained; it may be a mild form of anterior tibial compartment syndrome" (*Stedman's* 1990, 1413).

2. "An inflammatory condition characterized by exercise-induced pain localized to the posteromedial or anterior crest of the tibia, or both" (Bouche, Sullivan, & Ichikawa 1994, 248).

3. "Diffuse areas of increased tenderness over the anterior or posterior bony attachments of the tibialis anterior muscles to the tibia. . . . This relatively mild condition must be distinguished from its two more disabling cousins, tibial stress fracture and chronic exertional compartment syndrome" (Kibler & Chandler 1994, 549).

4. "Pain in the shin may be related to overuse or stress of the muscles within the extensor or flexor groups, stress fracture, or induced ischemia within muscular compartments leading to compartment syndrome" (Ciullo & Shapiro 1994, 661).

O'Donoghue (1984, 591) astutely noted, "As with many names in common use, there is considerable and often heated argument as to what is actually meant by the term. As is usual in these circumstances, the term 'shin splints' is a wastebasket one including many different conditions. The authors of various articles on the subject are inclined to state very definitely that it is caused by one particular thing to the exclusion of all others, which causes great confusion." We recommend relegating *shinsplints* to the "land of diction fiction" and selecting terms that are clinically correct, specific, and useful.

---

distal thirds of the tibia. Athletes in jumping sports (e.g., basketball and volleyball) tend to experience proximal fractures. Dancers, in contrast, sustain more midshaft fractures.

Traumatic Fractures of the Tibia and Fibula

High-energy insult to the lower leg often results in traumatic fracture of the tibia, fibula, or both. The sources of the applied force vary, but the usual suspects are: vehicle-pedestrian accidents and sports-related movements.

The mechanism of tibiofibular fracture can be direct impact, torsion, or bending, or a combination of the three. Motor vehicle accidents account for the majority of direct impact, or crushing, fractures. Torsional loading occurs when the lower leg is twisted about its long axis (see chapter 5), as in skiing when the ski provides an extended moment arm for applying torques to the tibial shaft. Details of a case of bilateral spiral fracture are presented in the sidebar on page 166. Bending loads are created when parallel and oppositely directed forces are applied simultaneously to the bone. The classic boot-top fracture illustrates this bending mechanism (figure 6.27).

A recent study identified baseball bats as a causal agent in tibial fractures. This is disturbing because the fractures did not occur during athletic competition, but rather resulted from the bats being used as weapons. Levy, Bromberg, and Jasper (1994) reported 47 such bat-induced fractures during a one-year period at an urban trauma center. Eleven of these fractures were to the tibia, and many involved extensive comminution and complications (e.g., delayed union, compartment syndrome).

Whatever the specific mechanism, tibiofibular fracture must be considered a serious injury because of the injured bone's compromised ability to carry

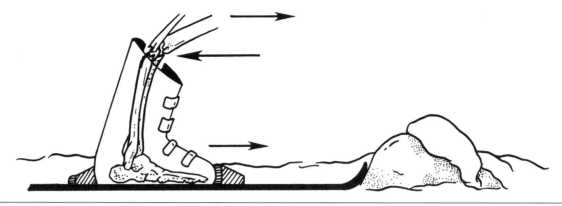

Figure 6.27 Tibial boot-top fracture. The top of the ski boot acts posteriorly as the middle fulcrum point in creating a three-point bending mechanism.

Case Study: Bilateral Spiral Fracture

Many thousands of skiing-related injuries occur every year, sometimes because of excessively tight bindings or binding release malfunctions (Hull & Mote 1980). Zernicke (1981) reported the case of a skiing-related injury in which a skier, on his first run of the day on the beginner's slope, unintentionally began to snowplow uncontrollably. Both of his legs were forced into extreme internal rotation. Failure of the bindings to release resulted in spiral fractures in both tibias. Subsequent testing of the skis, boots, and bindings using a biomechanical model (figure 6B.2) provided quantitative estimates of the torques transmitted to the lower leg as lateral

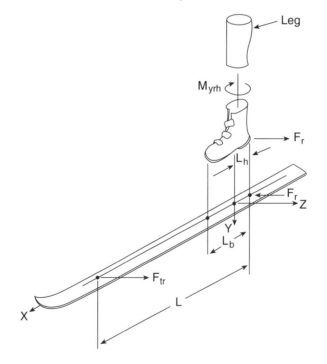

Figure 6B.2 Schematic diagram of leg-boot-ski binding system. M_{yrh} = torque transmitted to skier's lower leg; F_r = lateral release force applied to heel; L_h = distance from vertical axis of the tibia to the heel point; L_b = distance from the heel to the toe pivot point (i.e., length of the boot); F_{tr} = lateral force applied to the ski at a distance (L) in front of the heel-release point.

Reprinted from Zernicke 1981.

(continued)

(continued)

forces were applied to the skis. The data showed that the bindings placed the skier at high risk of injury, since "for nearly all applications of lateral loads to the ski, this skier's bindings would not have released prior to exceeding the torsional elastic threshold of the tibia" (Zernicke 1981, 243).

Fortunately, poor bindings such as the ones in this case are no longer in use. This example nonetheless demonstrates the potential for injury in skiing and points to the importance of proper equipment selection and maintenance in reducing the risk of musculoskeletal injury.

loads in its role as a critical link in the lower extremity's kinetic chain.

Foot and Ankle Injuries

Given its numerous bones, ligaments, and articulations, the foot and ankle region is arguably the human body's most complex area. The ankle joint is formed by the articulation of the tibia, fibula, and talus. The tibia and fibula create a deep socket, or mortise, that contains the talus. In a dorsiflexed position, the talus fits snugly within the mortise and is quite stable. As the ankle plantar-flexes, the narrower posterior section of the talus rotates into the area between the malleoli. This looser fit compromises joint stability, resulting in a relatively unstable ankle in the plantar-flexed position.

Many ligaments reinforce the ankle. Medially, the strong deltoid ligament complex provides resistance to forceful eversion. On the lateral aspect, three ligaments are primarily responsible for restricting inversion. The weakest of the three, the anterior talofibular ligament (ATFL), extends anteromedially from the fibular malleolus to the neck of the talus. The calcaneofibular ligament (CFL) passes posteroinferiorly from the tip of the fibular malleolus to the lateral surface of the calcaneus. The posterior talofibular ligament (PTFL) connects the fibular malleolar fossa to the lateral tubercle of the talus (figure 6.28).

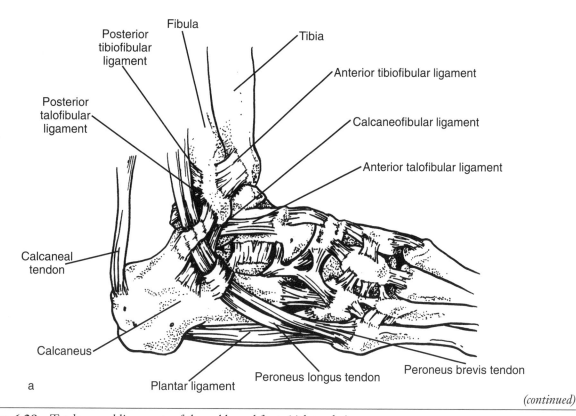

Fibula

Posterior tibiofibular ligament

Tibia

Anterior tibiofibular ligament

Posterior talofibular ligament

Calcaneofibular ligament

Anterior talofibular ligament

Calcaneal tendon

Calcaneus

Plantar ligament

Peroneus longus tendon

Peroneus brevis tendon

a

(continued)

Figure 6.28 Tendons and ligaments of the ankle and foot: (*a*) lateral view.

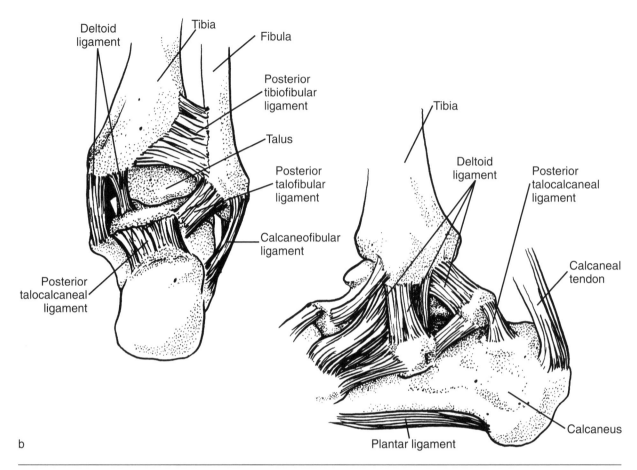

Figure 6.28 *(continued)* Tendons and ligaments of the ankle and foot: *(b)* posterior and medial views.

Each foot contains 26 bones (figure 6.29a). The largest of these, the calcaneus, serves as the attachment for the calcaneal (Achilles) tendon, which transmits the force of the triceps surae muscles in plantar-flexing the ankle. The articulation of the calcaneus with the talus forms the subtalar (talocalcaneal) joint, an articulation essential to proper function of the foot and ankle complex during load bearing. The subtalar joint axis runs obliquely, as shown in figure 6.29b.

The bones of the foot are arranged to form two primary arches: the longitudinal arch, running from the calcaneus to the distal ends of the metatarsals, and the transverse arch, which extends from side to side across the foot (figures 6.30 & 6.31b). The longitudinal arch is divided into a medial portion that includes the calcaneus, talus, navicular, three cuneiforms, and the three most medial metatarsals. The lateral portion is much flatter and is in contact with the ground during standing. The transverse arch is formed by the cuboid, cuneiforms, and bases of the metatarsals.

During weight bearing, the arches compress to absorb and distribute the load. Several ligaments assist in this force distribution. These include the plantar calcaneonavicular ligament (spring ligament), the short plantar ligament, and the long plantar ligament. The integrity of the arches and their ability to absorb loads is maintained by the tight-fitting articulations between foot bones, the action of intrinsic foot musculature, the strength of the plantar ligaments, and the plantar aponeurosis (plantar fascia).

Calcaneal Tendon: Tendinitis and Rupture

Ever since the Greek warrior Achilles was felled by an arrow judiciously aimed at his unprotected heel, the calcaneal region has been associated with susceptibility to injury. The calcaneal (Achilles) tendon, the largest and strongest tendon in the body, transmits substantial loads from the triceps surae group to its attachment on the posterior calcaneus. Forces in the tendon, for example, have been estimated to be as high as 10 times body weight during running (Burdett 1982). Frequent and

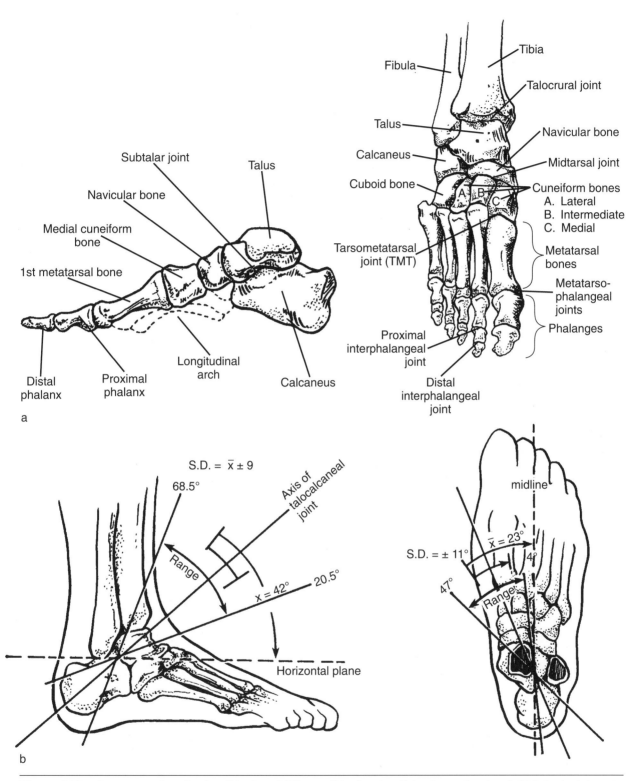

Figure 6.29   Anatomy and mechanics of the foot. (*a*) Bones of the foot (medial and superior views). (*b*) Subtalar joint axis. Part (*b*) from Sangeorzan 1991.

repeated loading of the calcaneal tendon predisposes it to overuse pathologies, most commonly peritenonitis (inflammation of the peritenon), insertional disturbances (e.g., bursitis, insertion tendinitis), myotendinous junction injury, or tendonopathies (Kvist 1994).

The etiology of calcaneal tendonopathies is multifactorial; contributing factors include training

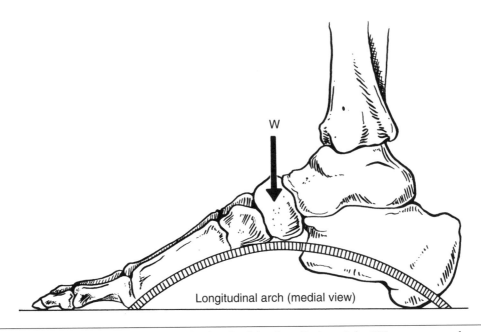

Figure 6.30 Schematic drawing of the longitudinal arch of the foot. Body weight (*W*) compresses the arch.

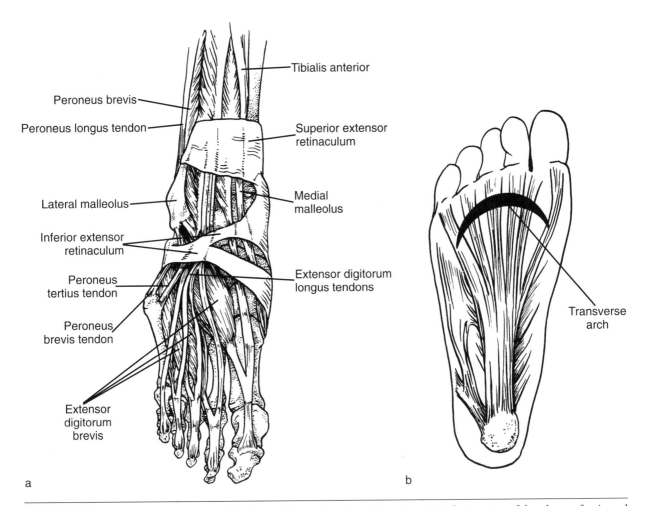

Figure 6.31 Tendons and ligaments of the foot. (*a*) Superior view of the foot. (*b*) Inferior view of the plantar fascia and transverse arch.

errors, malalignments and biomechanical faults, improper footwear, trauma, age, gender, anthropometrics, environment, psychological factors, and psychomotor factors.

Tendon degeneration may eventually lead to complete tendon rupture. Calcaneal tendon ruptures typically happen in men between 30 and 40 years old who suddenly exert themselves in a sporting task that involves rapid change of direction. In most instances these spontaneous tendon ruptures seem to "just happen." Postinjury assessment, however, has shown evidence of degeneration in the substance of the ruptured tendon. Tendon rupture thus seems to be secondary to degenerative processes rather than a primary injury that happens spontaneously. Tendon rupture usually occurs about two to six cm proximal to the calcaneal insertion in a region known to be hypovascular. This fact, combined with decreased blood flow associated with age, largely explains the frequency of rupture in middle-aged people.

As a side note of interest, it seems there may be a relation between blood type and increased incidence of tendon rupture. People with type O blood seem to be more likely to suffer from tendon rupture in general (Jozsa et al. 1989) and calcaneal tendon rupture in particular (Kujala et al. 1992), suggesting a genetic link between one's ABO blood group and the molecular structure of tendon tissue.

Four primary mechanisms have been implicated in calcaneal tendon rupture (Mahan & Carter 1992; figure 6.32): (1) sudden dorsiflexion of a plantarflexed foot (e.g., a football quarterback dropping back and planting his rear foot as he throws), (2) pushing off the weight-bearing foot while extending the ipsilateral knee joint (e.g., a basketball player executing a rapid change of direction), (3) sudden excess tension on an already taut tendon (e.g., catching a heavy weight), and (4) a taut tendon struck by a blunt object (e.g., baseball bat).

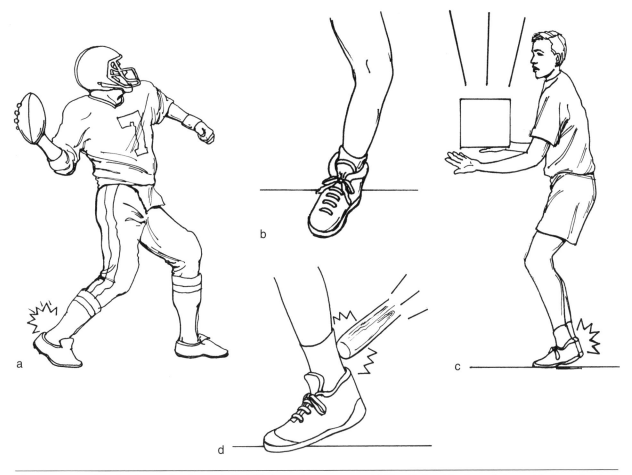

Figure 6.32 Mechanisms of calcaneal (Achilles) tendon rupture. (*a*) Rapid dorsiflexion of the ankle by a football quarterback. (*b*) Cutting maneuver with rapid change of direction. (*c*) Catching a falling weight. (*d*) Blunt trauma to a taut tendon.

Plantar Fasciitis

Plantar fasciitis (PF) has been described as an inflammatory condition of the plantar fascia in the midfoot or at its insertion on the medial tuberosity of the calcaneus that involves microtears or partial rupture of fascial fibers. Once again we encounter a catch-all term, plantar fasciitis, which has become entrenched in the literature as a general descriptor of pain in the plantar area of the posterior foot. The more appropriate nonspecific designation is heel pain syndrome, with PF reserved for inflammatory pathology to the plantar fascia alone.

In most cases, PF develops in response to repeated loading (e.g., running) in which compressive forces flatten the longitudinal arch of the foot. Forces in the plantar fascia during running have been estimated to be 1.3 to 2.9 times body weight (Scott & Winter 1990). This flattening of the arches stretches the fascia and absorbs the load in much the same way as a leaf spring bends to accommodate heavy weights. Extension of the toes puts added stress on the structures by way of a windlass mechanism, as depicted in figure 6.33.

Plantar fasciitis is hastened or worsened by lack of flexibility. Tightness of the calcaneal tendon, for example, limits ankle dorsiflexion and results in greater plantar fascial stress. Ankle strength and flexibility deficits have been observed in the symptomatic limbs compared with the unaffected limbs and with an asymptomatic control group (Kibler, Goldberg, & Chandler 1991).

In addition to strength and flexibility, other factors are associated with PF, including overtraining, leg length discrepancies, fatigue, fascial inextensibility, and poor movement mechanics. Excessive pronation during running provides a good example of how a pathological movement pattern contributes to PF.

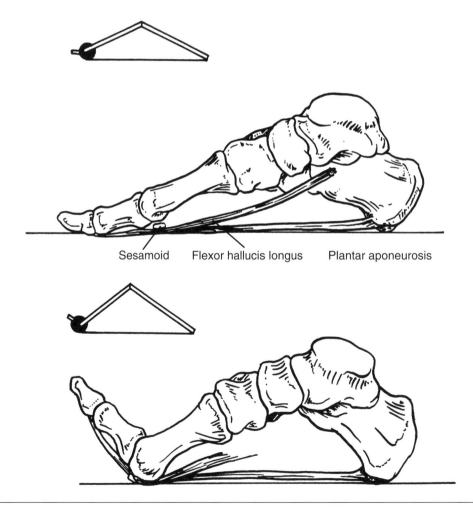

Sesamoid   Flexor hallucis longus   Plantar aponeurosis

Figure 6.33 Windlass mechanism created by extension of the toes (*bottom*). This mechanism tends to raise the longitudinal arch and resist the effect of compression in flattening the arch.

During pronation the subtalar joint everts, causing plantar fascial elongation and increased tissue stress. Repetition of this pathological loading leads to microdamage and attendant inflammation.

Ankle Sprain

As a result of its relative anatomical instability and its supportive function, the ankle joint is frequently injured. In certain sports (e.g., basketball) ankle sprains are the most common injury.

To present a meaningful discussion of ankle injury mechanisms, we must review several anatomical structures and their functional characteristics. As briefly described earlier, the ankle joint is formed by the articulation of the tibia, fibula, and talus. The talar body is wedge-shaped, with its anterior portion being wider than its posterior. This irregularity contributes directly to the joint's positional stability. In dorsiflexion the wider part wedges between the malleoli, lending stability to the joint. The narrow portion of the talus, however, moves between the malleoli in plantar flexion, permits talar translation and tilt, and results in lateral instability. The juxtaposition of the tibia and fibula is maintained by an interosseous ligament (syndesmosis) passing transversely between the two bones. This junction is further secured by the anterior and posterior tibiofibular ligaments.

Technically speaking, ankle sprain is a misnomer since the injury typically involves both the ankle and subtalar joints. These two joints move in concert to execute what must be correctly viewed as combined ankle-foot movement. Our movement conventions are described and illustrated in figure 6.34.

The determining factors in ankle injury, as in most injuries, are the joint position at the time of injury; the magnitude, direction, and rate of the applied forces; and the resistance provided by joint structures. The vast majority (85%) of ankle sprains result from what are termed inversion injuries. According to our nomenclature, the mechanism is actually supination (i.e., a combination of ankle plantar flexion, subtalar inversion, and internal rotation of the foot in which the longitudinal midline of the foot deviates, or rotates, medially). The term *inversion sprain* is so entrenched in the literature, however, that we do not suggest or recommend its extinction.

The joint motions commonly involved in ankle-foot injuries are precipitated by walking on uneven surfaces, stepping in holes, rolling the ankle during a cutting maneuver, or landing on another player's foot when descending from a jump in sporting events (figure 6.35). Resulting injuries range from fracture-dislocation to ligamentous damage (sprain).

In most cases there is an orderly sequence of ligament failure. The anterior talofibular ligament (ATFL) fails first because of its orientation at the instant of loading and its inherent weakness (Siegler, Block, & Schneck 1988). The calcaneofibular ligament (CFL) is next injured, followed by

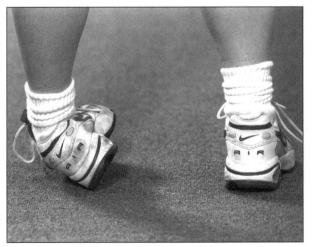

a

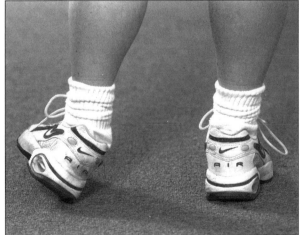

b

Figure 6.34 Foot and ankle movements. (*a*) Supination (combined motions of subtalar inversion, ankle plantar flexion, foot internal rotation). (*b*) Pronation (combined motions of subtalar eversion, ankle dorsiflexion, foot external rotation).

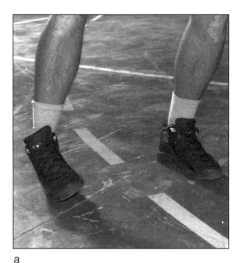
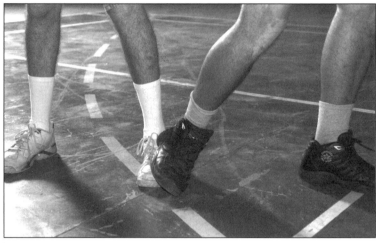

a   b

Figure 6.35 Ankle sprain caused by (*a*) rolling the ankle while in contact with the ground and (*b*) landing on an opponent's foot during descent from a jump.

rare failure of the posterior talofibular ligament (PTFL).

Occasionally the anterior portion of the deltoid ligament (DL) suffers injury during an inversion injury. At first glance, this may appear incongruous. Why would a medial structure incur damage from forcible inversion? The answer lies in the complexity of joint action, specifically the fact that the anterior portion of the DL is taut in ankle plantar flexion. Since the ankle is plantar-flexed at the time of injury, the anterior portion of the deltoid ligament becomes a candidate for injury. As an inherently strong ligament, however, the DL is rarely injured in so-called inversion sprains.

The opposite movement pattern creates eversion sprain (pronation by our definition); the injury mechanism involves ankle dorsiflexion, subtalar eversion, and lateral rotation of the foot. Given the inherent strength of the medial collateral (deltoid) ligament group, injuries resulting from this mechanism are both less frequent (about 5%) and less severe. In this mechanism the talus is forced against the lateral malleolus. Since the lateral malleolus is longer and thinner than the medial malleolus, the talus cannot rotate over the lateral malleolus. This may result in malleolar fracture. Rupture of the deltoid ligament may occur, though this is rare and is always seen in conjunction with other ligament tears. In some cases the forces drive the fibula away from the tibia with sufficient force to tear the interosseous membrane and tibiofibular ligaments.

Toe Injuries

Jacques Lisfranc, a field surgeon in Napoleon's army, described amputation through the tarsometatarsal joint of a gangrenous foot (Vuori & Aro 1993). While his description did not include reference to fracture-dislocation of the joint, his name is now given to these injuries to the tarsometatarsal region. The circumstances of Lisfranc joint injury vary and include both low-energy injuries (e.g., tripping or stumbling) and high-energy trauma (e.g., fall from a height, direct crush, vehicular crash). Several mechanisms have been suggested to explain Lisfranc fracture-dislocations. One relatively uncommon mechanism is direct force, as when a heavy object is dropped on the foot. Direct force applied to the metatarsal pushes the bone down and causes plantar dislocation and possible accompanying fracture. Force applied proximal to the tarsometatarsal joint results in dorsal dislocation.

A second mechanism involves axial loading of the region when indirect forces (e.g., ground reaction force) are applied to a foot in extreme plantar flexion. This occurs when a person is in a tip-toe position at the instant of load application. A similar loading may occur in dorsiflexion as well. In both cases the metatarsal is forcibly pushed out of joint. Such injury is typically accompanied by capsular rupture and metatarsal fracture.

Violent abduction, induced by a twisting mechanism, is another causal mechanism of Lisfranc injury. This is classically illustrated by an equestrian injury in which the rider's foot is fixed in the stirrup while the rider falls. The force of the fall pushes the metatarsals into extreme abduction.

While Lisfranc fracture-dislocations have instructive value in demonstrating mechanisms of injury, their incidence is actually quite low. A review of nearly 700 cases of metatarsal fracture found that less than 10% involved Lisfranc joint injuries (Vuori & Aro 1993).

Other foot and toe injuries are more prevalent. Among these is *turf toe*, an injury involving damage to the capsuloligamentous structures of the first metatarsophalangeal (MP) joint. Multiple mechanisms have been implicated in turf toe injuries, with hyperextension the most common. This injury typically occurs when the foot is planted on the ground with the first MP joint in extension. A load, such as another player falling on the foot, forces the joint into hyperextension and damages joint structures (figure 6.36a). Less frequently, hyperflexion is the mechanism of injury (figure 6.36b). Turf toe also occurs in response to excessive valgus and varus loading of the first MP joint. While once thought to be a relatively minor injury, turf toe is now recognized as a condition with significant short-term effects and potentially serious long-term consequences.

Concluding Comments

Lower-extremity injuries often compromise our ability to perform movements essential to effective daily living. The lower extremities accept the ground forces of walking and running, and these forces can easily reach several times body weight. High force levels multiplied by the thousands of steps we take daily result in a staggering load volume. Excessive load volume can result in chronic injuries as detailed in this chapter.

Suggested Readings

Hip

Steinberg, M.E. (Ed.). (1991). *The Hip and Its Disorders*. Philadelphia: Saunders.

Knee

Finerman, G.A.M., & Noyes, F.R. (1992). *Biology and Biomechanics of the Traumatized Synovial Joint: The Knee as a Model*. Rosemont, IL: American Academy of Orthopaedic Surgeons.

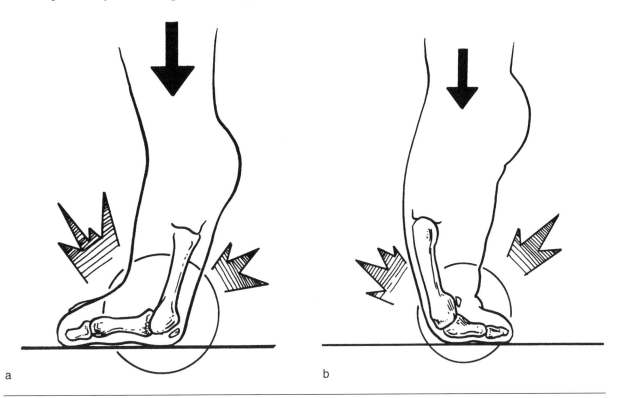

a   b

Figure 6.36   Turf toe injury caused by (*a*) hyperextension of the hallux (big toe) or (*b*) hyperflexion of the hallux (both with simultaneous compressive loading).

Scott, W.N. (1991). *Ligament and Extensor Mechanism Injuries of the Knee: Diagnosis and Treatment*. St. Louis: Mosby-Year Book.

Foot and Ankle

Baxter, D.E. (1995). *The Foot and Ankle in Sport*. St. Louis: Mosby-Year Book.

General Sources

Browner, B.D., Jupiter, J.B., Levine, A.M., & Levine, P.G. (1992). *Skeletal Trauma*. Philadelphia: Saunders.

Feliciano, D.V., Moore, E.E., & Mattox, K.L. (Eds.). (1996). *Trauma* (3rd ed.). Stamford, CT: Appleton & Lange.

Fu, F.H., & Stone, D.A. (1994). *Sports Injuries: Mechanisms, Prevention, Treatment*. Baltimore: Williams & Wilkins.

Nicholas, J.A., & Hershman, E.B. (Eds.). (1995). *The Lower Extremity and Spine in Sports Medicine*. St. Louis: Mosby-Year Book.

Rockwood, C.A., Jr., Green, D.P., Bucholz, R.W., & Heckman, J.D. (Eds.). (1996). *Rockwood and Green's Fractures in Adults* (4th ed.). Philadelphia: Lippincott-Raven.

Woo, S.L.-Y., & Buckwalter, J.A. (Eds.). (1988). *Injury and Repair of the Musculoskeletal Soft Tissues*. Park Ridge, IL: American Academy of Orthopaedic Surgeons.

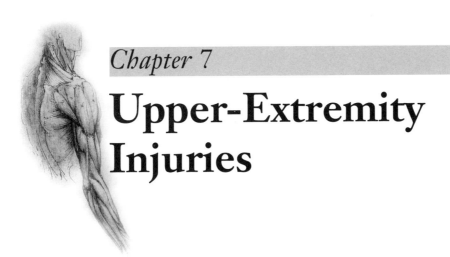

Chapter 7

Upper-Extremity Injuries

Whoever undertakes to hew wood for the master carpenter
rarely escapes injuring his own hands.
Lao Tzu (6th century B.C.)

A day rarely passes without media reports of some notable musculoskeletal injury. Headlines such as "Child Injures Hand Severely in Fireworks Accident," or "High Incidence of Carpal Tunnel Syndrome Found in Keyboard Operators," or "World Series Pitcher Suffers Rotator Cuff Tear" are all too common. Upper-extremity injuries are of special concern since they impair one's ability to manipulate the environment. Even simple tasks such as opening a jar become difficult for a person with impaired dexterity. Significant injury to the shoulder, elbow, wrist, or fingers can end a career or mandate a change of one's occupation or recreational involvement.

Effective diagnosis, treatment, and rehabilitation of upper-extremity injuries depend on a sound understanding of injury mechanisms. Only when the causal relations between applied forces and resultant injury are established and understood can appropriate programs of intervention and prevention be designed and implemented.

Shoulder Injuries

The shoulder, or pectoral girdle, comprises two bones: the scapula and clavicle. The clavicle attaches medially to the sternal manubrium (sternoclavicular joint) and laterally to the acromion process of the scapula (acromioclavicular joint) (figure 7.1). The acromioclavicular (AC) joint is a plane synovial joint with articular surfaces separated by an articular disk. The acromioclavicular ligament supports the AC joint superiorly, with inferior support provided by the coracoclavicular ligament.

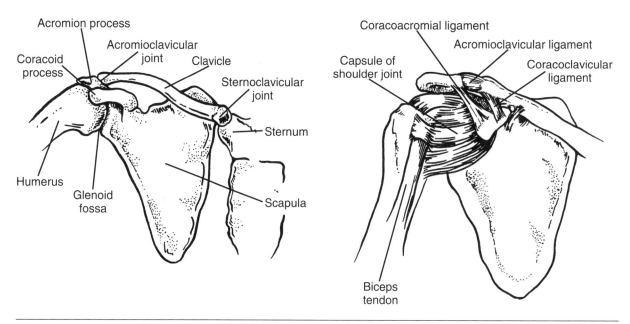

Figure 7.1 Bones and ligaments of the shoulder girdle.

The humerus of the upper arm articulates with the scapula at the glenohumeral (GH) joint (also called shoulder joint), the body's most mobile joint, where the humeral head fits loosely into the shallow glenoid fossa of the scapula. The glenoid labrum attaches to the rim of the glenoid fossa and improves the bony fit. Two ligaments strengthen the GH joint: the glenohumeral ligament (a thickening of the anterior joint capsule) and the coracohumeral

ligament, which anchors the humerus to the coracoid process of the scapula. The GH joint's ball-and-socket structure permits triplanar motions referred to as flexion/extension (sagittal plane), abduction/adduction (frontal plane), and internal/external rotation (transverse plane). The muscles responsible for producing and controlling movements at the GH joint are shown in figure 7.2 and summarized in table 7.1. Among the most impor-

Table 7.1 Muscles of the Shoulder

Muscle	Action
Biceps brachii	Flexes the arm
Coracobrachialis	Flexes and adducts the arm
Deltoid	Abducts the arm; posterior fibers extend and laterally (externally) rotate the arm; anterior fibers flex and medially (internally) rotate the arm
Infraspinatus*	Laterally rotates and slightly adducts the arm
Latissimus dorsi	Adducts, extends, and medially rotates the arm
Pectoralis major	Adducts, flexes, and medially rotates the arm
Subscapularis*	Medially rotates the arm
Supraspinatus*	Abducts the arm
Teres major	Adducts, extends, and medially rotates the arm
Teres minor*	Laterally rotates, slightly adducts, and extends the arm
Triceps brachii (long head)	Extends the arm

*Muscles included in the rotator cuff group.

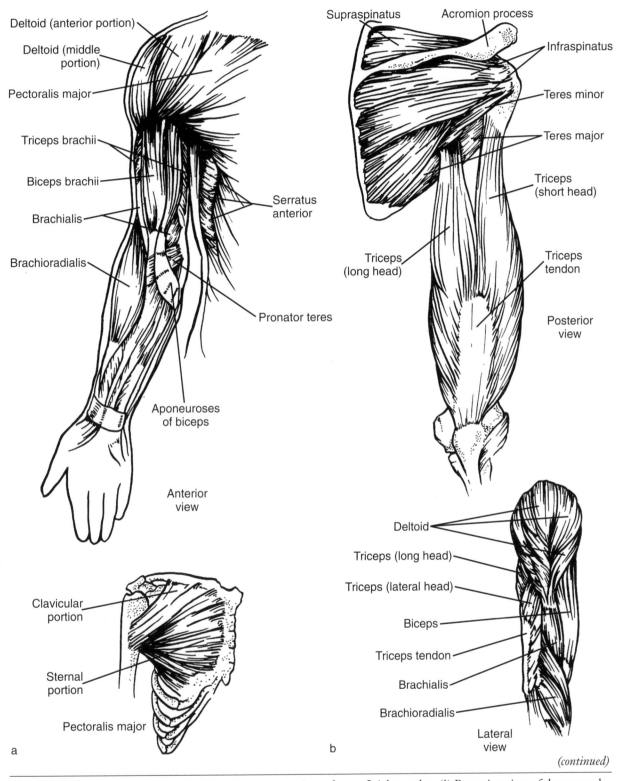

Figure 7.2   Musculature of the shoulder: (*a*) Anterior view of superficial muscles. (*b*) Posterior view of deep muscles and lateral view.

tant (and often injured) GH muscles are the four muscles of the rotator cuff group (subscapularis, supraspinatus, infraspinatus, teres minor). These muscles assist in stabilizing the GH joint by forming a "cuff" around the humeral head and pulling the humerus into the glenoid fossa.

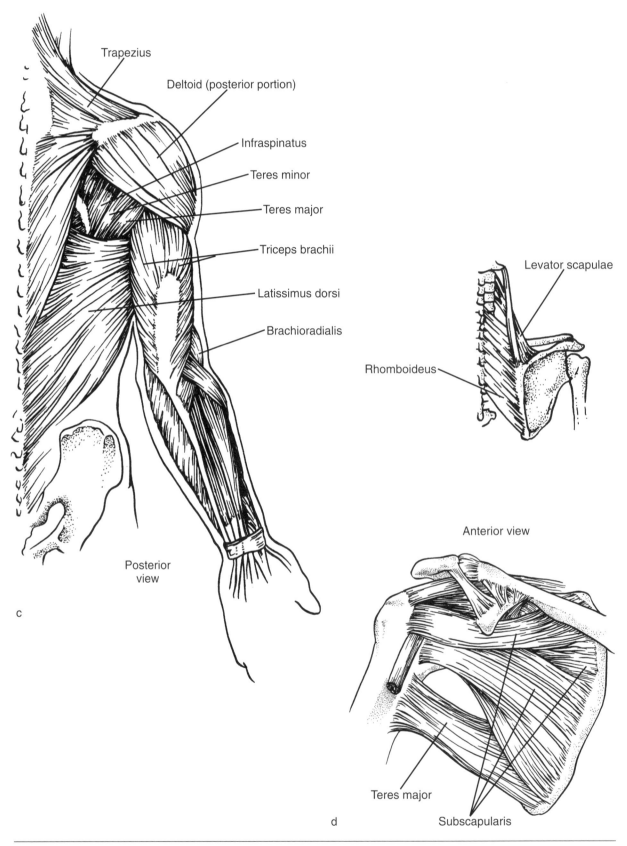

Trapezius

Deltoid (posterior portion)

Infraspinatus

Teres minor

Teres major

Triceps brachii

Latissimus dorsi

Brachioradialis

Posterior view

c

Levator scapulae

Rhomboideus

Anterior view

Teres major

Subscapularis

d

Figure 7.2 *(continued)* Musculature of the shoulder. (*c*) Posterior view of superficial muscles. (*d*) Anterior view of deep muscles.

Acromioclavicular Sprain

Acromioclavicular (AC) sprain results from applied forces that tend to displace the scapular acromion process from the distal end of the clavicle. This injury is commonly referred to as a *shoulder separation* and should not be confused with a shoulder dislocation. The synovial AC joint is classified as a plane-type joint and contains an intraarticular disk that normally degenerates with age (Horvath & Kery 1984). Superior and inferior AC ligaments provide horizontal stability, with vertical stability provided by the coracoclavicular ligaments.

Acromioclavicular injury results from either direct or indirect forces. Direct force applied to the point of the shoulder with the arm in an adducted position is the most common cause of AC injury. This mechanism is seen when a person collides with a solid object or surface (figure 7.3a). The impact force drives the acromion inferiorly relative to the clavicle. In the absence of fracture, increasing force levels cause AC injury progression from (1) mild sprain of the AC ligament, to (2) moderate AC ligament sprain with coracoclavicular ligament involvement, to (3) complete AC dislocation with tearing of clavicular attachments of the deltoid and trapezius muscles and complete rupture of the coracoclavicular ligament.

Less frequently, AC injuries result from indirect forces, as when a person falls on an outstretched arm. In this mechanism, contact forces are transmitted up the arm, through the humerus, and to the acromion. These superiorly directed loads force separation of the acromion and clavicle. On rare occasions, extreme traction forces applied to the arm may separate the acromion from its clavicular attachment (Rockwood, Williams, & Young 1996).

AC injuries are classified as six types of AC sprain and dislocation (Williams, Nguyen, & Rockwood 1989). The mechanism and resulting injuries for each of the six types are illustrated in figure 7.4.

Type I to III injuries are most common; incidence of types IV to VI is low. In type IV injuries, the clavicle is driven posteriorly by a severe force applied to the anterior aspect of the clavicle. Type V injuries are similar to type III but involve more drastic inferior displacement of the scapula. Type VI injuries occur when extreme forces are applied to the superior aspect of the clavicle and drive it inferiorly into a subacromial or subcoracoid position.

Glenohumeral Instability and Luxation

The ability of any joint to resist dislocation is directly related to its inherent stability. What the shoulder gains in mobility, it sacrifices in stability. As discussed in chapter 6, joints such as the hip, with good bony fit and extensive surrounding musculature, rarely luxate. The glenohumeral joint, in contrast, is prone to dislocation due to its relatively poor bony fit and limited supporting musculature. The shallowness of the glenoid fossa and limited contact area between the fossa and the humeral head contribute to the joint's instability. The glenoid labrum improves the joint fit to a limited extent by increasing surface area and deepening the fossa, but the fact remains that the glenohumeral joint is perhaps the least stable articulation in the body—a dubious distinction substantiated by its frequent dislocations. The factors contributing to its stability, therefore, must be understood to adequately discuss the mechanisms of glenohumeral luxation.

At the extremes of joint movement, tension in the capsuloligamentous structures provide resistance to dislocation. The laxity in these structures necessary for the exceptional movements at the glenohumeral joint precludes their involvement as stabilizers throughout normal ranges of motion. During normal ranges, other stabilizing mechanisms are necessary. These include the combined effects of limited joint volume and negative intraarticular pressure, and the mechanisms of concavity compression and scapulohumeral balance.

In a normal (undamaged capsule) glenohumeral joint, a small negative intracapsular pressure helps stabilize the joint (Speer 1995). While not especially large, this force (only 90-140N) nonetheless contributes to maintaining glenohumeral stability throughout its range of motion.

The mechanisms of concavity compression and scapulohumeral balance contribute significantly more to joint stabilization. Concavity compression refers to the stability created when a convex object is pressed into a concave surface (Lippitt & Matsen 1993). When the surfaces are pressed together, there is greater resistance to translational movement between the surfaces. At the surface between the humeral head and the glenoid fossa, numerous muscle forces increase the articular pressure and stabilize the joint. Translational resistance at the glenohumeral articulation is greater in the superior-inferior direction than in the anterior-posterior

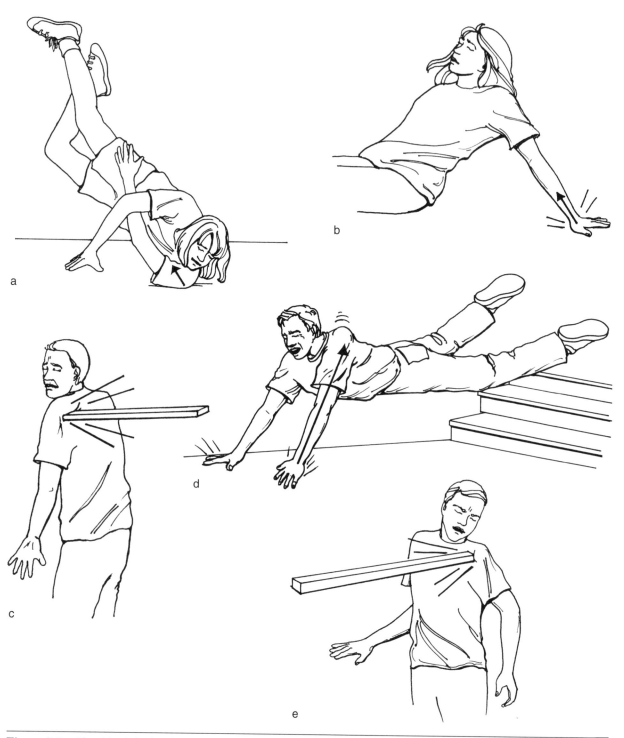

Figure 7.3 Shoulder injuries. (*a*) Acromioclavicular sprain (separated shoulder) caused by direct impact on the point of the shoulder. (*b*) Anterior glenohumeral dislocation from indirect force applied through the arm in an extended, abducted, and externally rotated position. (*c*) Anterior glenohumeral dislocation from direct force applied to the posterior aspect of the shoulder. (*d*) Posterior glenohumeral dislocation from indirect force applied through the arm in a flexed, adducted, and internally rotated position. (*e*) Posterior glenohumeral dislocation from direct force applied to the anterior aspect of the shoulder.

Parts (*a, d, e*) from *Rockwood and Green's Fractures in Adults* (4th ed.) (Fig. 20-11, p. 1351; Fig. 19-94, p. 1280; Fig. 19-93, p. 1279) by C.A. Rockwood, D.P. Green, R.W. Bucholz, & J.D. Heckman (Eds.),1996, Philadelphia: Lippincott-Raven Publishers. Copyright 1996 by Lippincott-Raven. Adapted by permission.

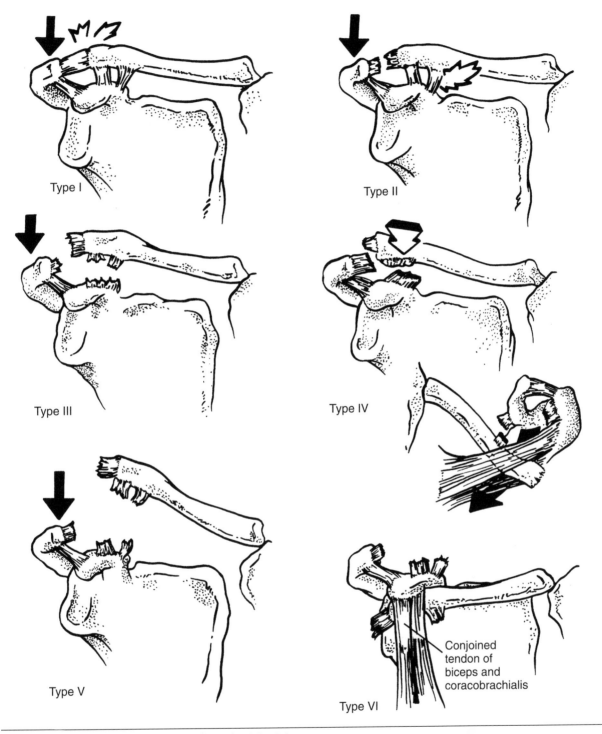

Figure 7.4   Mechanisms of acromioclavicular joint injury.

From *Rockwood and Green's Fractures in Adults* (4th ed.) (Fig. 20-14, p. 1354) by C.A. Rockwood, D.P. Green, R.W. Bucholz, & J.D. Heckman (Eds.),1996, Philadelphia: Lippincott-Raven Publishers. Copyright 1996 by Lippincott-Raven. Adapted by permission.

direction and increases with greater compressive loads (table 7.2). Despite the resistance, translation does occur with combined abduction, extension, and external rotation of the glenohumeral joint.

Harryman et al. (1990), using a three-dimensional position sensor, and force and torque transducers, reported translation of the humeral head with passive glenohumeral motion. They found

Table 7.2 Effect of Increasing Compressive Load on Glenohumeral Joint Stability

Direction	Compressive load (N)	Maximum translating force (N)
Superior: 0°	50	29 ± 7
	100	51 ± 9
Anterior: 90°	50	17 ± 6
	100	29 ± 5
Inferior: 180°	50	32 ± 4
	100	56 ± 12
Posterior: 270°	50	17 ± 6
	100	30 ± 12

From "Mechanisms of glenohumeral joint stability" by S. Lippitt & F. Matsen, 1993, *Clinical Orthopaedics and Related Research, 291* (Table 1, p. 24). Copyright 1993 by Lippincott-Raven. Adapted by permission.

significant anterior translation during glenohumeral flexion and cross-body movement, and posterior translation with extension and external rotation. Their results have clinical relevance since they indicate that the glenohumeral joint does not function purely as a ball-and-socket mechanism and that even passive manipulation of the joint causes significant translation of the humeral head across the glenoid fossa.

Scapulohumeral balance refers to the coordinated muscle action that maintains the net joint reaction force within the fossa. As seen in figure 7.5, when the reaction-force line of action is directed into the glenoid, the joint is stable. The joint becomes unstable as the line of action moves away from the geometric center of the glenoid and beyond the surface boundary. Muscular responsibility for maintaining appropriate glenohumeral congruity lies most immediately with the rotator cuff group and secondarily with the deltoid, trapezius, serratus anterior, rhomboids, latissimus dorsi, and levator scapulae. Fatigue in any of these muscles (e.g., from repeated throwing) compromises the compensatory capability of the musculoskeletal complex at the shoulder and predictably results in increased potential for injuries such as tendinitis, impingement, rotator cuff pathology, joint instability, and glenohumeral luxation.

Individuals with congenitally lax shoulders may experience atraumatic luxations in which minimal forces cause glenohumeral dislocation. Most cases of shoulder luxation, however, arise from traumatic insult to the glenohumeral complex. In the vast majority of these cases (> 90%) dislocation occurs anteriorly. Anterior luxation occurs most often from indirect forces when axial loads are applied to the abducted, extended, and externally rotated arm (figure 7.3b). Less frequently, anterior dislocation results from direct forces applied to the posterior aspect of the humerus (figure 7.3c).

Mechanisms of posterior dislocation essentially reverse those just described for anterior luxation. Indirect forces transmitted through a flexed, adducted, and internally rotated arm drive the humerus posteriorly (figure 7.3d). Posterior dislocation also results from direct trauma to the anterior aspect of the humerus (figure 7.3e). Cases have been reported in which violent muscle contractions during electrical shock or seizures have caused posterior dislocations. In such cases, the substantial forces of fully activated internal rotators (subscapularis, latissimus dorsi, pectoralis major) overwhelm the external rotators (infraspinatus, teres minor) and leverage the humeral head from the glenoid fossa. Occasional inferior dislocations occur from a hyperabduction mechanism that creates a fulcrum between the femoral neck and the acromion process, and levers the head out inferiorly.

Impingement Syndrome

In general, an impingement syndrome exists when pressure increases within a confined anatomical space and the enclosed tissues are deleteriously affected. With respect to the glenohumeral joint, impingement syndrome is an ill-defined term. It generally refers to arm abduction that results in suprahumeral structures (most notably the supraspinatus tendon and the subacromial bursae) being forcibly pressed against the anterior surface of the acromion and the coracoacromial ligament (coracoacromial arch).

Impingement pathologies fall in to two broad age-based categories. Impingement in those under 35 years usually involves sports (e.g., swimming, water polo, baseball, football) or occupations (e.g., carpenter, painter) involving extensive overhead movements. Older individuals are more likely to suffer from the effects of degenerative processes

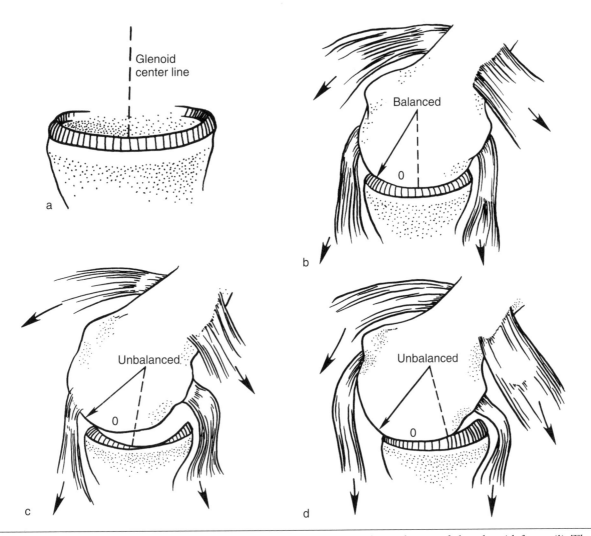

Figure 7.5   (*a*) Glenoid center line is defined as a perpendicular to the midpoint of the glenoid fossa. (*b*) The glenohumeral joint is stable in positions where the net joint reaction force is balanced within the glenoid fossa. (*c*) The glenohumeral joint is unstable in positions where the net joint reaction force is not balanced within the glenoid fossa. (*d*) Abnormal orientation of the glenoid fossa can contribute to an unbalanced and therefore unstable joint.

From "Mechanisms of glenohumeral joint stability" by S. Lippitt & F. Matsen, 1993, *Clinical Orthopaedics and Related Research* (Fig. 7, p. 26). Copyright 1993 by Lippincott-Raven. Reprinted by permission.

that lead to bone spur formation, capsular thinning, decreased tissue perfusion, and muscular atrophy.

Repeated abduction places large stresses on the musculotendinous and capsuloligamentous structures and eventually leads to tissue microtrauma. Continued mechanical loading further weakens the tissues and hastens their failure. Tissue failure, in turn, contributes to glenohumeral instability and greater joint movement. This increases the chance of humeral subluxation that further aggravates the impingement condition. Thus, the person is trapped in an unfortunate loop of joint deterioration and compromised function.

Jobe and Pink (1993) proposed an injury classification based on these age-based differences. Correct classification of the injury mechanism assists in proper diagnosis and treatment. Group I injuries are characterized by isolated impingement with no joint instability and are usually found in older recreational athletes. Group II injuries result from overuse, typically in young "overhead" athletes, and present primarily as glenohumeral instability with secondary impingement. Group III injuries also are common to young overhead athletes and are closely associated with group II. They are differentiated from group II by the presence of generalized ligamentous laxity at the elbow, knee, and fingers. The last category, group IV, includes injuries resulting from a traumatic event such as a fall or direct trauma.

The mechanisms underlying rotator cuff impingement pathologies are the subject of ongoing debate. In a broad sense, the mechanisms can be either extrinsic (forces acting outside the rotator cuff) or intrinsic (inflammatory changes within the cuff), or both. Extrinsic factors include structural characteristics of the subacromial space such as the

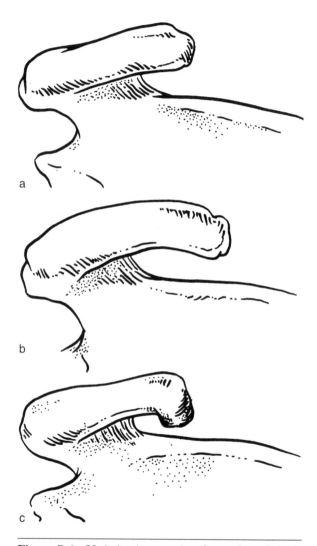

Figure 7.6   Variation in acromion shapes (lateral view). (*a*) Type I, flat. (*b*) Type II, curved. (*c*) Type III, hooked.

shape and size of the acromion. For example, a hook-type (type III) acromion (figure 7.6c) has been associated with higher incidence of rotator cuff tears. Additional extrinsic elements include bone spurs in the spaces that serve as stress risers. They

focus forces on the supraspinatus tendon and produce a functionally smaller supraspinatus outlet (Fu, Harner, & Klein 1991).

Intrinsic mechanisms have long been implicated in rotator cuff lesions due to impingement. The theory behind these mechanisms posits that the degenerative process is inherent to the supraspinatus itself, largely due to the compromised blood flow resulting from impingement pressures and regions of relative avascularity in the supraspinatus near its humeral attachment. Convincing evidence supports this concept. First, rotator cuff lesions are often seen in the absence of any extrinsic involvement. Second, studies have shown that degeneration first occurs on the articular surface of the tendon rather than on the bursal side. Support for the role of hypovascularity in impingement pathologies, however, is not universal. In light of the evidence, there is likely no single mechanism of impingement injury, rather a variety of factors specific to each individual's morphological characteristics and history of joint loading.

Risk factors for glenohumeral impingement syndrome are the same as those associated with cumulative trauma disorders of the shoulder (e.g., bicipital tendinitis, subacromial bursitis, thoracic outlet syndrome). These factors include awkward or static postures, heavy work, direct load bearing, repetitive arm movements, working with hands above shoulder height, and fatigue resulting from lack of rest.

Impingement syndrome affects special populations as well. Wheelchair athletes, for example, suffer a high incidence of rotator cuff impingement. It is suggested that muscle imbalance is a causal mechanism, and that the typical pattern of imbalance in wheelchair athletes differs from that in overhead athletes such as baseball pitchers, swimmers, and water polo players. Muscle imbalance in the overhead athlete appears as a relative weakness in the abductors and external rotators. Wheelchair athletes, in contrast, typically exhibit relative weakness in the adductors and overall rotator strength deficiency. The resulting abductor dominance exaggerates superior movement of the humeral head and leads to impingement in the subacromial space (Burnham et al. 1993).

We stress the importance of recognizing the integral relation among glenohumeral impingement, joint instability, and rotator cuff lesions. Discussion of shoulder pathology should not involve any one of these factors at the exclusion of the others.

Rotator Cuff Rupture

Rupture of musculotendinous structures in the rotator cuff is typically the final result of a chain of events that begins with minor inflammation progressing with continued overuse to advanced inflammation, microtearing of tissue, and finally partial or complete rupture. Compromised tissue integrity and muscle fatigue contribute to altered movement mechanics, and these modified movements further stress the involved tissues and hasten their eventual failure. The supraspinatus is the most commonly injured muscle in the rotator cuff group. Less frequently, other cuff muscles suffer damage. Supraspinatus injury, in particular, is associated with repeated, and often violent, overhead movement patterns (e.g., throwing, striking, hammering, painting).

The specific muscles involved depend on the shoulder movement pattern. Burkhart (1993) identified four distinct patterns of rotator cuff kinematics associated with specific cuff lesions. These patterns are summarized in table 7.3. All of the patterns involved injury to the supraspinatus. Type I (stable fulcrum kinematics) lesions showed tears of the supraspinatus and part of the infraspinatus, but not to a level that disrupted essential force couples. Patients had normal motion and near-normal strength levels.

Patients with type II lesions (unstable fulcrum kinematics, posterior cuff tear pattern) exhibited massive tears of the superior and posterior portions of the rotator cuff, which resulted in an uncoupling of the essential force couples and led to an unstable fulcrum for glenohumeral motion. Type II patients could perform little more than a shoulder shrug.

Type III (captured fulcrum kinematics) and type IV (unstable fulcrum kinematics, subscapularis tear pattern) lesions both involved tears of the subscapularis. The less-severe type III patterns had partial subscapularis tears (accompanying superior and posterior damage). Muscle damage in type III patients prevented the humeral head from centering in the glenoid fossa, and the humerus subluxated superiorly and formed a captured acromiohumeral fulcrum that restricted humeral elevation. Type IV lesions involved tears of the supraspinatus and subscapularis, with the posterior cuff muscles remaining intact. This essentially created a reversal of the type II pattern in which an unstable glenohumeral fulcrum due to the force couple imbalances was created by the muscle tears. Shoulder elevation in the type IV patients was poor (Burkhart 1993).

Many of the complex movements at the shoulder stress the muscles of the rotator cuff group. The throwing motion, in particular, places exceptional loads on the shoulder. As a result of these loads, the rotator cuff is especially susceptible to injury. The entire rotator cuff synergistically resists distraction forces that tend to pull the humeral head from the glenoid. Injury or fatigue to any of these muscles leads to altered throwing mechanics and increases the chance of additional tissue damage.

Upper-Arm Injuries

The upper arm (also called arm) spans the shoulder and elbow joints and contains the humerus, which is surrounded by two muscle compartments. The anterior compartment contains the biceps brachii, brachialis, and coracobrachialis; the posterior compartment houses only the triceps brachii, a muscle complex with three heads: the long head, medial head, and lateral head (figure 7.2). The humerus

Table 7.3 Kinematic Patterns Related to Rotator Cuff Tear Location

Kinematic pattern	Tear location
I. Stable fulcrum kinematics	Supraspinatus + part of infraspinatus
II. Unstable fulcrum kinematics (posterior cuff tear pattern)	Supraspinatus + all of posterior cuff (infraspinatus and teres minor)
III. Captured fulcrum kinematics	Supraspinatus + major posterior cuff + at least 50% subscapularis
IV. Unstable fulcrum kinematics (subscapularis tear pattern)	Supraspinatus + complete subscapularis

Adapted from Burkhart 1993.

articulates proximally with the scapula and distally with the radius and ulna at the elbow joint.

Humeral Fracture

Fractures of the humerus account for only 7% of all fractures (Praemer, Furner, & Rice 1992). Despite their low incidence, humeral fractures illustrate several important injury concepts and mechanisms. Humeral fractures result from either direct or indirect trauma. Direct injuries typically are high energy and exhibit extensive comminution and soft tissue disruption, while indirect trauma involves less energy and minimal bony displacement. The pattern of bone fracture varies: Compressive forces lead to proximal and distal end disruption; bending results in transverse shaft fracture; torsional loads create spiral fractures, and combined torsion and bending theoretically causes oblique fracture or butterfly fragmentation.

Humeral fracture results from mechanisms involved in falls on an outstretched arm, motor vehicle accidents, and direct loading of the arm. Fractures also occur in response to violent muscular contractions. The pattern of fracture depends on the magnitude, location, and direction of applied forces, with segment movement determined by the action of muscles in the area. For example, when fracture occurs proximal to the pectoralis major attachment site, the distal segment is displaced medially by the pectoralis major, while the proximal segment is abducted and internally rotated by the rotator cuff (figure 7.7a). If the fracture site is between the attachments of the pectoralis major and the deltoid, the distal segment is abducted through action of the deltoid, while the proximal segment is pulled medially by the pectoralis major, latissimus dorsi, and teres major (figure 7.7b). In fractures distal to the deltoid attachment, the proximal segment is abducted and flexed, with the distal segment displaced superiorly (figure 7.7c).

As with most injuries, age plays a prominent role in determining the nature and extent of tissue damage. Humeral fracture in older people commonly results from falls, while in younger individuals the usual culprits are direct impact or vigorous throwing. Humeral fractures have been documented as a result of throwing objects as varied as baseballs, javelins, and hand grenades. Various theories have been proposed to explain throwing-related fractures, including factors of antagonistic muscle action, violent uncoordinated muscle action, poor throwing mechanics, excessive torsional forces, and fatigue.

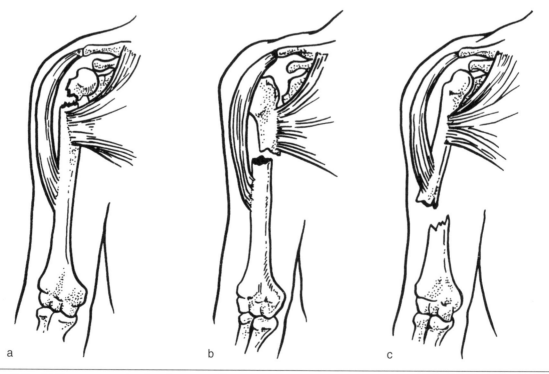

Figure 7.7   (a) Fracture proximal to the pectoralis major insertion. (b) Fracture distal to the pectoralis major insertion and proximal to the deltoid insertion. (c) Fracture distal to the deltoid insertion.

A report on a series of 12 spontaneous humeral fractures in baseball players (average age 36) who played regularly in an over-30 league, notes that the injured players had been generally inactive for years prior to joining the league. The prolonged layoff period may have contributed to disuse atrophy in the humerus and may have predisposed the athletes to both sudden and stress fractures. Four risk factors for fracture were identified: age, prolonged absence from pitching activity, lack of a regular exercise program, and prodromal (precursory) arm pain (Branch et al. 1992). As with many injuries, an individual's condition and activity pattern play an important role in determining their susceptibility to injury.

Biceps Tendon Injuries

The long head of the biceps brachii attaches proximally to the supraglenoid tuberosity in conjunction with the superior aspect of the glenoid labrum. From this attachment the biceps tendon courses through the rotator cuff interval in the bicipital groove of the humerus. Distally, the biceps brachii attaches to the radial tuberosity. The primary action of the biceps is to flex the elbow (with lesser involvement at the glenohumeral joint). It is predisposed to injury at its proximal tendon because of its intimate involvement with the action of the rotator cuff. Injuries to the biceps tendon include acute and chronic tenosynovitis, subluxation, dislocation, and rupture.

The etiology of biceps injury is unclear, in large part due to the complex interaction of impingement and instability pathologies and considerable anatomical variability. Biceps peritenonitis (tenosynovitis) is commonly associated with repeated overhead tasks such as throwing. Acutely, peritenonitis manifests as swelling and inflammation. With repeated insult, chronic peritenonitis progresses to include tendon fraying, synovial proliferation, fibrosis, and eventual tendon rupture or dislocation (Ptasznik & Hennessy 1995). The biceps tendon typically dislocates medially, often in conjunction with rotator cuff lesions and acute trauma. The mechanisms of biceps dislocation include abduction with external rotation, falls onto an outstretched hand, direct lateral impact, hyperextension, and anterior glenohumeral dislocation. Anatomical features, most notably the depth and angulation of the bicipital groove, have been implicated as predisposing factors in biceps tendon dislocation. The tendon is more likely to dislodge from a shallow or low-angled groove.

Given the integral relation between rotator cuff and biceps tendon pathologies, it is not surprising that the mechanisms that encourage cuff lesions (e.g., impingement) are strongly associated with biceps tendon degeneration as well. Rupture of the biceps tendon may be a logical consequence of progressive tissue degradation. Biceps tendon rupture has been associated with distal traction and active biceps contraction, as seen when a person is actively pulling and has his or her arm suddenly jerked distally.

The structural congruity of the glenoid labrum and biceps tendon often results in combined injuries at the bicipital-labral junction. This injury has been termed a SLAP (superior labrum anterior-posterior) lesion. While the exact mechanism of injury remains unresolved, both biceps tendon traction and humeral head traction may be involved.

Elbow Injuries

The elbow joint is structurally classified as a synovial hinge joint and is formed by dual articulations of the capitulum (humerus) with the head of the radius, and the trochlea (humerus) with the trochlear notch of the ulna (figure 7.8a). The radius and ulna articulate at the proximal radioulnar joint. Normal elbow motion is confined to uniplanar flexion/extension, with forearm pronation/supination produced by the combined rotations of the proximal and distal radioulnar joints. As a synovial joint, the elbow is surrounded by a thin fibrous capsule that runs from its proximal humeral attachment to become continuous distally with the synovial capsule of the proximal radioulnar joint.

The elbow is reinforced by the lateral (radial) collateral ligament (LCL) complex, which extends from the lateral epicondyle of the humerus to the annular ligament of the radius. It is also reinforced by the medial (ulnar) collateral ligament (MCL) complex, which connects the medial epicondyle with the coronoid process and olecranon of the ulna (figure 7.8b). The LCL complex consists of three ligaments (radial collateral ligament, annular ligament, lateral ulnohumeral ligament) and provides primary restraint against varus loading (i.e., laterally directed force on the medial aspect of the elbow). The MCL comprises three distinct bundles (anterior, posterior, transverse). The anterior and

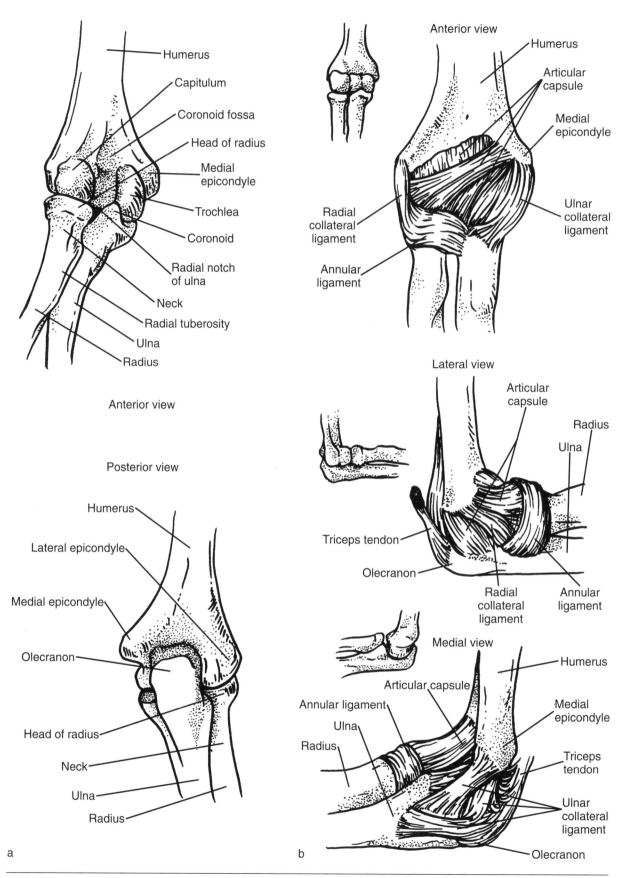

Figure 7.8 (*a*) Bones and (*b*) ligaments of the elbow joint.

posterior bundles resist valgus loading (i.e., medially directed force on the lateral aspect of the elbow), while the transverse bundle plays a minimal role in joint stabilization. Muscles controlling elbow motion are shown in figure 7.2 and summarized in table 7.4.

Table 7.4 Muscles of the Elbow

Muscle	Action
Anconeus	Extends the forearm
Biceps brachii	Flexes the forearm; also supinates the forearm and flexes the arm
Brachialis	Flexes the forearm
Brachioradialis	Flexes the forearm
Triceps brachii	Extends the forearm; long head also extends the arm

Before considering specific injuries, we will dispense up front with several pervasive "wastebasket" terms used to describe elbow injuries. The most common of these is the ubiquitous *tennis elbow*, a term with varied meanings, ranging from a general descriptor of any pain in and around the elbow to the specific designation of lateral epicondylitis. In the latter case, tennis elbow is doubly confusing since it can be interpreted to mean that tennis is solely responsible for epicondylitis or that epicondylitis is the only injury seen in tennis players. Neither of these suppositions is correct. As with previously noted terms of this type, we refrain from using the colloquial *tennis elbow* and its cousins, *Little League elbow*, *golfer's elbow*, and *climber's elbow* (Safran 1995) and instead focus on specific clinical descriptors.

Significant injuries to the elbow include epicondylitis, tendinitis, myotendinous strain, osteochondritis dissecans, osteochondrosis, dislocation, bursitis, ligamentous sprain, and fractures of the humerus, ulna, and radius. Many of these injuries are common in athletes and are specific to athletic tasks (table 7.5).

Epicondylitis

Most elbow injuries are overuse conditions characterized by progressive tissue degeneration. As with most chronic injuries, repeated loading produces tissue microtrauma before the condition becomes symptomatic. Even in asymptomatic individuals, evidence of intracytoplasmic calcification, collagen fiber splitting and kinking, and abnormal fiber cross links have been reported (Kannus and Jozsa 1991). The causes of these histopathologies have not been clearly established but may be mechanical or vascular in nature.

Continued loading worsens the microscopic damage and eventually leads to symptomatic tissue involvement in the form of inflammation, inflexibility, and tissue weakness. At the elbow these events often manifest as epicondylitis, an inflammation of soft tissue attachments on humeral epicondyles. Task specificity determines whether the medial or lateral epicondyle is involved. Lateral epicondylitis is characterized by pain of the lateral aspect of the elbow and is most often attributed to inflammation of the proximal attachment of the extensor carpi radialis brevis (ECRB).

Lateral epicondylitis is prevalent in tennis players (hence the term *tennis elbow*), with between 40% and 50% of players experiencing this injury at some time during their years of playing. The injury is most common in middle-aged players between 30 and 50 years old. The suspected causal mechanisms include faulty stroke mechanics, off-center

---

Not-So-Funny Bone

The so-called funny bone is neither a bone, nor particularly funny. The name is derived from the transient sensation of numbness and tingling experienced when you strike the posteromedial aspect of the elbow. In this area, the *ulnar nerve* passes by the posterior aspect of the humeral epicondyle on its way from the shoulder to the forearm and hand. Violent compression on the ulnar nerve against the humerus causes a temporary blockage of the flow of nerve impulses. This creates the "funny" sensation you feel upon striking this nerve.

Table 7.5   Sport-Specific Elbow Injuries

Sport	Injury
Archery	Extensor muscle fatigue, lateral epicondylitis of bow arm
Baseball	Valgus stress of pitching, medial traction, lateral compression, posterior abutment
Basketball	Posterior compartment syndrome with follow-through on jump shot
Bowling	Flexor-pronator soreness
Canoeing, kayaking	Distal bicipital tendinitis
Football	Valgus stress with throwing a pass; hyperextension and dislocation, olecranon bursitis with direct trauma
Golf	Medial epicondylitis on downswing with trailing arm; lateral epicondylitis at impact with leading arm on backhand
Gymnastics	Radiocapitellar overload, posterior impingement, dislocation, olecranon bursitis with direct trauma
Javelin	Valgus extension overload of throwing, medial traction, posterior abutment, lateral compression
Racquet sports	Lateral epicondylitis with backhand
Rock climbing	Brachialis or distal biceps tendinitis
Shot put	Posterior impingement with follow-through
Volleyball	Valgus stress at impact of spiking
Waterskiing	Valgus extension overload of posterior compartment
Weight training	Ulnar collateral ligament sprain, ulnar nerve irritation

From "Elbow injuries in athletes: A review" by M.R. Safran, 1995, *Clinical Orthopaedics and Related Research, 310* (p. 258). Copyright 1995 by Lippincott-Raven. Adapted by permission.

ball contact, grip tightness, and racquet vibration. Repeated impact of the racquet and ball stresses the muscles that stabilize and control movement of the wrist. These stresses can result from both concentric and eccentric muscle action.

The mechanics of the backhand stroke in particular have been associated with the incidence of lateral epicondylitis (Priest, Braden, & Gerberich 1980). Electromyographic studies have shown high levels of wrist extensor activity, especially in the ECRB, during the backhand stroke (Giangarra et al. 1993; Morris et al. 1989). When a player (usually a novice) leads with the elbow, greater forces are generated in the wrist extensors. These loads are transferred through the active and stiffened musculature to the proximal attachment on the lateral humerus. Use of a two-handed backhand stroke has been associated with a lower incidence of lateral epicondylitis because the simplified and coordinated action of trunk rotation and arm movement imposes fewer mechanical demands on the musculoskeletal system.

Lateral epicondylitis is not an injury exclusive to tennis. Other striking sports such as racquetball and golf are implicated, as are occupations involving repetitive motions of the wrist and elbow (e.g., carpenters and surgeons). Research has shown that pinching and grasping of the fingers and hand always produce flexor moments at the wrist and that extensor moments are generated to maintain equilibrium. Overuse of the extensor mechanism in repeated pinching and grasping, such as in chronic work with hand tools or writing, increases the susceptibility to lateral epicondylitis (Snijders et al. 1987).

Medial epicondylitis occurs infrequently compared with lateral epicondylitis in tennis. Medial epicondylitis results from excessive loading during the forehand and service strokes. These motions, especially by advanced players, involve forcible extension of the wrist. The eccentric action of the wrist flexor muscles in controlling wrist extension places considerable stress on these muscles and their attachments on the medial aspect of the humerus. Medial epicondylitis occurs more often in throwers (e.g., baseball, javelin) whose movement patterns include a high-velocity valgus extension mechanism (Wilson et al. 1983).

Valgus Extension Loading Injuries

Numerous studies have examined the kinematics, kinetics, and muscle involvement at the elbow during the throwing motion. The throwing motion is divided into five phases: windup, cocking, acceleration, deceleration, and follow-through. A sixth phase, stride, is sometimes included between windup and cocking.

Several studies (e.g., Fleisig et al. 1995) have quantified elbow kinetics during throwing, and reported large and potentially injurious forces and moments. Near the end of the cocking phase when the elbow is approaching terminal extension, the elbow experiences valgus loading that is resisted by a varus torque produced by musculotendinous and periarticular tissues (figure 7.9). Varus torques at this point have been estimated as ranging from 64 to 120 N·m, with predicted joint force between the

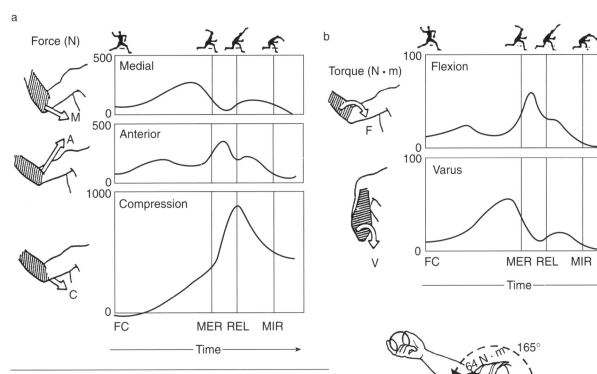

Figure 7.9   Kinetics of baseball pitching. (*a*) Force applied to the forearm at the elbow in the medial (M), anterior (A), and compression (C) directions. The instants of front foot contact (FC), maximum external rotation (MER), ball release (REL), and maximum internal rotation (MIR) torque are shown. (*b*) Torques applied to the forearm at the elbow in the flexion (F) and varus (V) directions. (*c*) Shortly before maximum external rotation, the arm was externally rotated 165°, and the elbow was flexed 95°. At this instant there were 67 N·m of internal rotation torque, 310 N of anterior force at the shoulder, and 64 N·m of varus torque at the elbow.

Adapted from Fleisig et al. 1995.

radius and humerus of approximately 500 N (Fleisig et al. 1995; Werner et al. 1993).

The coupling of valgus torque and elbow extension produces a so-called valgus extension overload mechanism that can lead to medial elbow injuries, including epicondylitis, ulnar collateral ligament rupture, avulsion fracture, and nerve damage. In addition, the valgus stress in extension causes impingement of the medial aspect of the olecranon on the olecranon fossa and radial head impingement on the capitulum. Repeated impingement leads to inflammation, chondromalacia, and osteophyte formation.

We see in throwing, as in other dynamic movements, that the largest loads are developed during eccentric actions that resist and control high-velocity motion. Repeated application of these high loads may lead to progressive degeneration and eventual tissue failure. We emphasize that although this process is common, it is not inevitable. Some athletes and workers are able to repeatedly load their tissues with minimal, if any, symptomatic response. Why does a particular loading history cause injury in one person but not in another? The answer likely lies in the fact that injury is a multifactorial puzzle and that some individuals are more susceptible to injury than others. To define this susceptibility, Meeuwisse (1994) recently proposed a model that incorporates both intrinsic (e.g., age, strength, flexibility, previous injury) and extrinsic (e.g., biomechanics of movement skills, equipment, environmental conditions, schedule, inherent demands) factors.

Throwing, by its repetitive nature, provides an instructive example of chronic injury development and the interactive nature of these intrinsic and extrinsic factors. Kibler (1995) characterized progressive degeneration as a negative feedback cycle in which five complexes interact to create a downward spiral, or vicious cycle, leading to tissue failure. The five complexes are: (1) tissue overload, (2) clinical symptoms, (3) tissue injury, (4) functional biomechanical deficit, and (5) subclinical adaptation (Kibler 1995).

Applying this model to the throwing motion, for example, we see how the complexes interactively contribute to elbow injury. During the late cocking phase, the valgus extension mechanism causes tissue overload on the medial aspect of the elbow in the form of asymptomatic microtrauma. Repeated mechanical insults lead to clinical symptoms of point tenderness over the medial epicondyle and tissue injury to flexor-pronator group attachments and ulnar collateral ligaments. The elbow then suffers functional biomechanical deficits in the form of flexor-pronator inflexibility and weakness, coupled with elbow inflexibility and muscle imbalance. The thrower then alters his or her technique (subclinical adaptation) in an attempt to compensate for the deficits. These compensations further overload the tissues, and the insidious cycle continues until ultimate tissue failure. Appropriate rehabilitation must address all five complexes to break the negative feedback cycle.

Elbow Dislocation

Given the elbow's relative stability, it is not surprising that the elbow is more than three times less likely than the shoulder to become dislocated (Praemer, Furner, & Rice 1992). Elbow dislocation, nonetheless, is not uncommon. Joint luxations are rarely isolated, but rather they are accompanied by extensive soft tissue damage as the bones are forcibly displaced. Elbow dislocations follow this pattern and typically involve complete rupture or avulsion of both the ulnar and radial collateral ligaments. Elbow dislocation is most prevalent in younger individuals and in conjunction with sport activities.

The elbow's bony configuration provides exceptional resistance to anterior dislocation. In fact, the majority of dislocations are posterior. The most likely mechanism of injury involves axial force application to an extended or hyperextended elbow. This force effectively levers the ulna out of the trochlea and causes capsular and ligament rupture that then allows joint dislocation (Hotchkiss 1996). During the forcible hyperextension, the joint's alignment also creates valgus stresses that can lead to rupture of the medial collateral ligament and sometimes rupture at the origin of the flexor-pronator group on the medial aspect of the humerus.

Elbow Fractures

Fractures can occur to any of the three bones (humerus, ulna, radius) of the elbow. The involvement of each depends on the applied forces' nature, magnitude, location, and direction. Humeral fractures can involve various areas of the distal humerus including the supracondylar, intercondylar (Y- and T-fractures), condylar, epicondylar, and articular regions. Ulnar fractures commonly involve the olecranon and result either from direct and violent impact to the posterior aspect of the elbow or indirectly from falls that load the elbow joint. Radial head fractures most often result from either longitudinal loading of the radius as a result of a fall (figure 7.10) or accompanying elbow dislocation. Radioulnar fractures are more fully described in the following section.

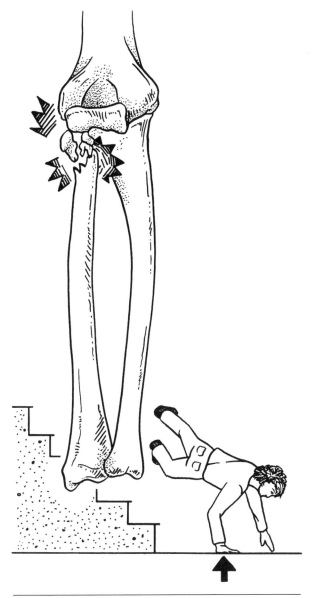

Figure 7.10   Mechanism of proximal radius fracture. The forces at impact are transmitted through the radius to the radial head.

Forearm Injuries

The forearm spans the elbow and wrist joints and consists of two longitudinally aligned bones, the radius (lateral) and ulna (medial), surrounded by numerous muscles that function at the elbow, radioulnar, and wrist joints and whose distal tendons continue to the hand to control finger movements. The forearm muscles are divided into two major groups: the flexor-pronator group and extensor-supinator group. Specific muscles in each of these groups are presented in table 7.6.

The radius and ulna articulate with one another at the proximal radioulnar joint, a synovial pivot joint between the head of the radius and the ulnar radial notch, and at the distal radioulnar joint, a synovial pivot joint articulating the head of the ulna with the ulnar notch of the radius. Coordinated action of these two joints creates the forearm motions of pronation and supination. In pronation, the radius rolls over a relatively fixed ulna. The reverse occurs in supination when the radius returns to its anatomical position (figure 7.11).

Diaphyseal Fractures of the Radius and Ulna

Fractures of the radius and ulna can occur in isolation or combination, with numerous suggested injury mechanisms. Identification of the specific mechanism involved in a given injury is important since it suggests the location and type of fracture. Combined injury to both the radius and ulna typically involves direct, high-energy trauma, such as motor vehicle accidents or gunshot wounds, or the lower-energy impact of a fall.

Isolated fractures of the upper two thirds of the radius (proximal fractures) are rare because of the protection offered by the overlying musculature. Forces sufficient to cause radial fracture in this region most often fracture the ulnar shaft as well. Fracture at the junction between the middle and distal thirds of the radius is more common and is often associated with injury to the distal radioulnar joint. Fractures of the distal third of the radius are termed *Galeazzi fractures* (after Galeazzi 1934) and result most often from a fall on an outstretched arm or a direct blow on the dorsolateral side of the wrist.

Isolated fracture of the ulna arises from various mechanisms. Injury from direct trauma is colloquially termed a *nightstick fracture*, referring to the situation in which a person, in response to an impending overhead blow, raises his or her arm and exposes the medial surface to impact. Another mechanism of isolated ulnar fracture involves dislocation of the radial epiphysis. This mechanism was originally suggested in 1814 by Monteggia, who

Table 7.6 Muscles of the Forearm

Flexor-pronator group	Extensor-supinator group
Superficial group	Extensors, abductors, and adductors of the wrist
Pronator teres	Extensor carpi radialis longus
Flexor carpi radialis	Extensor carpi radialis brevis
Palmaris longus	Extensor carpi ulnaris
Flexor carpi ulnaris	
Flexor digitorum superficialis	Extensors of the four medial digits
	Extensor digitorum
Deep group	Extensor indicis
Flexor digitorum profundus	Extensor digiti minimi
Flexor pollicis longus	
Pronator quadratus	Extensors and abductors of the thumb
	Abductor pollicis longus
	Extensor pollicis brevis
	Extensor pollicis longus

described fracture of the proximal ulna associated with anterior dislocation of the radial head. Bado (1967) proposed the term *Monteggia lesion* and enlarged the scope of the injury to include all ulnar fractures resulting from radial epiphyseal luxation. Bado suggested a classification system consisting of four types of injury. These types I through IV are depicted in figure 7.12. Type I Monteggia fractures are the most common, resulting from forced pronation that causes ulnar fracture and eventual anterior displacement of the radial head. Type IV injuries have a similar mechanism with the added presence of radial fracture.

Type II fractures are a result of posterior elbow dislocation in which the ulnar shaft fractures before ulnar collateral ligament failure. Recently four subtypes of type II injuries have been identified based on the location and loading mechanism (bending, shearing, compression) of the ulnar fracture (Jupiter et al. 1991). Type III lesions occur from laterally directed forces causing forearm abduction.

Given the importance of the forearm in mediating movement between the elbow and fingers, accurate assessment of injury mechanisms and attention to the details of diagnosis and treatment are of primary importance.

Fracture of the Distal Radius

Fractures of the distal radius are common, accounting for up to one sixth of all fractures. Young males and older females greatly outnumber their opposite-gender counterparts in the incidence of fracture.

The literature is replete with eponyms for fractures of the distal radius. These include *Colles'*, *Smith's*, and *Barton's fractures*, each with their own distinguishing characteristics. Here, we will use the clinical descriptions with parenthetical reference to corresponding eponymic designations.

Many classification systems have been proposed to describe distal radial fractures. The most useful system groups these fractures according to their mechanisms of injury rather than by radiological characteristics (Jupiter & Fernandez 1996). Five types are included: type I, bending fractures; type II, shearing fractures of the joint surface; type III, compression fractures of the joint surface; type IV, avulsion fractures; and type V, combined fractures (figure 7.13).

Type I bending fractures result from landing on an outstretched arm. Axial compressive loads cause bending of the radius with a fracture pattern (Colles' fracture) showing volar (anterior) metaphyseal cortex failure in tension and varying degrees of comminution on the dorsal (posterior) surface. These type I injuries constitute the majority of distal radial fractures. An opposite bending results from a fall on either a flexed wrist or an outstretched and supinated arm. The compressive loading then results in tensile failure (Smith's fracture) on the dorsal aspect of the metaphysis and compressive comminution on the volar aspect. This fracture pattern also is seen

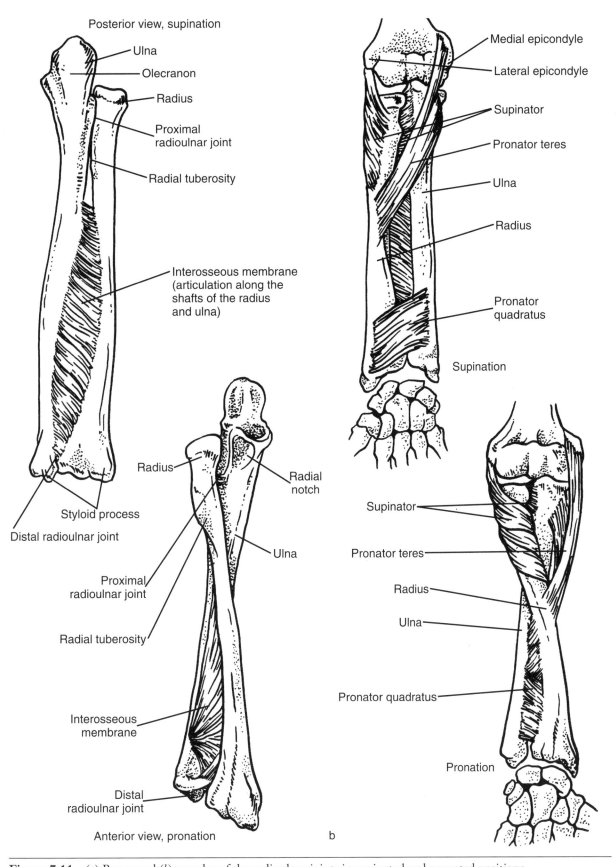

Figure 7.11 (*a*) Bones and (*b*) muscles of the radioulnar joints in supinated and pronated positions.

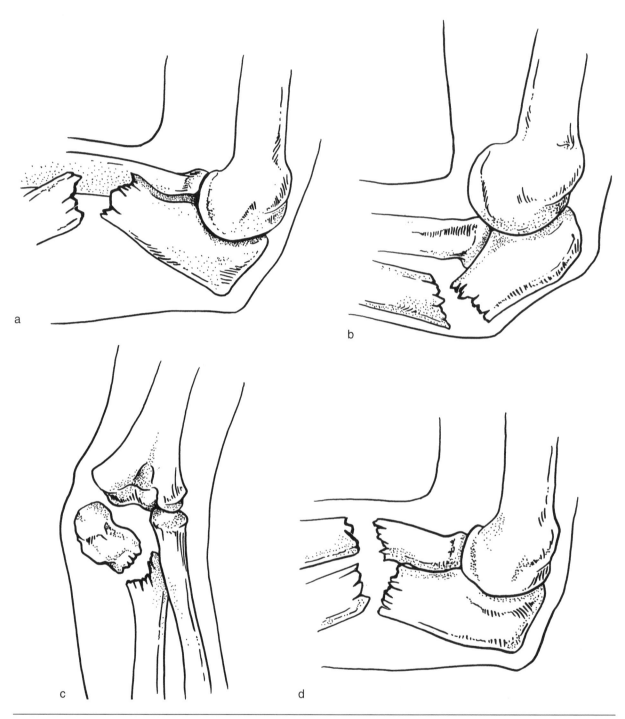

Figure 7.12 Classification of Monteggia fractures. (*a*) Type I, anterior dislocation of radial head and fracture of ulnar diaphysis with anterior angulation. (*b*) Type II, posterior or posterolateral dislocation of radial head and fracture of ulnar diaphysis with posterior angulation. (*c*) Type III, lateral or anterolateral dislocation of radial head and fracture of ulnar metaphysis. (*d*) Type IV, anterior dislocation of radial head and fracture of proximal third of radius and ulna.

when a slightly flexed clenched fist impacts on a rigid surface.

High-energy loading, particularly in young individuals, produces type II shearing fracture (Barton's fracture) in which the volar lip of the radial articular surface is sheared off. In type III fractures, high compressive loads (such as those generated in landing from a high fall) cause intraarticular fractures of

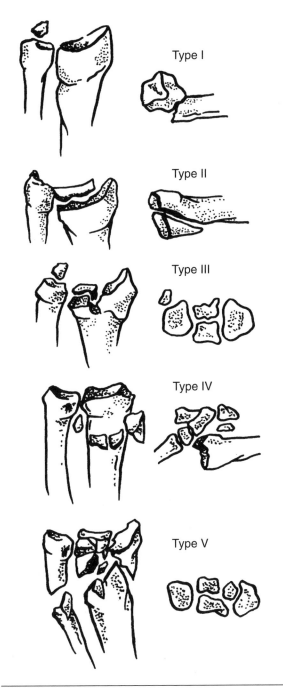

Type I

Type II

Type III

Type IV

Type V

Figure 7.13 Fractures of the distal radius (see text for explanation).

From *Fractures of the Distal Radius* (Table 2.3, p. 49) by D.L. Fernandez & J.B. Jupiter, 1996, New York: Springer-Verlag. Copyright 1996 by Springer-Verlag. Adapted by permission.

the joint surface with disruption of the subchondral and cancellous bone.

Mechanical loading that creates high stresses on the osteoligamentous attachments, as in exaggerated torsion, produces avulsion (type IV) fractures. The most complex mechanism of distal radial frac-

ture is type V, or combined fracture, that usually results from high-energy injuries including combinations of bending, compression, shearing, or avulsion mechanisms.

Ulnar Variance

The relative lengths of the ulna and radius play an important role in forearm and wrist mechanics. This length difference is referred to as ulnar variance (UV). If the two bones are the same length (within 1 mm), UV is zero. When the ulna is longer than the radius, there exists a positive ulnar variance. Conversely, a negative ulnar variance exists when radial length exceeds ulnar length. Measures of UV vary, with reported means ranging from –0.84 mm to +0.2 mm (Nakamura et al. 1991; Kristensen, Thomassen, & Christensen 1986). Caution is warranted in interpreting mean values since UV varies by age, ethnicity, and possibly gender.

Ulnar variance is determined by age, genetics, elbow pathology, and loading history (De Smet 1994). The last of these factors is most relevant to our discussion of injury mechanisms. Though the wrist is not designed to function as a load-bearing joint, certain activities (e.g., gymnastics) expose the wrist to considerable loads. These compressive loads are transmitted through the carpals to the radius and ulna, with the radius accepting approximately 80% of the load. In cases of repetitive compressive loading in the skeletally immature individual, this loading differential dictates premature closure of the radial growth plate. Continued growth of the ulna then creates an acquired ulnar variance. Gymnasts are especially prone to UV. The dual risk factors of early onset (beginning training at a relatively young age) and repetitive upper-extremity load bearing account for the prevalence of wrist lesions in this population.

Certain gymnastic skills place the athlete's wrist at particular risk. The back handspring, for example, loads the wrist with forces up to 2.4 times body weight, with the radius accepting most of the load (Koh, Grabiner, & Weiker 1992). For men, the pommel horse is the main culprit. Joint forces of up to two times body weight and loading rates of up to 219 times body weight per second have been reported (Markolf et al. 1990). Clearly, the gymnast's wrist assumes a load-bearing role for which it is ill designed. The consequences manifest in an ulnar impaction syndrome, characterized by progressive degeneration of the triangular fibrocartilage complex and the ulnar carpus.

With respect to joint loading, the critical question is: How much is too much? Due to the multifactorial nature of the problem, the question remains problematic and unresolved. Some guidance is provided by a recent study that examined factors associated with wrist pain in young gymnasts. Training intensity, relative to the age of the participant and the age when training began, seems to be a critical determinant of wrist pain development (DiFiori et al. 1996).

Wrist and Hand Injuries

The wrist is not a single joint, but rather a group of articulations that includes the distal radioulnar, radiocarpal, and intercarpal joints. The hand contains numerous articulations, namely the carpometacarpal (CM), metacarpophalangeal (MP), and interphalangeal (IP) joints (figure 7.14). All of these are synovial joints. Structurally, the MP joints are condyloid, while the IP joints are hinge joints. Both MP and IP joints are strengthened by palmar and collateral ligaments.

Muscles in the forearm primarily control wrist and finger motion with assistance from intrinsic muscles of the hand. The distal tendons of most flexor muscles in the forearm pass along the ventral aspect of the wrist, where they are held firmly in place by the flexor retinaculum, a thick and relatively inextensible fascial sheath. These tendons, along with neurovascular structures, pass through the so-called carpal tunnel formed by the carpal bones and the flexor retinaculum (figure 7.15). The distal tendons of the extensors are secured similarly between the carpal bones and the extensor retinaculum.

Carpal Tunnel Syndrome

Injuries resulting from repeated tissue stress are collectively known as cumulative trauma disorders (CTDs; also called repetitive strain injury, chronic microtrauma, overuse syndrome, cumulative trauma

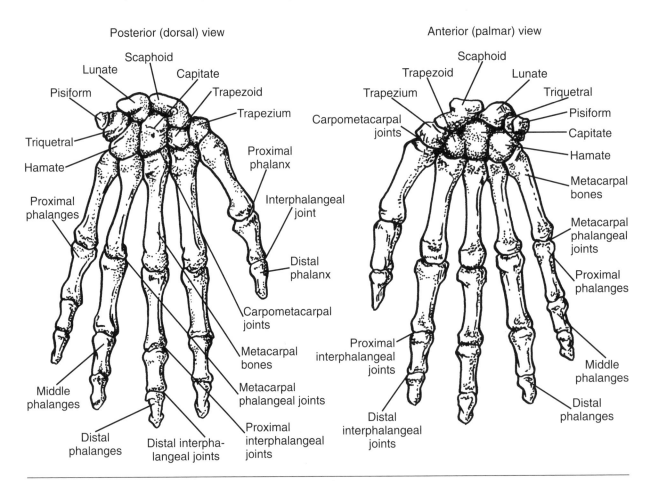

Figure 7.14 Bones and articulations of the wrist and hand.

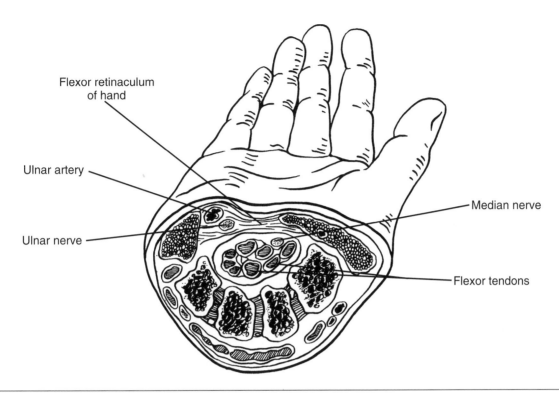

Flexor retinaculum
of hand

Ulnar artery

Ulnar nerve

Median nerve

Flexor tendons

Figure 7.15 Structure of the carpal tunnel. Neurovascular structures, including the median nerve, pass through the carpal tunnel bounded by the flexor retinaculum and the carpal bones.

syndrome). These chronic injuries have been increasing at an alarming rate, especially in occupational settings, and account for 64% of all new occupational illnesses (Bureau of Labor Statistics estimate for 1994; National Safety Council 1996). CTDs are prevalent in many occupations and prove costly in both economic and human terms.

One of the most debilitating chronic disorders is carpal tunnel syndrome (CTS), a condition characterized by swelling within the carpal tunnel that creates a compressive neuropathy affecting the median nerve (figure 7.15). As with other entrapment syndromes, CTS is characterized by increased pressure within a confined space. The inextensible borders formed by the carpal bones and the flexor retinaculum preclude an increase in tunnel size. Inflammation and edema in response to repeated loading compresses neurovascular tissues and compromises their function. Of greatest consequence is compression of the median nerve, which results in sensory symptoms of numbness, tingling, burning, and pain in the wrist and radial 3 1/2 fingers. Sensory deficits from CTS are more pronounced than reductions in motor function.

Symptoms of CTS are associated with specific movement patterns (e.g., wrist flexion/exten-

sion), and tasks (e.g., assembly work, typing, playing a musical instrument, polishing, sanding, scrubbing, hammering). Carpal tunnel syndrome has also been documented in workers across a diverse range of jobs, including keyboard operators, sheet metal workers, supermarket checkers, sheep shearers, fish-processing workers, and sign language interpreters. Making a causal connection in all cases warrants caution, however, since discrimination between work-related and non-work-related cases of CTS sometimes is tenuous. The prevalence of self-reported CTS in the general population has been estimated at about 1.5%, with confirmed cases less frequent. CTS is more common among women than men.

The etiology of CTS is complex since many mechanisms and risk factors play a contributing role. Accurate diagnosis of CTS is sometimes difficult initially since repetitive stress is implicated in other hand and wrist pathologies such as tendinitis. Once diagnosed, CTS remains mechanically problematic due to the multiple risk factors. These include forceful exertions, repetitive or prolonged activities, awkward postures, localized contact stresses, vibration, and cold temperatures.

Silverstein, Fine, and Armstrong (1987) evaluated 652 workers to assess the role of force and repetition on the prevalence of CTS in workers. They found the lowest prevalence (0.6%) in those with low-force, low-repetition jobs and the highest occurrence (5.6%) in workers in high-force, highly repetitive jobs. Of the two factors, they concluded that high repetitiveness appeared to be a greater risk factor than high force. Though studies such as this shed some light on the relation among CTS risk factors, unraveling the interrelations and relative contributions of all risk factors remains a challenge.

Carpal Fractures

Wrist fractures encompass osseous injury to the radius and ulna (discussed earlier) and fractures to any of the eight carpal bones. The most common mechanism of injury is a compressive load applied to a hyperextended (dorsiflexed) wrist (figure 7.16). Other, less-common mechanisms have been implicated in carpal fracture. These mechanisms include hyperflexion and rotational loading against a fixed object or surface.

The vast majority of carpal fractures occur when axial loads are transmitted through a hyperextended

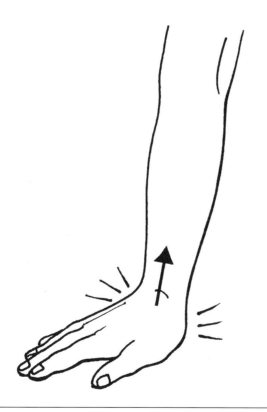

Figure 7.16 Mechanism of injury due to compressive load applied to a hyperextended wrist at impact.

wrist. With the wrist in this position, compressive forces are transmitted through the carpals to the distal radioulnar complex. Predictably, certain carpals are more likely to suffer injury than others. Mitigating influences include the degree of radial or ulnar deviation, amount of energy absorbed, point of application and direction of the applied forces, and relative strength of the bones and ligaments.

Given an 80:20% load distribution between the radius and ulna, respectively, the scaphoid and lunate are the most likely to be fractured because of their articulations with the radius. Scaphoid fractures alone account for 60% to 70% of all carpal fractures (Botte & Gelberman 1987). Scaphoid fractures are most likely to occur when the wrist is hyperextended past 95° and the radial portion of the palm accepts most of the load (Weber & Chao 1978).

Lunate fractures are second in frequency and typically result from compressive forces applied through the capitate, which push the lunate ulnarly and exacerbate the dorsal rotation caused by wrist hyperextension. The forces resisting these movements tend to cause transverse lunate fractures. Fractures of the other carpals are relatively rare, with injury mechanisms ranging from a direct blow to impingement caused by hyperflexion or hyperextension.

Thumb Injuries

The thumb is essential to our prehensile abilities, as it is the digit that opposes the four other fingers. Injury to the thumb can severely impair a person's manual dexterity. We describe three common thumb injuries (sprain, fracture, and neural lesion) to illustrate injury mechanisms that can cause significant impairment of thumb function.

The most common sprain in the hand damages the ulnar collateral ligament of the first metacarpophalangeal joint (figure 7.17a). This injury, colloquially referred to as *gamekeeper's thumb* or *skier's thumb*, can involve chronic tensile loading (stretching) of the ligament or acute loading that result in any level of sprain, including complete rupture (figure 7.17b). This injury most commonly occurs when a skier falls onto an outstretched hand with the thumb in an abducted position. The ski pole handle effectively holds the thumb in abduction as the compressive load of the fall is accepted by the hand. The forceful abduction places excessive tensile loads on the ulnar collateral ligament and hastens its failure.

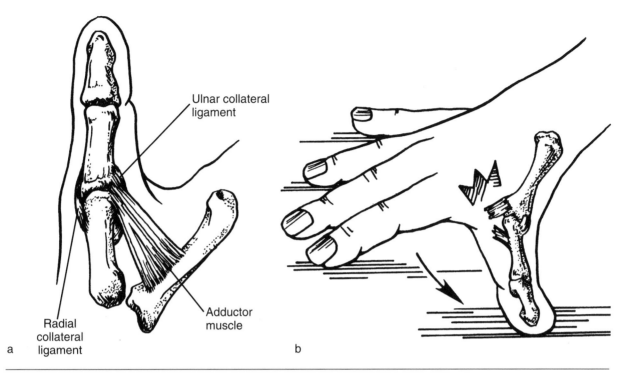

Figure 7.17   Mechanism of first metacarpophalangeal (MCP) sprain. (*a*) Collateral ligaments of the first MCP joint. (*b*) Abductor mechanism causing severe sprain (rupture) of a skier's thumb.

Ulnar collateral sprain also can result from hyperextension of the first metacarpophalangeal joint, such as when a collision occurs between two athletes. A softball player tagging an opponent who is sliding into second base may have her thumb forcibly hyperextended by the contact force between her thumb and the foot or leg of the incoming base runner.

Fracture subluxation of the trapeziometacarpal joint (Bennett's fracture) is an intraarticular fracture of the first metacarpal (thumb) resulting from axial force applied when the metacarpal bone is in flexion. Many circumstances can cause this injury, but it is classically observed as a result of a poorly delivered punch in a boxing match or fistfight.

Our third injury is a neural lesion characterized by perineural fibrosis of the ulnar digital nerve of the thumb. Known as *bowler's thumb*, this injury most commonly involves symptoms of paresthesia (tingling) and, to a lesser extent, tenderness and hyperesthesia (pathological sensitivity). The injury mechanism is repeated blunt trauma to the thumb's ulnar digital nerve caused by the gripping and release of a bowling ball. This condition can be treated conservatively or prevented by redrilling the bowling ball or modifying the grip mechanics to lessen the repetitive trauma to the nerve.

Metacarpal and Phalangeal Conditions

The pattern of fracture and dislocation involving the metacarpals and phalanges directly depends on the circumstances of injury (direct impact, crushing, indirect trauma) and the nature of the force application (e.g., magnitude, location, direction). Among the implicated injury mechanisms are direct trauma caused by an implement or fall, forcible hyperextension or hyperflexion, twisting forces, violent distraction, forced leverage, crushing, or a combination of these mechanisms.

Concluding Comments

We use our upper extremities primarily to interact with our immediate environment in intricate and exquisite ways. Impairment to any structural component of the upper limb compromises our ability to effectively manipulate things within our reach. This loss of dexterity can have profound effects on our ability to efficiently perform activities of daily living. People with severe arthritis of the hands, for example, may experience great difficulty in performing even simple grasping or manipulative tasks.

Acute or chronic injuries to any of the upper-extremity joints can cause a person to adjust his or her work or recreational activities. In cases of severe injury, the victim may have to cease certain activities altogether. If these activities serve as his or her means of survival, injury can cause drastic hardships.

Suggested Readings

Shoulder

Andrews, J.R., & Wilk, K.E. (Eds.). (1994). *The Athlete's Shoulder.* New York: Churchill Livingstone.

Burkhead, W.Z., Jr. (Ed.). (1996). *Rotator Cuff Disorders.* Baltimore: Williams & Wilkins.

Elbow

Morrey, B.F. (Ed.). (1993). *The Elbow and its Disorders* (2nd ed.). Philadelphia: Saunders.

Wrist and Hand

Gilula, L.A. (Ed.). (1992). *The Traumatized Hand and Wrist.* Philadelphia: Saunders.

General Sources

Browner, B.D., Jupiter, J.B., Levine, A.M., & Levine, P.G. (1992). *Skeletal Trauma.* Philadelphia: Saunders.

Feliciano, D.V., Moore, E.E., & Mattox, K.L. (Eds.). (1996). *Trauma* (3rd ed.). Stamford, CT: Appleton & Lange.

Fu, F.H., & Stone, D.A. (1994). *Sports Injuries: Mechanisms, Prevention, Treatment.* Baltimore: Williams & Wilkins.

Nicholas, J.A., & Hershman, E.B. (Eds.). (1995). *The Upper Extremity in Sports Medicine* (2nd ed.). St. Louis: Mosby-Year Book.

Richards, R.R. (1995). *Soft Tissue Reconstruction of the Upper Extremity.* New York: Churchill Livingstone.

Rockwood, C.A., Jr., Green, D.P., Bucholz, R.W., & Heckman, J.D. (Eds.). (1996). *Rockwood and Green's Fractures in Adults* (4th ed.). Philadelphia: Lippincott-Raven.

Woo, S.L.-Y., & Buckwalter, J.A. (Eds.). (1988). *Injury and Repair of the Musculoskeletal Soft Tissues.* Park Ridge, IL: American Academy of Orthopaedic Surgeons.

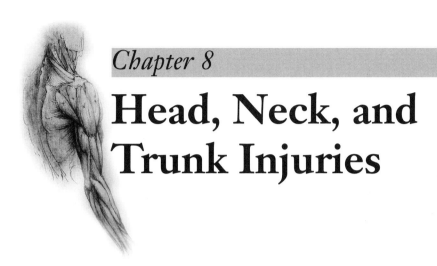

Chapter 8

Head, Neck, and Trunk Injuries

The doctors X-rayed my head and found nothing.
Dizzy Dean, Hall of Fame baseball pitcher, after being hit
on the head by a ball during the 1934 World Series

Of all the body's regions, the head, neck, and trunk are of paramount importance in controlling life-sustaining processes. Trauma to structures in these regions (e.g., brain, spinal cord, heart) poses the greatest danger to our physical well-being. In the preceding two chapters we discussed numerous injuries to the extremities that result in disability but rarely with fatal consequences. Injuries to the head, neck, and trunk, in contrast, have real and immediate potential to be fatal. An understanding of the mechanisms responsible for these injuries can assist with their proper diagnosis, treatment, and prevention.

Head Injuries

The head comprises the skull, brain, meninges, cranial nerves, and sense organs. Structures in the head are protected by an intricate collection of 29 bones. The brain and its protective meningeal covering are contained in a cranial vault composed of eight cranial bones: frontal, occipital, ethmoid, and sphenoid bones, and paired temporal and parietal bones (figure 8.1). The anterior and anterolateral aspects of the head are formed by 14 facial bones: paired nasal, maxillae (upper jaw), zygomatic (cheek), lacrimal, palatine, and inferior nasal conchae bones and singular mandible (lower jaw) and vomer bones. Of the seven remaining bones of the head, six are housed in the ear. These bones are collectively referred to as auditory ossicles (paired incus, stapes, and malleolus bones). The final bone is the hyoid, which is suspended from the styloid process of the temporal bone by ligaments and muscles.

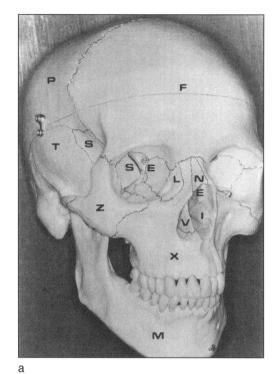
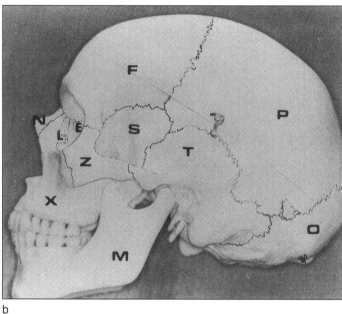

a   b

Figure 8.1   Bones of the skull from (*a*) frontal and (*b*) lateral views. Bones: ethmoid (E), frontal (F), inferior nasal concha (I), lacrimal (L), mandible (M), nasal (N), occipital (O), parietal (P), sphenoid (S), temporal (T), vomer (V), maxilla (X), zygomatic (Z).

Parts (*a, b*) reprinted with permission from SAE P-276 © 1994 Society of Automotive Engineers, Inc.

The brain is composed of the cerebrum, cerebellum, and brain stem (figure 8.2). The cerebrum, largest and most superior of the brain structures, appears as two hemispheres of highly convoluted nervous tissue. Each hemisphere is divided into regions, or lobes (frontal, parietal, temporal, occipital), each with unique and often complementary roles in sensorimotor processing. The cerebrum (and spinal cord) are covered by three layers of protective tissue known as meninges. The outermost layer is the dura mater, a tough connective tissue that in the cranium splits into two sheets. The outer (endosteal) sheet adheres tightly to the bone and is separated from the inner sheet in some areas by cavities known as venous sinuses. The middle meningeal layer (arachnoid) appears as a weblike membrane and is separated from the innermost layer (pia mater) by the subarachnoid space. The subarachnoid space contains cerebrospinal fluid (CSF) that circulates around the brain and spinal cord and provides supportive, protective, and nutritive functions.

Located just inferior to the cerebrum is the brain stem. The three structures of the brain stem (midbrain, pons, and medulla oblongata) serve as pathways for most sensory and motor information passing between the cerebrum and spinal cord and also house numerous vital reflex centers essential for basic life-supporting functions such as heart rate, respiration, blood pressure, and levels of consciousness. The brain stem also contains the nuclei for most of the 12 cranial nerves (table 8.1).

The second largest brain structure, the cerebellum, is located inferior to the cerebrum and posterior to the brain stem. Among its functions are coordination of the subconscious movements of skeletal muscles, movement error detection, maintenance of equilibrium and posture, and prediction of the future position of the body during a particular movement. The cerebellum also plays a role in emotional development by modulating sensations of pleasure and anger.

Principles of Head Injury

Head injuries sometimes are epidemiologically associated with their causal events (e.g., motor vehicle accidents). While some authors refer to these events as the "mechanism" of injury, we prefer to view them as the causal circumstances associated with the

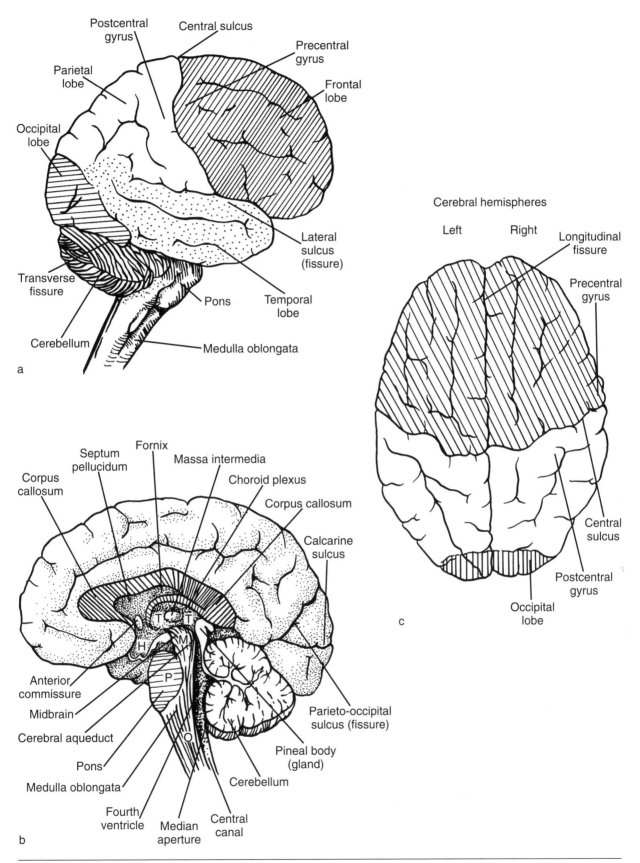

Figure 8.2 Anatomy of the brain. (*a*) Lateral view. (*b*) Median section: hypothalamus (H), midbrain (M), medulla oblongata (O), pons (P), thalamus (T). (*c*) Superior view.

207

Table 8.1 Cranial Nerves

Nerve	Name	Sensory functions	Motor functions
I	Olfactory	Olfaction	None
II	Optic	Vision	None
III	Oculomotor	Proprioception	Movement of eyeball and eyelid, lens accommodation, pupil constriction
IV	Trochlear	Proprioception	Movement of eyeball
V	Trigeminal	Proprioception, sensations of touch, pain, and temperature for opthalmic, maxillary, and mandibular regions	Mastication
VI	Abducens	Proprioception	Movement of eyeball
VII	Facial	Proprioception, taste	Facial expression, saliva and tear secretion
VIII	Vestibulocochlear	Balance, hearing	None
IX	Glossopharyngeal	Taste, blood pressure regulation, proprioception	Secretion of saliva
X	Vagus	Sensations from many organs, proprioception	Visceral muscle movement, speech, swallowing, decreases heart rate
XI	Accessory	Proprioception	Swallowing, head movements
XII	Hypoglossal	Proprioception	Tongue movement during speech and swallowing

injury and reserve the term *mechanism* for the physical processes directly causing an injury. The prevalence of causal events is shown in figure 8.3. These statistics, while of general interest, are of limited usefulness for determining risk or understanding specific factors that cause head injury.

Head injuries occur in response to the sudden application of forces to the head or its connected structures. Numerous interrelated factors combine to determine the exact mechanism of injury. Several of these factors involve the type of force and its magnitude, location, direction, duration, and rate.

The forces causing head injuries are characterized as direct or indirect. Direct (contact) loading results from impact, as exemplified by a boxer's punch. Indirect (inertial) loading occurs when forces are transmitted to the head through adjacent structures such as the neck (e.g., whiplash mechanism). Whether direct or indirect, an applied force either accelerates or decelerates the head. Forces applied to a stationary head will tend to accelerate its mass, while forces

acting in opposition to the head's motion will decelerate it (figure 8.4). A forceful blow to the head typifies an acceleration mechanism. The deceleration mechanism is involved when the head's motion is abruptly stopped by an unyielding surface. These acceleration and deceleration mechanisms often are implicated in brain injury caused by head trauma.

The effects of forces also are categorized by the type of head motion that occurs in response to loading. Forces directed through the head's center of mass cause linear translation of the head (figure 8.5a), while forces acting eccentrically (off center) from the center of mass result in rotation of the head in any or all of the three primary planes (figure 8.5b). In many situations the applied forces cause combined translational and rotational, or general, motion of the skull and its contents.

The mechanical properties of the head's constituent tissues play an important role in determining the location and severity of injury. The skull forms a stiff, yet slightly compressible container

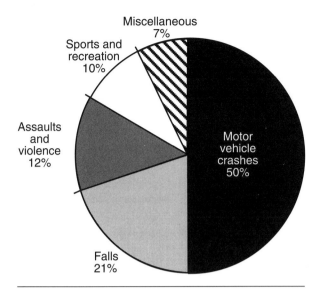

Figure 8.3   Causes of head injury.
Adapted from McGehee 1996.

housing the brain and its covering structures. The brain, in contrast, is more compliant. The different mechanical responses and relative mobility of these tissues must be considered in describing potential injury mechanisms. When a load is applied to the head, the acceleration/deceleration profiles of each structural component dictate a complex, and not completely understood, response.

The brain and other intracranial tissues develop internal stresses in response to loading and usually are deformed, or strained. Each of the three principal stresses and strains (compression, tension, shear) can be present. Injury occurs when the strain exceeds the capacity of the tissue to withstand the applied load. Tissue damage may be restricted to a limited area (focal injury) or pervade a large region of neural tissue (diffuse injury).

In terms of general structural damage, head injuries are categorized either as closed head injuries or penetrating injuries. Closed head injuries (e.g., concussion, cerebral edema, diffuse axonal injury) result from rapid translational or rotational acceleration of the head with attendant damage to the brain or its covering structures but with no exposure to the external environment. Penetrating injuries, in contrast, occur when an object (e.g., bullet, javelin, arrow) directly penetrates the skull and its neurovascular contents.

It is important to note that the factors just described are not mutually exclusive aspects of injury mechanisms. Rather they are complementary in the sense that two or more of them may be used to characterize any given injury. For example, the unfortunate recipient of an upper-cut punch in boxing might experience an acceleration injury that creates violent hyperextension (figure 8.5c). In

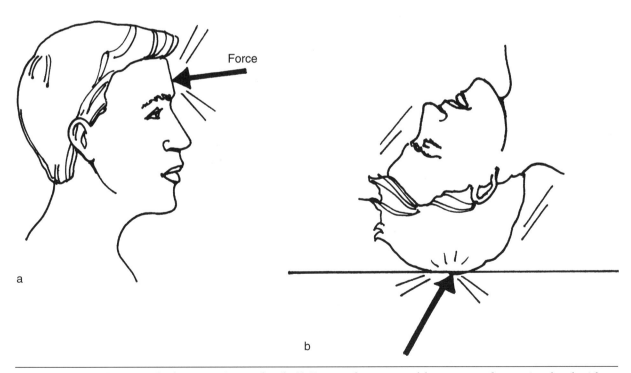

Figure 8.4   (*a*) Force applied to a stationary head. (*b*) Impact force created by contact of a moving head with an unyielding surface.

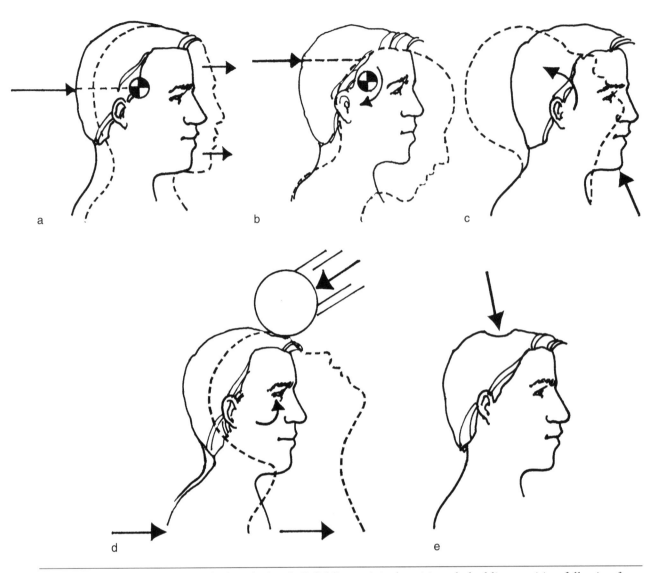

Figure 8.5 Effect of forces applied to the head. (Solid line, original position; dashed line, position following force application.) (*a*) Force applied through the center of mass causes linear translation of the head. (*b*) Force applied eccentrically (off center) causes rotation of the head. (*c*) Upper-cut punch to a boxer's chin causes rotation of the head. (*d*) Simultaneous impact by a soccer ball to the head and contact force to the back produce both rotation of the head and translation of the body. This combination accentuates the hyperextension mechanism in the cervical spine. (*e*) Blunt trauma to the superior aspect of the head causes a depressed skull fracture.

another example, a soccer player who, while heading the ball, is simultaneously contacted in the back by an opponent (figure 8.5d) would experience the combined effects of forward linear translation of the trunk and hyperextension of the neck caused by the impacting ball.

We offer two final observations before considering specific head injuries. First, head injuries often are insidious, in that evidence at the time of primary injury may provide little, if any, indication of associated secondary injuries that will subsequently de-

velop. Second, injury to superficial structures does not necessarily and invariably result in intracranial damage to the brain and its coverings. Evidence of extensive superficial damage (e.g., copious bleeding), for example, does not always predict cerebral injury. Conversely, extensive brain injury can occur in the absence of superficial damage. In most cases the overall severity of a head injury is best judged by the degree of internal damage to neural structures since these are responsible for effective cognitive, sensory, and motor function.

Boxing: Heavyweight Issues

The sport of boxing presents complex social and medical issues. No other sport generates more controversy, condemnation, and passion than boxing. On purely medical grounds, the discontinuance of boxing easily could be justified. The sport, however, does not exist in a vacuum; it is surrounded by complex sociological, psychological, moral, and financial considerations. While some vehemently argue that boxing should be banned, the sport's historical and contemporary complexity make it more amenable to compromise than to abolition.

From a physical perspective, boxing raises many interesting issues. Boxers participate in perhaps the most vigorous of all sports, one that requires an efficient combination of strength, speed, agility, coordination, and stamina. To a greater degree than any other athletes, boxers subject themselves to unprotected physical abuse. Boxing-related injuries range from minor cuts and abrasions to more severe damage, such as head and neck trauma. At particular risk of injury are the hand and wrist (e.g., carpometacarpal fracture, first metacarpophalangeal ulnar collateral ligament tear), face (e.g., ocular injuries, lacerations, facial fractures), and brain (e.g., concussion, subdural hematoma, intracerebral hemorrhage, diffuse axonal injury). In their most severe form, boxing injuries can lead to sudden death. Though other sports (e.g., college football, scuba diving, motorcycle racing, hang gliding, skydiving, horse racing) have higher fatality rates than boxing, it nonetheless has accounted for more than 650 deaths worldwide in the 20th century.

Perhaps even more devastating than the acute injuries just noted are the cumulative neurological injuries that develop after repeated mechanical insult. These injuries have been described in both common terms (e.g., punch drunk) and medical terms (e.g., dementia pugilistica). The currently preferred term is chronic traumatic boxer's encephalopathy (CTBE; Ward 1994). The existence of these chronic sequelae is beyond dispute. The current controversial issues revolve around questions of how much is too much and who is at risk. Recent evidence suggests that some boxers may be predisposed to severe chronic brain injury, while others can receive innumerable blows over many years and exhibit limited, if any, discernible neurological deficits.

Skull Fracture

Fractures of the cranium usually result from blunt trauma as the head impacts on an immediate surface or object (e.g., falls or motor vehicle accidents) or from a direct blow to the head (e.g., by a baseball bat). Deleterious consequences of the fracture itself are typically minimal. The greater concern is that skull fractures are commonly associated with injury to underlying intracranial structures (brain and meninges). These injuries include cerebral contusions, intracranial hemorrhage, and in cases of exposure to contaminants (as with scalp laceration or exposure to the nasal cavity and paranasal sinuses), infection of the cerebrospinal fluid (meningitis or cerebritis). Skull fracture is strongly predictive of intracranial hemorrhage. The absence of fracture, however, should not be interpreted as preclusive of brain injury since 20% to 30% of fatal head injuries show no evidence of skull fracture (Adams & Victor 1993).

In head injuries it is not uncommon for the intracranial damage to occur some time after the actual instant of injury. Computer tomography (CT) scans taken immediately after an injury may indicate no intracranial contusion or hemorrhage. Evidence of injury may not appear for several days. Continued monitoring of head injury patients therefore is strongly advised.

Skull fractures can occur along the convexity, or vault, of the skull or through the skull base. The mechanism causing convexity fractures is typically low-velocity, blunt trauma, while the mechanism in basilar fractures is usually high-velocity acceleration.

In severe cases the compressive force of blunt trauma can cause depression of a skull fragment into the subcranial space in what is termed a depressed skull fracture (figure 8.5e). These fractures usually cause cerebral contusion and tearing of the dura mater. The extensive meningeal vasculature increases the likelihood of hemorrhage between the layers. Most often hemorrhage occurs in the subarachnoid space. Subarachnoid hematoma usually is not associated with neurological dysfunction. Less common, but more serious, is bleeding in the subdural space. These subdural hematomas arise from rupture of surface veins of the brain and are much more likely to require surgical intervention.

Cerebral Concussion and Contusion

Cerebral concussion is one of the most common head injuries. Many definitions have been proposed for concussion. While they vary somewhat in their exact diction, they contain the basic elements of the classic characterization of concussion as "traumatic paralysis of neural function in the absence of lesions" (Denny-Brown & Russell 1941, 159). Symptoms of concussion include immediate loss of consciousness, suppression of reflexes, transient respirational arrest, a brief period of bradycardia (slow heart rate), and a fall in blood pressure. Concussive symptoms may also include disturbances of vision and equilibrium. While the symptoms are transient by definition, the time course of recovery varies considerably, ranging from several seconds to much longer.

Various scales have been devised to measure the degree of neural dysfunction from head injury. The most commonly used is the Glasgow Coma Scale. It measures a patient's auditory, motor, and visual response to stimulation and determines the level of brain dysfunction on a 13-point scale ranging from 3 to 15 (table 8.2). A summed score of 13 to 15 indicates mild brain injury, with lower scores suggesting more serious brain trauma and dysfunction.

Concussion results from a change in momentum of the head, and thus most often involves acceleration or deceleration mechanisms. In the vast majority of cases, direct impact to the head is implicated. A forceful blow, however, is not required. Rapid acceleration without direct impact also can cause concussion. Whether induced by direct impact or not, rotational (rather than linear) accelerations predominate and are associated with stronger forces. The importance of rotational acceleration as a mechanism of concussive injury has been reiterated

Table 8.2 Glasgow Coma Scale

Eye opening	Spontaneous	4
	To speech	3
	To pain	2
	None	1
Best motor response	Obeys	6
	Localizes	5
	Withdraws	4
	Abnormal flexion	3
	Extends	2
	None	1
Verbal response	Oriented	5
	Confused conversation	4
	Inappropriate words	3
	Incomprehensible sounds	2
	None	1
Total EMV score	Eye + motor + verbal	3-15

Adapted from Teasdale & Jennett 1974.

by many researchers, notably Ommaya & Gennarelli (1974), who suggested that rotational accelerations to the head cause diffuse and widespread injury, whereas translational accelerations mainly cause focal injuries only.

In addition to cerebral concussion, other injuries result from mechanical loading of the head (figure 8.6). These include skull fracture (discussed earlier), focal concussion (localized disruption of function in a restricted area of the cerebral cortex), and primary brain lesions. Cerebral contusion is one of the most important of such brain lesions. Bruises to the brain's surface can occur at the site of impact (coup lesion) or on the side opposite the site of impact (contrecoup lesion) as shown in figure 8.7.

Contusions and other traumatic brain lesions often are accompanied secondarily by brain swelling, a serious and potentially fatal condition in which the contents of the cranial vault increase in volume. This growth in volume increases intracranial pressure (ICP), which in turn can result in compromised neurovascular function, cerebral ischemia, or herniation into adjacent intracranial spaces.

Brain swelling may be due to cerebral hyperemia (increased blood volume) or cerebral edema, a specialized condition characterized by increased tissue fluid content. Five different types of cerebral edema have been identified: vasogenic, hydrostatic, cytotoxic, hypo-osmotic, and interstitial (Miller 1993). Each type is summarized in table 8.3.

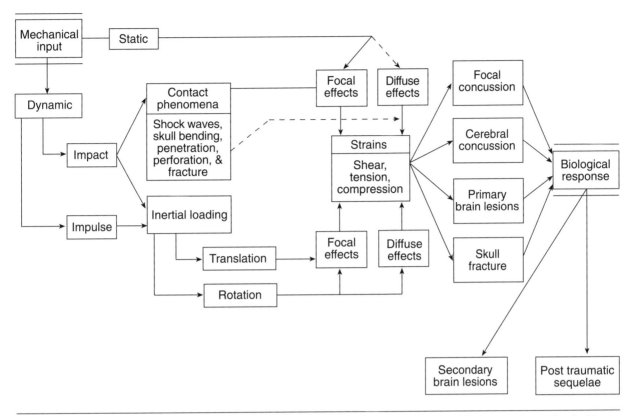

Figure 8.6 Flow chart illustrating the critical factors in the mechanics of head injury. The traumatic mechanical input is shown at the top left.

Reprinted from Ommaya & Gennarelli 1974.

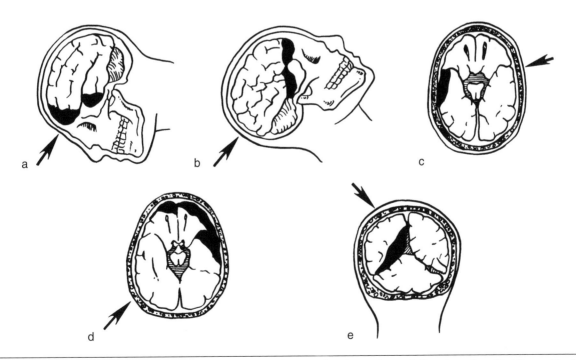

Figure 8.7 Mechanisms of cerebral contusion. Arrows show application point and direction of applied force. Shaded areas indicate location of contusion. (*a*) Frontal impact with frontotemporal contusion. (*b*) Occipital impact with frontotemporal contusion. (*c*) Lateral impact with contralateral temporal lobe contusion. (*d*) Temporo-occipital impact with contralateral frontotemporal contusion. (*e*) Vertex impact with diffuse medial temporo-occipital contusion.

To *Coup* or *Contrecoup?*

Head impact often results, not surprisingly, in contusion of the cerebral cortex. Explaining the observed location of the resulting lesion, however, is not a simple task. Contusion can occur directly beneath the site of impact (*coup* injury) or opposite to the impact location (*contrecoup* injury). The mechanisms responsible for each type of injury are complex and have been the source of considerable debate in the medical literature.

Early accounts set the stage for this ongoing debate. Holbourn (1943, 438) noted that "the idea that the brain is loose inside the skull, and that when the head is struck it rattles about like a die in a box, thereby causing coup and contrecoup injuries, is erroneous." Courville (1942) implicated force wave transmission through the brain to account for contrecoup lesions and explained the localization of injury to "anatomic conformation of the skull and the relation of the cranial cage to the brain" (Courville 1942, 20).

The mechanism of coup and contrecoup lesions has been described in the literature. Adams and Victor (1993, 755) state that "inertia of the malleable brain, which causes it to be flung against the side of the skull that was struck, to be pulled away from the contralateral side, and to rotate against bony promontories within the cranial cavity explain[s] these coup-contrecoup contusions."

Valsamis (1994, 176-177) notes that "the rates of acceleration and deceleration will determine whether contact will be made at the initiation or cessation of skull movement. Thus, fast acceleration and relatively slow deceleration will result in a coup lesion. Relatively slow acceleration coupled with rapid deceleration will result in a contrecoup lesion. If both the components are rapid, a 'coup-contrecoup' lesion will be produced, and, if both components are relatively slow, no contusion will result."

Several principles have emerged from the years of observation (i.e., autopsy findings), theorizing, and debate. Dawson and colleagues (1980) summarized these principles as follows. (1) Contrecoup contusions result from the impact of a moving head against an unyielding surface and occur most commonly in the temporal and frontal regions (figure 8B.1) and only rarely in the occipital area. (2) Blunt force applied to a resting yet movable head results in coup injury at the point of impact and only rarely causes contrecoup injury. (3) With few exceptions, coup lesions are not seen in the rapid deceleration of a moving head, and contrecoup injuries do not result from a direct blow to a resting head. (4) Contusions resulting

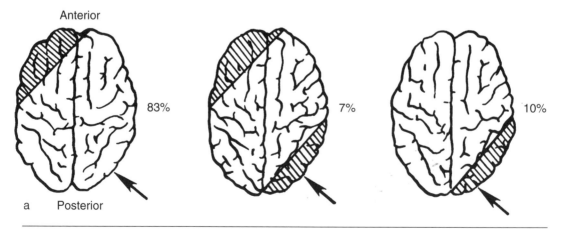

Figure 8B.1   Location of coup and contrecoup lesions in 63 cases in which patients died as a result of head injuries. (Arrows indicate location of impact force. Shaded areas indicate areas of cerebral lesions.) (*a*) Occipital impacts.

(continued)

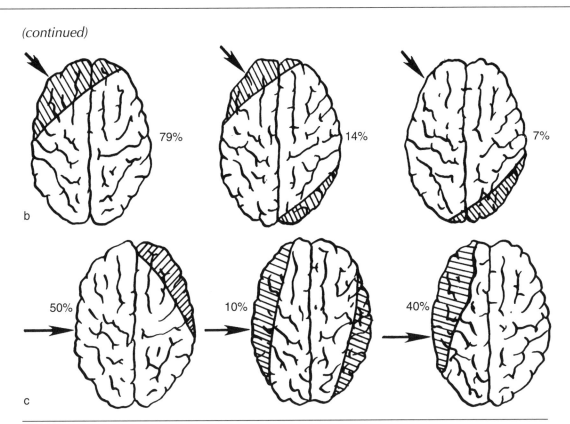

Figure 8B.1 *(continued)* *(b)* Frontal impacts. *(c)* Lateral impacts.

Adapted from Sano et al. 1967.

from transient displacement of skull fracture margins are not associated with coup-contrecoup mechanisms. (5) Cerebral lacerations, rather than contusions, are more likely in falls from considerable heights and the crushing of the head between an applied force and a firm surface that shatters the skull.

With respect to specific head motions involved in cerebral injury, the importance of head rotation, rather than translation, in the development of shearing loads in cerebral tissue has been appreciated for many decades. Holbourn (1943), for example, noted that the shear strains produced by linear acceleration of the head are small compared to those developed in response to rotational accelerations. This fact was experimentally verified by Ommaya, Grubb, and Naumann (1971, 515), who discounted the role of linear motion ("pure head translation has never been demonstrated as an injury producing factor for the brain") and submitted that "skull distortion and head rotation . . . explains a greater number of observations on coup and contrecoup injuries."

While much has been learned about the mechanisms of coup and contrecoup head injuries, many questions remain regarding this complex set of cerebral contusion injuries.

Diffuse Axonal Injury

One of the distinguishing characteristics of mild cerebral concussion is an absence of detectable pathology. In cases of more severe injury, neural structures suffer damage. These lesions may be in the form of contusion, laceration, hemorrhage, or axonal damage. Axonal lesions have been described as diffuse degeneration of the white matter, diffuse white-matter shearing injury, and inner cerebral trauma. The most common current designation is diffuse axonal injury (DAI).

Table 8.3   Types of Cerebral Edema

Type	Cause
Vasogenic	Vascular damage, such as that resulting from contusion, laceration, intracerebral hematoma
Hydrostatic	Increase transmural vascular pressure, as from a loss of autoregulation after release of brain compression
Cytotoxic	Membrane pump failure due to insufficient energy, resulting in hypoxia, ischemia
Hypo-osmotic	Hyponatremia (low sodium concentration in circulating blood), as from altered secretion of antidiuretic hormone
Interstitial	High-pressure hydrocephalus (excessive fluid accumulation in the cerebral ventricles)

Reprinted from Miller 1993.

In diffuse axonal injury, violent forces applied to neural tissue cause structural axonal failure and severance of the axon into proximal and distal segments. The distal segment predictably experiences Wallerian degeneration (see chapter 5) and becomes deafferented (separated from its sensory components). Injury to a sufficient number of axons produces profound neural dysfunction. In these cases of severe trauma the mechanical insult may directly disrupt axonal structure. In milder injuries, direct mechanical disruption of the axon may not occur. It has been suggested that axonal damage in these cases may develop over time subsequent to the traumatic event.

Accurate diagnosis of DAI, especially in its mildest forms, remains problematic since its detection requires careful microscopic examination. Computed tomography (CT) scans may miss DAI since it sometimes occurs in the absence of intracranial hemorrhage, elevated intracranial pressure, or cerebral contusion. DAI is graded according to the localization of its lesions. Grade I lesions exhibit axonal injury in the white matter of the cerebral hemispheres, corpus callosum, brain stem and, less often, the cerebellum. More severe grade II lesions show added focal lesions in the corpus callosum, while grade III includes focal lesions in the brain stem. The importance of axonal damage is highlighted by the close association between axonal lesions and prolonged traumatic coma, its sequelae, and the effects of secondary complications such as hypoxia (tissue oxygen deficiency), ischemia, and metabolic pathologies.

Cerebral tissue is relatively incompressible and thus not readily susceptible to injury under compressive loading; however, the tissue has limited resistance to shearing loads. Shearing strains arising from angular acceleration of the head are now generally accepted as being responsible for most cases of DAI. More specifically, the plane of angular acceleration largely determines the extent of injury. In studies on nonhuman primates, angular acceleration in the sagittal plane resulted in only grade I lesions. Similar levels of angular acceleration in the transverse (horizontal) plane typically caused grade II injuries. The most severe grade III lesions were associated with accelerations in the coronal (frontal) plane.

Penetrating Injuries

In general, *penetrating injuries* occur when structural damage results in exposure of the intracranial space to the external environment. The term is sometimes used in this broad sense to describe injuries from any cause, including motor vehicle accidents, occupational and sports injuries, and an object penetrating the skull. More commonly, penetrating injuries are limited to those in which an object pierces the cranium and exposes the contents of the cranial vault. These injuries can be divided into missile (or penetrating) injuries, caused by bullets or shrapnel fragments, and nonmissile (or perforation) injuries resulting from penetration by weapons (e.g., knives) or other implements (e.g., javelin).

In recent decades, cases of nonmissile injury have been relatively few, with most reports being case studies or anecdotal accounts. The variety of penetrating objects makes a curious list, including nails, keys, sewing needles, car antennas, arrows, and javelins. One notably remarkable case of a penetrating injury is described in the sidebar on page 217.

The Curious Case of Phineas Gage

Tragically, most of today's head-penetration injuries result from gunshot wounds. In contrast to these all-too-common contemporary tragedies stands the peculiar case of Phineas Gage, a 25-year-old railroad construction foreman in mid-19th century Vermont. As colorfully described by Damasio (1994, 3-10), Gage was working late one hot summer afternoon placing explosives to blast stone from the planned path of the Rutland & Burlington Railroad. By tragic accident the explosive powder in a hole drilled in the stone detonated prematurely and launched the iron rod Gage was using to tamp the powder into the hole. The rod (weighing more than 13 lb [5.9 kg] and measuring 1 1/4 in. [3.2 cm] in diameter and more than 3 1/2 ft [1.1 m] in length) penetrated Gage's head. As graphically described by Damasio (p. 4), "The explosion is so brutal. . . . The bang is unusual, and the rock is intact. The iron enters Gage's left cheek, pierces the base of the skull, traverses the front of his brain, and exits at high speed through the top of the head. The rod has landed more than a hundred feet away, covered in blood and brains. Phineas Gage has been thrown to the ground. He is stunned, in the afternoon glow, silent but awake." Miraculously, Gage survived and was "able to talk and walk and remain coherent immediately afterward" (p. 5).

Gage was pronounced fully cured (at least physically) within two months of the accident and had no difficulty walking, touching, hearing, or speaking. It seems that the areas of his brain responsible for language, perception, and motor function had survived the accident relatively unaffected. Gage, however, suffered from devastating and progressive alterations in his personality; his social reasoning skills were forever changed.

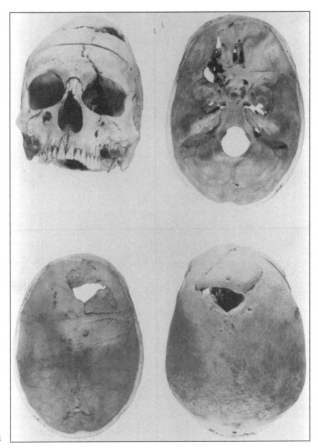

a

Figure 8B.2 (*a*) Photographs of several views of the skull of Phineas Gage.

(continued)

(continued)

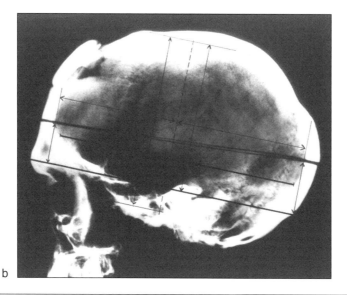

b

Figure 8B.2   *(continued)* (*b*) An X ray of his skull.

Parts (*a, b*) reprinted with permission from Damasio H, Grabowski T, Frank R, Galaburda AM, Damasio AR: The return of Phineas Gage: Clues about the brain from the skull of a famous patient. *Science, 264:* 1102-1105, 1994. Department of Neurology and Image Analysis Facility, University of Iowa. Copyright 1994 American Association for the Advancement of Science.

The implications of Gage's response to injury are profound. "Gage's story hinted at an amazing fact: Somehow, there were systems in the human brain dedicated more to reasoning than to anything else, and in particular to the personal and social dimensions of reasoning. The observance of previously acquired social convention and ethical rules could be lost as a result of brain damage, even when neither basic intellect nor language seemed compromised" (Damasio 1994, 10).

The vast majority of penetrating head injuries are caused by gunshot wounds. Recent increases in shooting-related injuries (hastened by escalated drug use, gang involvement, domestic abuse, and interpersonal violence) have created an epidemic health problem.

Ballistics is the science dealing with the motion of projectiles, or missiles. In the case of bullets or shrapnel fragments, ballistic principles govern the path and mechanical characteristics that set the stage for head injury upon penetration. Missiles, by virtue of their motion, possess kinetic energy: $E_k = 0.5 \cdot m \cdot v^2$ [eq. (3.17)], where m = mass and v = linear velocity. The destructive potential of a bullet is given by the magnitude of its kinetic energy at the moment of impact. Clearly, the larger and faster the bullet, the greater its ability to injure. Of the two components constituting kinetic energy, velocity exerts a more potent influence because it is squared. Doubling a bullet's mass, for example, will double its kinetic energy. But by increasing its velocity twofold, the bullet's kinetic energy quadruples!

In mechanical terms, the destructive energy absorbed (E_a) by the tissues of the head is the amount of kinetic energy lost between bullet impact and exit:

$$E_a = E_i - E_e = 0.5 \cdot m \cdot (v_i - v_e)^2 \qquad (8.1)$$

where E_i = kinetic energy at impact, E_e = kinetic energy at exit, m = mass, v_i = impact velocity, and v_e = exit velocity. This relationship assumes, of course, that the bullet remains intact, maintains its mass, and does not fragment. In cases where the bullet does not exit the skull, all the kinetic energy is absorbed intracranially. Frequently, the bullet has sufficient energy to traverse the entire brain but not enough to pierce the skull a second time and exit the cranium. In these instances the bullet typically ricochets off the interior surface of skull, burrowing back into the brain and causing further damage.

With respect to the mechanisms of direct laceration, shock wave transmission, and cavitation associated with missile injury (Kim & Zee 1995), velocity is the critical variable. Missiles with low impact velocities (< 100 m·s⁻¹), such as those in stabbing injuries and handguns fired from a distance, typically exact limited damage, primarily in the form of direct laceration. As missile velocity increases, shock wave transmission and cavitation become more evident. Low-velocity firearms (muzzle velocities less than 320 m·s⁻¹, though the exact cutoff is somewhat arbitrary and varies in the literature) induce laceration injury and some shock wave damage. In high-velocity firearms (> 320 m·s⁻¹) the predominant mechanisms of injury are shock wave transmission and cavitation. At very high velocities, cavitation predominates. In cavitation the missile pushes away tissue in its path and creates a conical cavity in its wake. This cavity can be many times larger than the missile and has a subatmospheric pressure (partial vacuum) that suctions surrounding material into its space and causes extensive tissue damage.

Bullet characteristics such as caliber (diameter), construction, and configuration also contribute to the amount of energy absorbed by tissues. The size of the bullet and the shape of its nose determine the frontal area at the bullet-tissue interface and influence the amount of drag developed. Bullets designed and constructed to deform or fragment after impact enhance kinetic energy loss and increase the severity of tissue damage.

Finally, the extent of trauma is also influenced by tissue characteristics such as tissue strength, density, and elasticity. Denser tissues, for example, provide greater retarding resistance and contribute to greater energy loss.

All of the foregoing factors interact to determine the complex profile of energy transfer as energy dissipates from the missile and is absorbed by the tissue surrounding the missile's path. The resulting pattern of injury varies tremendously (figure 8.8). The regrettable trend toward firearms designed to use smaller, faster, and more deformable bullets portends an increase in destructive potential and inevitably greater levels of injury and catastrophic death.

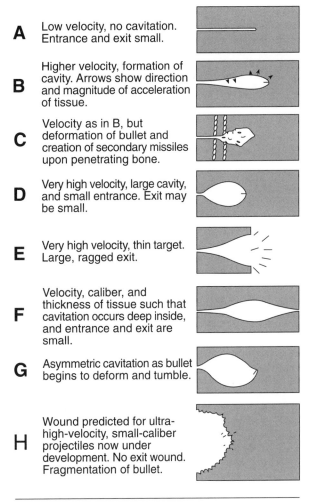

A Low velocity, no cavitation. Entrance and exit small.

B Higher velocity, formation of cavity. Arrows show direction and magnitude of acceleration of tissue.

C Velocity as in B, but deformation of bullet and creation of secondary missiles upon penetrating bone.

D Very high velocity, large cavity, and small entrance. Exit may be small.

E Very high velocity, thin target. Large, ragged exit.

F Velocity, caliber, and thickness of tissue such that cavitation occurs deep inside, and entrance and exit are small.

G Asymmetric cavitation as bullet begins to deform and tumble.

H Wound predicted for ultra-high-velocity, small-caliber projectiles now under development. No exit wound. Fragmentation of bullet.

Figure 8.8 Variations of ballistic effects on animal tissue. Adapted from Swan & Swan 1989.

Facial Fractures

Facial fractures are of particular concern due to the close proximity of the facial bones to vital neural and sensory structures. A recent survey of the literature, for example, found that neurological injury associated with facial fractures was as high as 76% (Haug et al. 1994). The mechanism of injury in the vast majority of cases is forceful blunt trauma. The impacting object takes a variety of forms. Collision with a part of another person's body (e.g., head, shoulder, elbow), an implement (e.g., hockey stick, baseball bat), a projectile (e.g., cricket ball, baseball, golf ball), or an unyielding surface (e.g., vehicle steering wheel) have all been reported as causing facial fractures.

The recent increase in facial fractures resulting from violent assault suggests a disturbing trend. One recent study reported that assault was the leading etiological factor, accounting for 51.2% of 839 facial fractures reviewed (Lim et al. 1993). Automobile crashes have also been cited as a common cause of facial fractures. The high energy of these vehicular collisions greatly increases the likelihood of accompanying injuries.

Evidence clearly shows that seat belt use has greatly reduced the incidence of chest injury in frontal car crashes. At impact, unrestrained drivers are launched chest first into the steering wheel. The restrained driver, in contrast, is more likely to sustain head injury as the cranium is thrown toward the steering wheel (figure 8.9). This unfortunate trade-off has resulted in an increased proportion of brain injuries in restrained passengers. At first glance, the increasing use of air bag restraints would appear an ideal answer to this problem. In most cases air bags do, in fact, prevent or reduce the severity of head injury. The air bag should not be considered a panacea, however, since substantial injury can still occur when crash speeds are insufficient to trigger air bag deployment. In addition, serious harm, or even death, can be caused by the explosive deployment of air bags into people of short stature and small body mass (e.g., children and small adults).

An interesting but unresolved controversy exists concerning the question of whether facial fractures absorb energy and therefore decrease the severity of neurological injury or serve to transmit force to underlying structures. On one hand, impact force may be attenuated by the tissue disruption of a fracture with energy transferred to the neural structures within the craniofacial vault. On the other hand, midfacial bones may actually transmit impact force to the cranium.

Because facial injury typically results from direct trauma, the risk of fracture depends largely on the strength of the bony tissue at the impact site. Hampson (1995) summarized craniofacial bone tolerances for the zygoma, zygomatic arch, mandible, maxilla, frontal bone, and nose. These data are depicted in figure 8.10.

Facial fractures are particularly problematic because they often cross disciplinary boundaries. Treatment of injuries associated with facial fractures frequently requires the combined expertise of orthopedists, neurologists, dentists, ophthalmologists, and other medical specialists.

Neck Injuries

The neck provides the structural link between the head and trunk. It contains components of many of

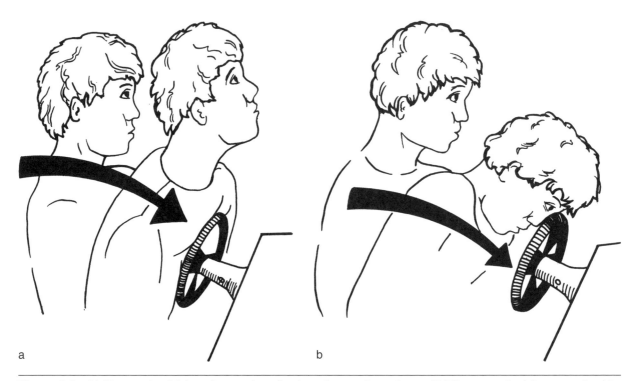

a   b

Figure 8.9   (*a*) Unrestrained driver thrown chest first into the steering column. (*b*) The torso of a driver restrained by a lap seat belt rotates forward and results in head impact with the steering wheel assembly.

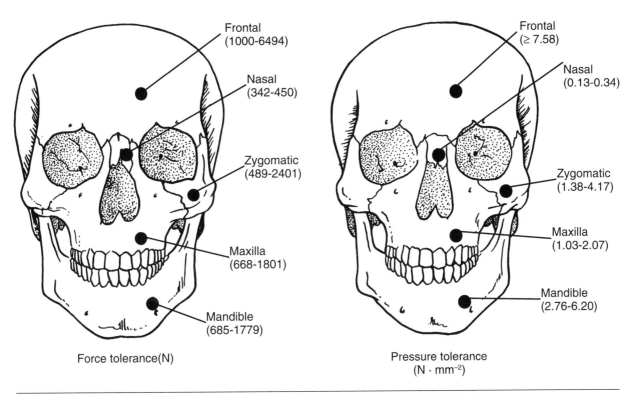

Frontal
(1000-6494)

Nasal
(342-450)

Zygomatic
(489-2401)

Maxilla
(668-1801)

Mandible
(685-1779)

Force tolerance(N)

Frontal
(≥ 7.58)

Nasal
(0.13-0.34)

Zygomatic
(1.38-4.17)

Maxilla
(1.03-2.07)

Mandible
(2.76-6.20)

Pressure tolerance
(N · mm⁻²)

Figure 8.10   Force and pressure tolerances for facial bones.
Reprinted from Ommaya & Gennarelli 1995.

the body's principal systems. Many essential structures emanate from the root of the neck (figure 8.11). Among these are the following important types of structures: vascular (common carotid arteries, subclavian arteries and veins, brachiocephalic trunk and veins), respiratory (trachea, larynx), digestive (esophagus), nervous (sympathetic trunk, phrenic nerve, vagus nerve), and endocrine (thyroid and parathyroid glands). The skeletal portion of the neck includes the cervical vertebrae (figure 8.12a). Among the more prominent muscles of the neck are the sternocleidomastoid and trapezius (figure 8.12b).

The vertebral column (spine) is a group of 33 vertebrae extending from the base of the skull to its inferior termination at the coccyx (tailbone). The spine is divided into five regions (figure 8.13): cervical (7 vertebrae), thoracic (12), lumbar (5), sacral (5 fused), coccygeal (4 fused). Vertebrae in the cervical, thoracic, and lumbar regions are separated by an intervertebral disk that is composed of a gelatinous inner mass (nucleus pulposus) surrounded by a layered fibrocartilage network (annulus fibrosus). Each vertebra consists of a body, vertebral arch, and processes arising from the arch (figure 8.14). The size and orientation of these structural elements differs between regions (figure 8.15). Just

posterior to the vertebral body is an open passage (vertebral foramen) that houses the spinal cord. Other passages (intervertebral foramina) between adjacent vertebrae allow the exit of spinal nerve roots on both sides of the vertebral column.

Of the many cervical structures susceptible to injury, the spinal cord is the one with the greatest catastrophic potential. The consequences of spinal cord damage range from mild, as in neurapraxia (transient loss of nerve conduction without structural degeneration), to severe instances of paralysis or death. In cases of severe injury, the level of spinal cord involvement is critical in determining the type and extent of sensorimotor deficit. Injury at the C3-C4 level, for example, may result in complete paralysis of the trunk and extremities and loss of unassisted respiration. Injury at C5-C6 may allow limited arm movement, while lower-level injury at C7-T1 may spare upper-extremity muscle function and limit paralysis to the lower extremities.

Cervical Trauma

The complex structure and intricate motion of the cervical region present special challenges in identifying and describing mechanisms of cervical injury.

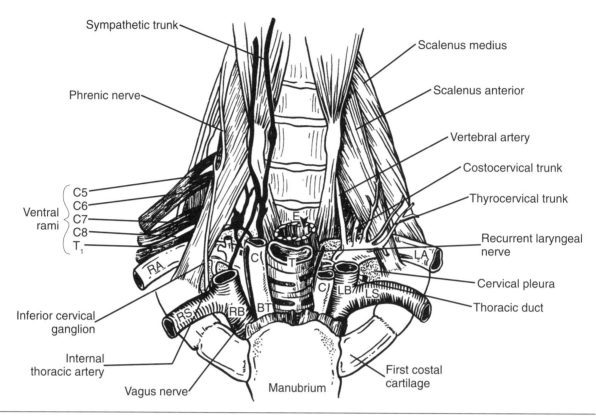

Figure 8.11   Root of the neck. Structures: esophagus (E), trachea (T), left and right common carotid arteries (C), right subclavian artery (RA), left subclavian artery (LA), right subclavian vein (RS), left subclavian vein (LS), right brachiocephalic vein (RB), left brachiocephalic vein (LB), brachiocephalic trunk (BT).

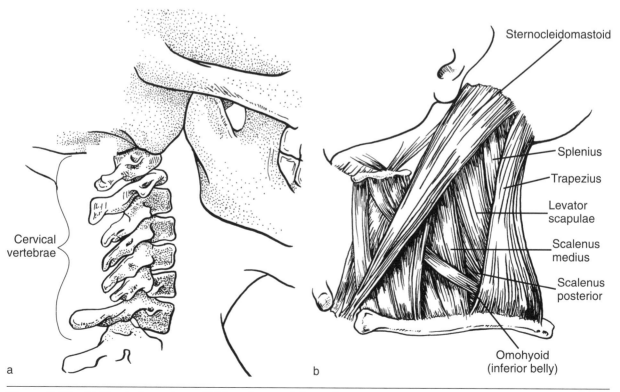

Figure 8.12   (*a*) Cervical vertebrae. (*b*) Musculature of the neck.

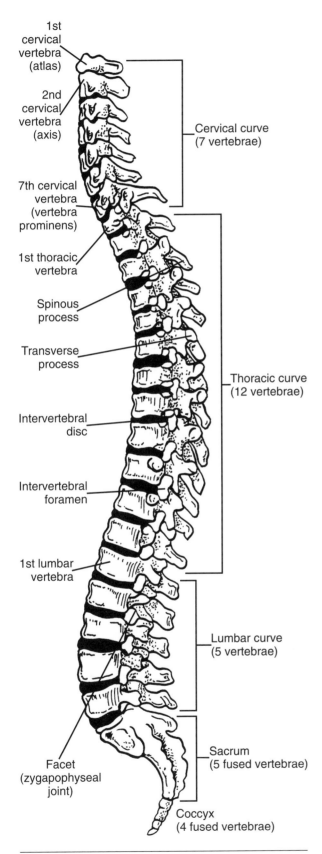

Figure 8.13   Skeletal structures of the vertebral (spinal) column.

Labels on figure 8.13:
- 1st cervical vertebra (atlas)
- 2nd cervical vertebra (axis)
- Cervical curve (7 vertebrae)
- 7th cervical vertebra (vertebra prominens)
- 1st thoracic vertebra
- Spinous process
- Transverse process
- Thoracic curve (12 vertebrae)
- Intervertebral disc
- Intervertebral foramen
- 1st lumbar vertebra
- Lumbar curve (5 vertebrae)
- Facet (zygapophyseal joint)
- Sacrum (5 fused vertebrae)
- Coccyx (4 fused vertebrae)

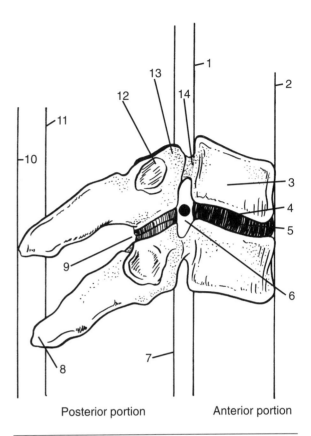

Posterior portion   Anterior portion

Figure 8.14   Sagittal view of a spinal motion segment formed by two adjacent vertebral bodies and the intervening disk. Structures: 1, posterior longitudinal ligament; 2, anterior longitudinal ligament; 3, vertebral body; 4, cartilaginous end plate; 5, intervertebral disk; 6, intervertebral foramen with nerve root; 7, ligamentum flavum; 8, spinous process; 9, intervertebral joint formed by the superior and inferior facets (joint capsule not shown); 10, supraspinous ligament; 11, interspinous ligament; 12, transverse process (intertransverse ligament not shown); 13, vertebral arch; 14, vertebral canal (spinal cord not shown).

The sometimes confusing mixture of engineering and medical terminology used to describe cervical mechanics further complicates the task.

Classification of cervical injury mechanisms requires great care and precision because: (1) the overall motion of the head relative to the trunk may not be indicative of local motion between adjacent segments, (2) small deviations (< 1 cm) in the point of force application or in head position can change the injury mechanism from compression-flexion to compression-extension, and (3) observed head motions may occur after the instant of injury and thus not reflect the true injury mechanism (Myers, McElhaney, & Nightingale 1994).

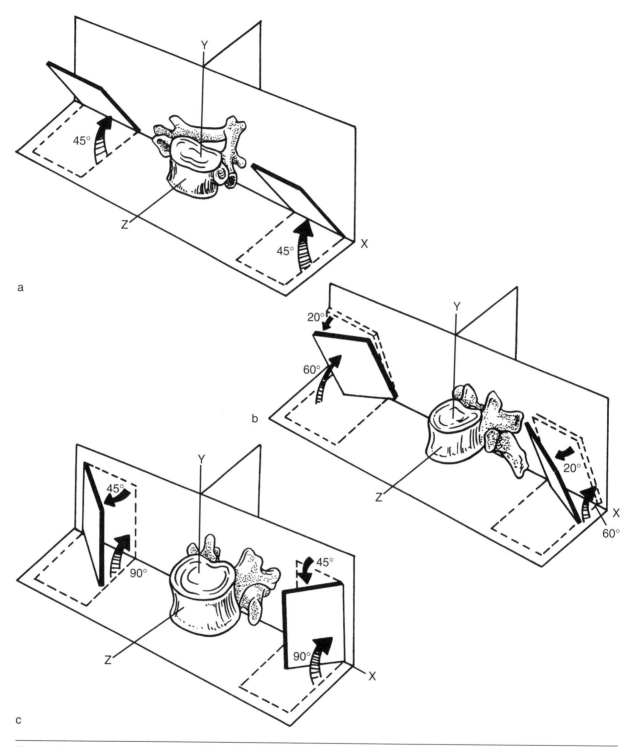

Figure 8.15 Orientation of the vertebral facet joints. (*a*) Cervical spine. The vertebral facets in the cervical spine are inclined at 45° above the horizontal plane and are parallel with the frontal plane. (*b*) Thoracic spine. The facets in the thoracic region are inclined at 60° above the horizontal plane and deviate 20° behind the frontal plane. (*c*) Lumbar spine. Facets in the lumbar spine are inclined at 90° above the horizontal plane and deviate 45° behind the frontal plane. These regional changes in facet orientation play an essential role in determining movement potential between adjacent vertebrae in each region. Angle values are rough estimates. Actual values vary within regions of the spine and among individuals.

From *Clinical Biomechanics of the Spine* (2nd ed.) (Fig. 1-19, p. 30) by A.A. White & M.M. Panjabi, 1996, Philadelphia: J.B. Lippincott Company. Copyright 1990 by Lippincott-Raven. Reprinted by permission.

While various classification systems have been proposed, we favor a system based on the principal loading applied to the cervical spine (figure 8.16 and table 8.4). Using this system, we present several example injuries and their mechanisms.

Cervical spinal cord injury (SCI) occurs in many activities. The reported incidence for specific activities depends on the location and circumstances of the population being studied. Motor vehicle accidents are the most common culprit, accounting for up to half of all SCIs. Societal conditions influence the statistics, though: In one study, gunshot wounds were the leading cause of SCI (36%), ranking ahead of motor vehicle accidents (25%) (Hart & Williams 1994). Spinal cord injuries also have been reported due to falls from heights, work-related tasks, and sporting and recreational activities. Despite their relative infrequency, sports-related SCIs often achieve notoriety in the media, usually in cases of American football injuries that result in paralysis.

Sporting activities provide instructive examples of cervical spine injury mechanisms. It was once thought that cervical injury in football was due to either a hyperflexion mechanism or a "guillotine" effect in which the posterior rim of the helmet acted as a pivot during cervical hyperextension. These mechanisms have been discounted as primary causes of cervical injury. The most common mechanism is accepted to be flexion-compression. When the neck

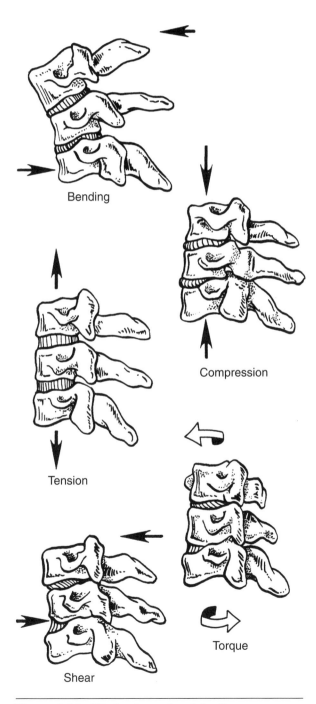

Figure 8.16 Mechanisms of neck loading.

Table 8.4 Mechanisms of Cervical Spine Injuries and Associated Injuries

Vertical compression (Jefferson fracture, multipart atlas fracture, vertebral-body compression fracture, burst fracture)

Compression-flexion (vertebral-body wedge compression fracture, hyperflexion sprain, unilateral facet dislocation, bilateral facet dislocation, teardrop fracture)

Compression-extension (posterior element fractures)

Tension (occipitoatlantal dislocation)

Tension-extension (whiplash, anterior longitudinal ligament tears, disk rupture, horizontal vertebral-body fracture, hangman's fracture, teardrop fracture)

Tension-flexion (bilateral facet dislocation)

Torsion (rotary atlantoaxial dislocation)

Horizontal shear (anterior and posterior atlantoaxial subluxation, odontoid fracture, transverse ligament rupture)

Lateral bending (nerve root avulsion, transverse process fracture)

Other fractures (e.g., clay shoveler's fracture)

From "Biomechanical aspects of cervical trauma" (p. 319) by J.H. McElhaney & B.S. Myers, 1993. In: A.M. Nahum & J.W. Melvin (Eds.), *Accidental Injury: Biomechanics and Prevention*, New York: Springer-Verlag. Copyright 1993 by Springer-Verlag. Adapted by permission.

is flexed slightly, the normal cervical lordosis disappears and the cervical vertebrae are aligned axially (figure 8.17a). In this position, the cervical spine becomes a segmented column that lacks the curvature required for energy-absorbing bending. The cervical structures then must absorb all of the loading energy (figure 8.17b). When this energy exceeds the capacity of the cervical structures, failure of the intervertebral disks, the body and processes of the vertebrae, or spinous ligaments may occur. Disruption of these structures permits further flexion or rotation of the cervical spine and associated vertebral dislocation. This dislocation carries the risk of impinging the spinal cord or spinal nerves. The flexion-compression mechanism is common to football, diving, and ice hockey and accounts for several cases of quadriplegia each year. The flexion-compression mechanism also has been implicated in

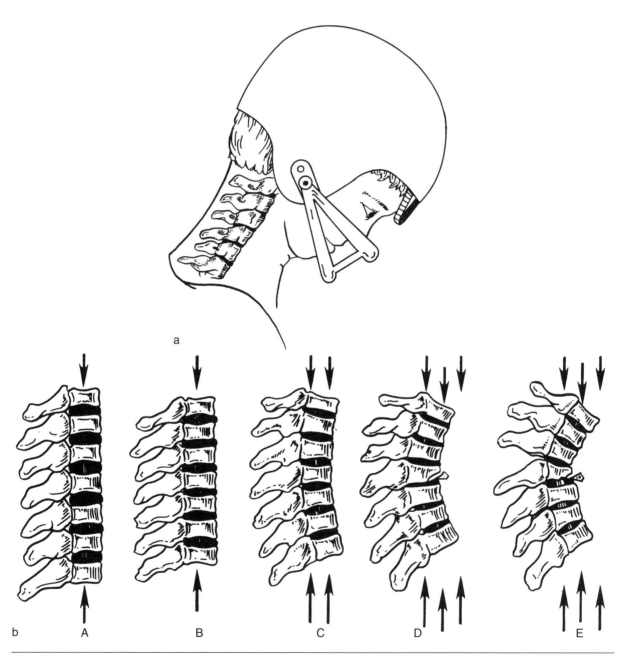

a

b   A   B   C   D   E

Figure 8.17   (*a*) With the neck slightly flexed (approximately 30°), the cervical spine is straightened and functions as a segmented column. (*b*) Axial compressive forces applied to a segmented column (A) initially compress the column (B). Increased loading causes angular deformation (C), buckling (D), and eventual fracture, subluxation, or dislocation (E).
Reprinted from Torg et al. 1990.

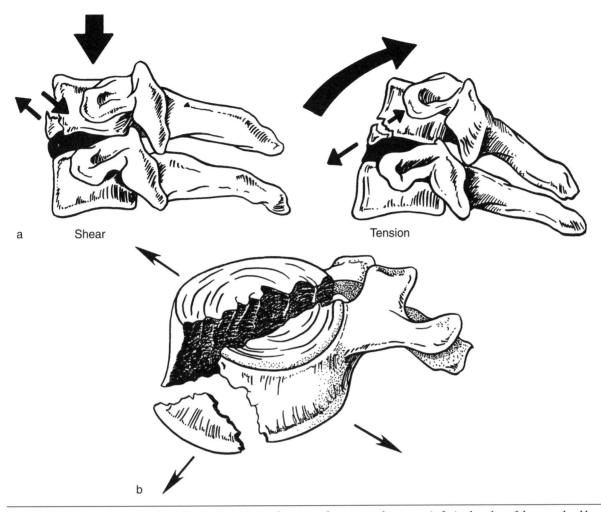

Figure 8.18   Teardrop vertebral fractures. (*a*) Bone fragment fracture at the anteroinferior border of the vertebral body resulting from compressive loading (*left*) that results in shearing at the fragment interface (dark arrows) or from spinal extension (*right*) that creates tensile loading at the fragment interface. (*b*) A three-part, biplanar teardrop fracture with an anteroinferior corner fracture fragment and a sagittal fracture through the vertebral body.

fracture at the anteroinferior corner of a cervical vertebral body in what is termed a *teardrop fracture* (figure 8.18).

Cervical injury also results from an extension-tension mechanism in which the head is forcibly hyperextended by posterior impact with forcible resistance applied to the chin (figure 8.19*a*), inertial forces resulting from posterior impact (figure 8.19*b*), or forces applied inferiorly to the posterior aspect of the head (figure 8.19*c*). This mechanism creates tension stresses in the anterior cervical structures and can involve disruption of the anterior longitudinal ligament, intervertebral disk, or horizontal fracture of the vertebral body. High-energy loading can also result in posterior vertebral displacement and risk of spinal cord injury.

Spinal cord injury, while catastrophic, is rela-

tively rare. More commonly, cervical injury manifests as a temporary sensorimotor lesion caused by pinching of cervical nerve roots or the brachial plexus. These so-called burners or stingers result in burning pain, with numbness and temporary weakness in the affected arm. Watkins & Dillin (1994a) describe two mechanisms associated with this injury. The first involves an off-center axial load applied while the neck is extended and laterally flexed. In this position the spinal canal and foramina narrow and allow the bony borders to impinge on the exiting nerve roots. This mechanism is most commonly seen in American football players during the impacts of blocking, tackling, and ground contact. In the second mechanism the shoulder on the involved side is depressed and the head is forcibly pushed away contralaterally. This motion violently

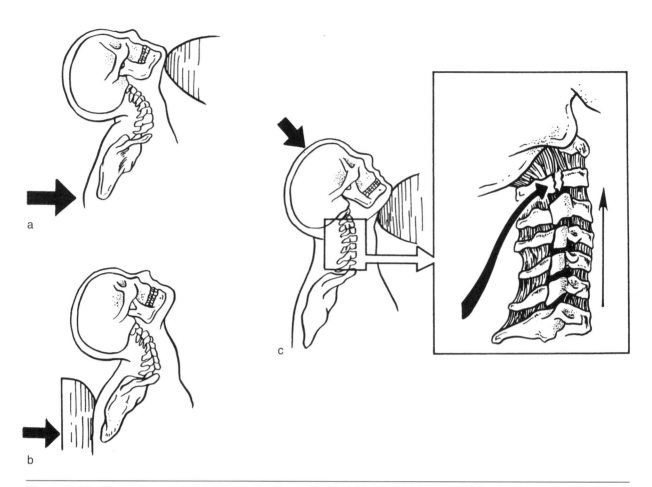

Figure 8.19 Extension-tension injury mechanisms. Cervical hyperextension caused by (*a*) posterior impact with forcible resistance on the chin, (*b*) inertial forces from posterior impact, and (*c*) forces applied inferiorly to the posterior aspect of the head with forcible resistance applied to the chin.

Reprinted, by permission, from SAE publication, *Head and Neck Injury* (P-276, p. 123). Copyright 1994 by Society of Automotive Engineers, Inc.

stretches the nerve roots and associated brachial plexus and results in transient neurological symptoms. In mild burners, sensorimotor function returns within several minutes and recovery is complete within a week or two. More severe injury can result in motor loss to muscles such as the biceps brachii and deltoid that persists for weeks or even months.

Of all cervical disorders, whiplash injuries are among the most common and most misunderstood. The very definition of whiplash is controversial. In one context whiplash describes an injury mechanism, while in another it refers to a clinical syndrome. This latter usage is inappropriate because of its lack of specificity. A useful definition of whiplash is "trauma causing cervical musculoligamental sprain or strain due to acceleration/deceleration of the head relative to the trunk in any plane" (Sturzenegger et al. 1994, 688).

In rear-end collisions there is sequential acceleration of the vehicle, the occupant's trunk and shoulders, and last the occupant's head (figure 8.20). At the instant of impact, the head remains stationary (according to Newton's first law) while the vehicle is violently pushed forward. When the occupant's trunk and shoulders are accelerated anteriorly, the head is forced into hyperextension. Once its inertia is overcome, the head is thrown ("whiplashed") forward into flexion.

While usually considered a sagittal plane injury caused by a rear-end impact, whiplash can also result from lateral or frontal forces that exact their own unique pattern of injury. In addition, motion of the neck sometimes is not confined to a single plane. If a driver is looking to the side at the instant of impact, for example, the injury mechanism involves a combination of hyperextension and rotation. In this case the rotation is enhanced by the impact

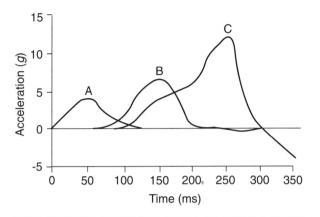

Figure 8.20 Idealized acceleration curves of (*A*) an impacted vehicle, (*B*) an occupant's shoulders, and (*C*) an occupant's head. As the vehicle is impacted (e.g., in an automobile rear-end collision), it accelerates first, reaching a peak acceleration of almost 5 *g*'s (i.e., five times the acceleration of gravity). The vehicle occupant's shoulders reach their peak acceleration of about 7 *g*'s 100 ms later. Finally, the occupant's head reaches its peak acceleration of greater than 12 *g*'s 250 ms after initial impact. This sequential progression of peak accelerations is evidence of both momentum and energy transfers.

Reprinted from Barnsley, Lord, & Bogduk 1994.

forces prior to cervical hyperextension, and cervical structures are prestretched and more predisposed to severe injury.

At first glance, whiplash might appear a simple injury mechanism. However, "in an individual accident there is likely to be a complex interaction between different forces depending upon the speed and direction of impact and the attitude of the head and neck" (Barnsley, Lord, & Bogduk 1994, 288). Many structures can be injured in whiplash accidents. These include structures in the brain, temporomandibular joint, muscles, spinous ligaments, intervertebral disks, vertebral bodies, and facet (zygapophyseal) joints. Various mechanisms and potential injury sites are shown in figure 8.21.

Cervical Spondylosis

The etiology of chronic cervical conditions, such as cervical spondylosis, stands in marked contrast with the potentially catastrophic traumatic injuries just described. While their onset is less dramatic, chronic injuries nonetheless can cause considerable dysfunction. Cervical spondylosis is a general term used to describe degenerative changes in the cervical intervertebral disks and surrounding structures.

As part of the normal aging process, disks lose vertical height and become less extensible, due in large part to reduced water content and degradation of the disk substance. Disk degeneration is accompanied by osteophyte (bony outgrowth) formation and increased stresses on articular cartilage. These structural alterations increase the risk of spinal stenosis (narrowed canal), impingement on neural tissue, and impaired blood perfusion of the spinal cord. Symptoms associated with cervical spondylosis include paresthesia, neck and arm pain, weakness, and sensory loss. Recent advances in imaging technologies (e.g., magnetic resonance imaging) have improved diagnostic accuracy. Considerable debate continues, however, on the advisability of surgical intervention in treating the lesions associated with cervical spondylosis.

Disturbance or disease of the spinal cord (myelopathy) associated with cervical spondylosis is a well-recognized clinical entity. Mechanical factors that may be causal agents in cervical spondylotic myelopathy include a narrowing of the spinal canal, kyphotic conditions causing cervical flexion, spinal cord compression and related ischemia, and ligamentous ossification. Despite the often insidious onset of cervical spondylosis, its sequelae have significant potential for causing severe neuromuscular dysfunction.

Trunk Injuries

The trunk (also called truncus or torso) extends from the base of the neck down to the pelvic girdle. As the largest body region, the trunk accounts for 45% to 50% of the body's mass and contains such vital organs as the heart (and its major vessels), spinal cord, lungs, stomach and intestines, kidneys, liver, and spleen. The sternum, ribs, and vertebrae of the axial skeleton protect these important organs.

Trunk musculature serves both movement and protective functions. The principal muscles of the anterior trunk are the pectoralis major, serratus anterior, rectus abdominis, external obliques, internal obliques, and transversus abdominis (figure 8.22b). Important posterior trunk muscles include the trapezius, latissimus dorsi, rhomboids (major and minor), and erector spinae (figure 8.22, a and c).

Vertebral Fracture

Spinal fractures are a major health concern, with more than 80,000 cases in the United States each

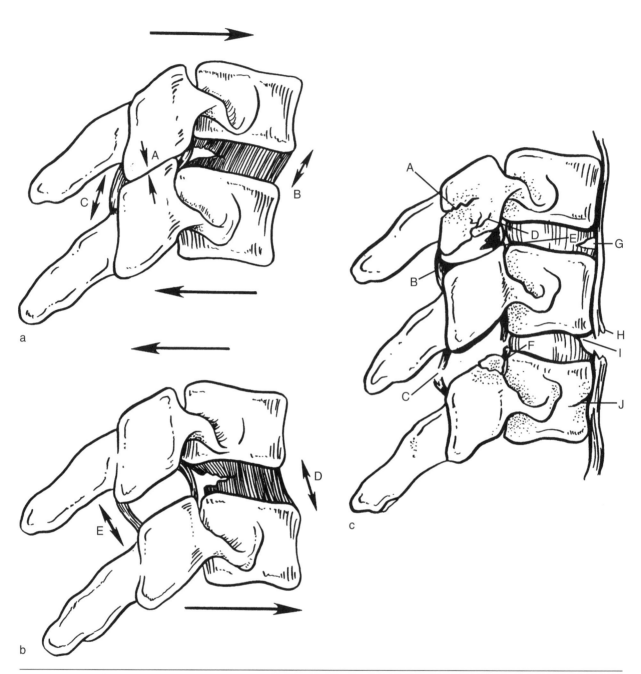

Figure 8.21 Shear forces affecting a spinal motion segment. (*a*) Translation of the superior vertebral body anteriorly relative to the inferior body. This movement stresses the articular surfaces of the zygapophyseal joints (A), the anterior annulus fibrosus (B), and the zygapophyseal joint capsule (C). (*b*) Translation of the superior vertebral body posteriorly relative to the inferior body, which stresses the intervertebral disk (D) and the zygapophyseal joint capsules (E). (*c*) Common lesions affecting the cervical spine following whiplash injury. A, articular pillar fracture; B, hemarthrosis (hemorrhage into a joint) of the zygapophyseal joint; C, rupture or tear of the zygapophyseal joint capsule; D, fracture of the subchondral plate; E, contusion of the intraarticular meniscus of the zygapophyseal joint; F, fracture involving the articular surface; G, tear of the annulus fibrosus; H, tear of the anterior longitudinal ligament; I, end-plate avulsion fracture; J, vertebral body fracture.

year (Praemer, Furner, & Rice 1992). Fractures of the vertebrae are of particular concern because of their close proximity to the spinal cord. In displaced spinal fractures, bone fragments may be forced into the spinal canal and impinge on the cord. This impingement can cause severe neural damage and attendant paralysis or even death. Vertebral fractures usually are caused by axial compressive loads and occur most commonly in the cervical and thoracolumbar regions. Vertebrae in the thoracolumbar region (variably defined to include vertebrae between T11 and L3) are especially susceptible to fracture because of the spine's relatively neutral alignment (minimal curvature) in this region, and because this region is a transition zone between the relatively rigid thoracic region and the more flexible lumbar region.

Roaf (1960) and Holdsworth (1963, 1970) provided early descriptions of the mechanism of compressive vertebral fracture. Holdsworth (1963) postulated a two-column model of the spine, consisting of an anterior column (region between the anterior longitudinal ligament and the posterior longitudinal ligament) and a posterior column (posterior bony complex bounded by the posterior longitudinal ligament and the posterior ligamentous complex that includes the supraspinous ligament, interspinous ligament, capsule, and ligamentum flavum). Holdsworth's two-column model was modified by Denis (1983), who proposed a three-column model (figure 8.23) to explain the pattern of thoracolumbar injuries (table 8.5).

In describing the mechanism of compressive vertebral fracture, Holdsworth (1970) coined the term *burst fracture*, noting that when a severe compression force is applied to either cervical or

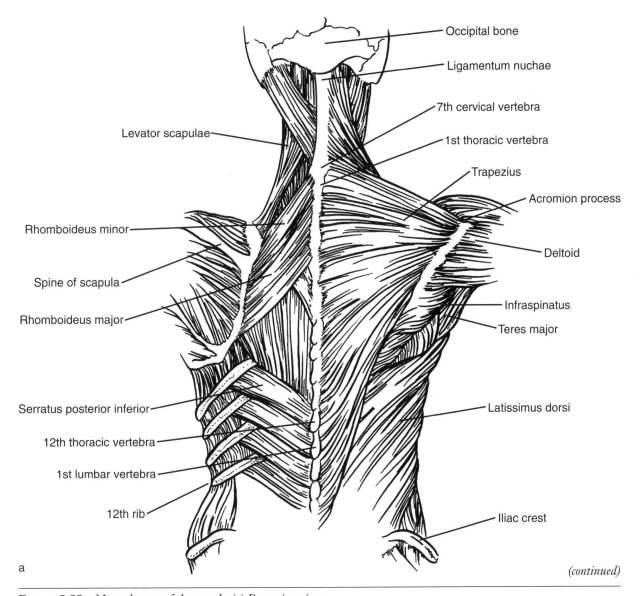

Levator scapulae

Rhomboideus minor

Spine of scapula

Rhomboideus major

Serratus posterior inferior

12th thoracic vertebra

1st lumbar vertebra

12th rib

Occipital bone

Ligamentum nuchae

7th cervical vertebra

1st thoracic vertebra

Trapezius

Acromion process

Deltoid

Infraspinatus

Teres major

Latissimus dorsi

Iliac crest

a

(continued)

Figure 8.22   Musculature of the trunk. (*a*) Posterior view.

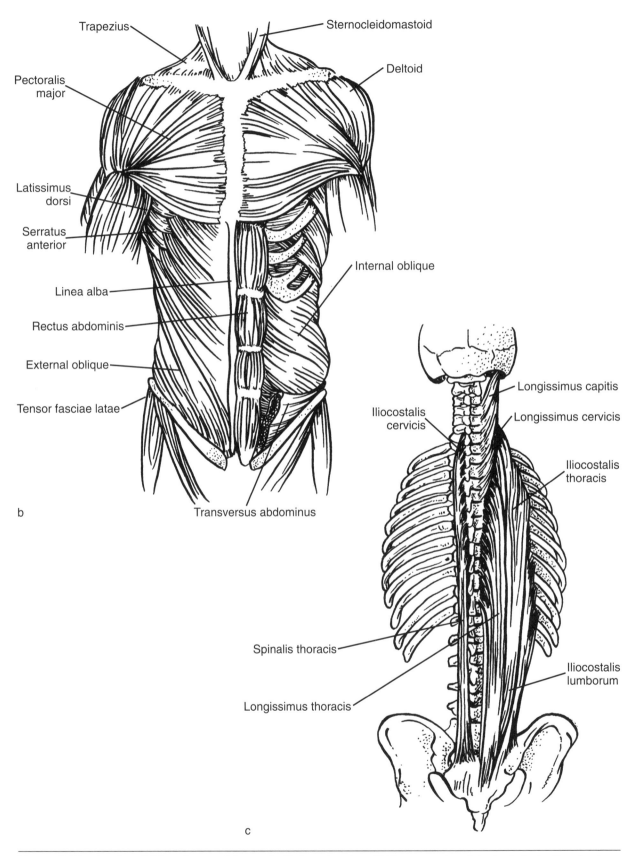

Figure 8.22 *(continued)* Musculature of the trunk. (*b*) Anterior view. (*c*) Deep muscles of the back, including the three subdivisions of the erector spinae group (iliocostalis, spinalis, longissimus).

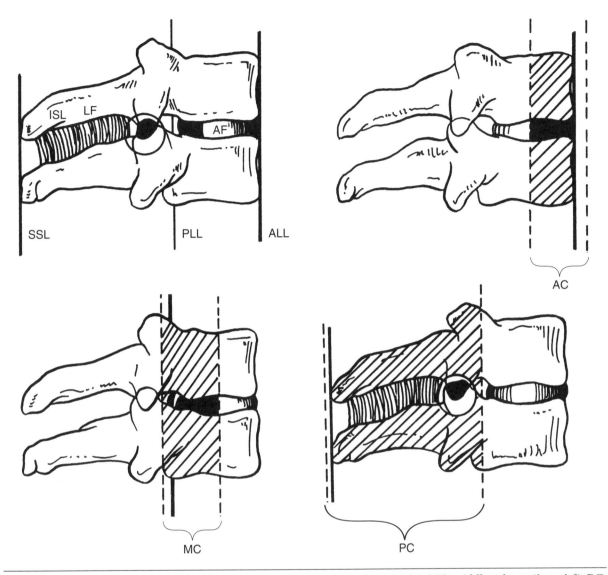

Figure 8.23   Three-column model of the spine: AC, anterior column (*upper right*); MC, middle column (*lower left*); PC, posterior column (*lower right*). Vertebral structures: SSL, supraspinous ligament; PLL, posterior longitudinal ligament; ALL, anterior longitudinal ligament; AF, annulus fibrosus; LF, ligamentum flavum; ISL, interspinous ligament.

From "The three column spine and its significance in the classification of acute thoracolumbar spinal injuries" by F. Denis, 1983, *Spine*, *8(8)*, (Fig. 1, p. 818). Copyright 1983 by J.B. Lippincott Company. Reprinted by permission.

Table 8.5   Failure Mechanisms Using a Three-Column Model of the Spine

| Type of fracture | Column | | |
	Anterior	Middle	Posterior
Compression	Compression	None	None or distraction (severe)
Burst	Compression	Compression	None
Seat-belt type	None or compression	Distraction	Distraction
Fracture dislocation	Compression rotation shear	Distraction rotation shear	Distraction rotation shear

From "The three column spine and its significance in the classification of acute thoracolumbar spinal injuries" by F. Denis, 1983, *Spine*, *8(8)* (Table 1, p. 818). Copyright 1993 by Lippincott-Raven. Adapted by permission.

lumbar vertebrae when they are aligned in a straight (noncurved) row, or column, the body of the vertebra can shatter from within (i.e., explode or burst).

The danger of spinal cord lesion due to fragment displacement depends on the rate of loading. In controlled conditions, with constant energy input and force direction, spine motion segments impacted at high loading rates fracture with significant encroachment into the spinal canal. Low loading rates, in contrast, produce minimal intrusion (Tran et al. 1995).

The level of instability created by burst fractures has been the subject of some controversy, especially in cases where there is an absence of neurological deficit associated with the fracture. A study by Panjabi and colleagues (1994) found multiaxial instabilities, especially in response to axial rotation and lateral bending. Their results suggest that treatment of burst fractures requires caution and that their fixation and stabilization should be approached conservatively.

The degree of disk degeneration confounds the mechanism of burst fracture. A finite-element computer model (figure 8.24; Shirado et al. 1992) showed that in motion segments with normal disks, the highest stresses were found under the nucleus and at the superoposterior portions of the trabecular body. In a severely degenerated disk, no stresses were seen under the nucleus and little stress at the middle of the end plate. Based on the computer model of thoracolumbar loading, the researchers concluded that with healthy disks, rapid axial compressive loading induces a burst fracture with bone fragments retropulsed into the spinal canal. In people with severely degenerated disks (e.g., elderly with osteoporosis), burst fractures would be much less likely and, should they occur, would involve the anterior column and thus not have associated neurological deficits (Shirado et al. 1992).

Spinal Deformities

Injury, disease, and congenital predisposition all can cause deformities of the spinal column that take the form of abnormal structural alignment or alteration of spinal curvatures. These deformities are not injuries, per se, but since they often result in abnormal force distribution patterns and pathological tissue adaptations, they may indirectly lead to or exacerbate other musculoskeletal injuries and thus deserve mention in our discussion.

There are three primary types of spinal deformity: scoliosis, kyphosis, and lordosis. These deformities are classified by their magnitude, location, direction, and cause and can occur in isolation or in combination. Spinal deformities have long been associated with cardiopulmonary dysfunction. Hippocrates, for example, noted that hunchbacks (those with kyphosis) had difficulty breathing, and that patients afflicted with scoliosis commonly exhibited dyspnea, or shortness of breath (Padman 1995).

Scoliosis is defined as a lateral (frontal plane) curvature of the spine, which is also usually associated with a twisting of the spine (figure 8.25a). Mild spinal deviations are well tolerated and usually are asymptomatic. Severe deformities, in contrast, can markedly compromise cardiopulmonary processes. Scoliotic curvatures exceeding 90° greatly increase the risk of cardiorespiratory failure through the cumulative effect of decreased lung and chest wall compliance, poor blood oxygenation (hypoxemia), increased work of breathing, reduced respiratory drive, enlarged heart (cardiomegaly), and pulmonary arterial hypertension (Padman 1995).

Treatment options for scoliosis are either nonoperative or operative. Nonoperative interventions include electrical stimulation, biofeedback, manipulation, and bracing. Of these, bracing has proved most successful (figure 8.25b). For severe scoliotic curvatures, the preferred treatment is operative vertebral fusion in which adjacent vertebrae are fused to forestall further progression of the deformity (figure 8.26).

The importance of early diagnosis and intervention should not be understated, since in many cases scoliotic deformity is progressive. Lack of early intervention can result in severe, even life-threatening, deformities later in life. While the causal mechanisms of scoliosis are often unknown, the mechanics of treatment in the form of braces or implanted spinal rods are well established and proven to be effective.

Kyphosis is a sagittal-plane spinal deformity characterized by excessive flexion and usually is seen in the thoracic region, where it produces a hunchback posture. Kyphosis is more severe in women than in men and is more prevalent with advancing age in both genders. Elderly, postmenopausal women are at particular risk, largely because of the strong association between kyphosis and osteoporosis (Bradford 1995). Kyphosis in these women is readily evident by the presence of a characteristic hump.

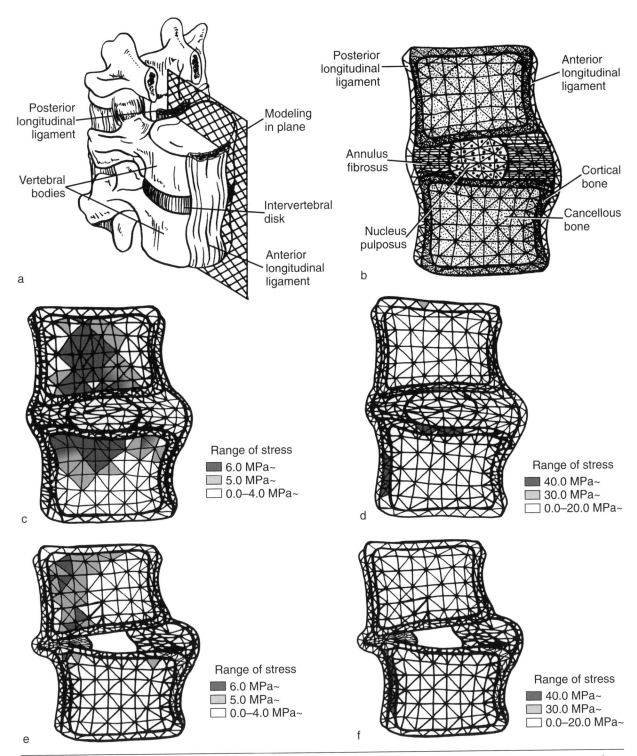

Figure 8.24 (*a*) Median (midsagittal) plane of modeling. (*b*) Finite-element plane model. (*c*) Stress distribution of one motion segment with a healthy disk under axial compression showing highest trabecular bone stresses under the nucleus pulposus and at the superoposterior regions, and (*d*) highest cortical shell stresses at the middle of the end plate and posterior wall cortex. (*e*) Stress distribution in a model of a severely degenerated disk shows no stresses in the trabecular bone under the nucleus, and (*f*) highest stresses in the cortical bone of posterior wall.

From "Influence of disc degeneration on mechanism of thoracolumbar burst fractures" by O. Shirado, K. Kaneda, S. Tadano, H. Ishikawa, P.C. McAfee, & K.E. Warden, 1992, *Spine, 17(3)* (Fig. 1, p. 287; Figs. 5 & 6, p. 291). Copyright 1992 by Lippincott-Raven. Adapted by permission.

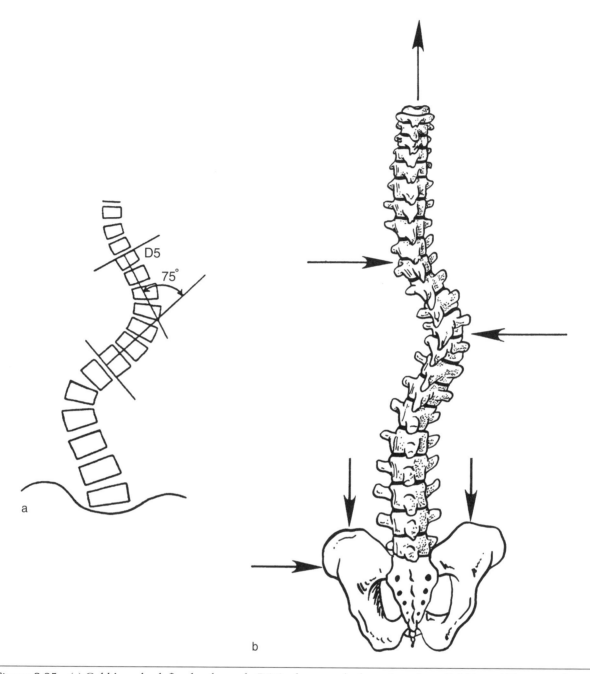

Figure 8.25   (*a*) Cobb's angle, defined as the angle (75° in the example shown here from Cobb's work) between the two lines that perpendicularly bisect the lines through the surfaces of the vertebrae at each end of the curvature. (*b*) Free-body diagram of the forces exerted on the spine by a brace to correct scoliosis deformity.

The degree of kyphosis is measured by the curvature of the spine in the sagittal plane (using a method similar to Cobb's angle, described in figure 8.25) or alternatively by the sum of the wedge angles between adjacent vertebrae (figure 8.27). The wedge angles of thoracic vertebrae T4-T12 increase exponentially as a function of age, up to 70 years (Puche

et al. 1995). This vertebral wedging and its attendant kyphosis affect rib mobility and pulmonary function. Specifically, the thoracic angle in kyphosis has a significant negative correlation with inspiratory capacity, vital capacity, and lateral expansion of the thorax (Culham, Jimenez, & King 1994). The best treatment for kyphosis may lie in prevention.

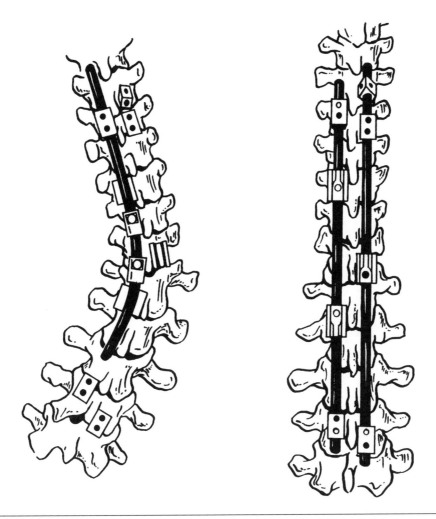

Figure 8.26   Variations of Harrington instrumentation used to correct spinal deformities.

Women with satisfactory exercise habits have a significantly lower index of kyphosis, suggesting that physical conditioning programs aimed at proper postural maintenance may delay or prevent the onset of kyphosis associated with aging (Cutler, Friedmann, & Genovese-Stone 1993).

Children may exhibit a special type of kyphosis, known as *Scheuermann's kyphosis*, in which structural changes are seen in the end plates of the growing vertebral bodies. Scheuermann's kyphosis is idiopathic, and mild cases are readily controlled by appropriate back extension exercises, with symptoms subsiding on completion of bone growth. More severe cases may require bracing or surgery as described earlier.

Lordosis is an abnormal extension deformity, usually seen in the lumbar region, that produces a hollow or swayback condition. Forward tilting of the pelvis accentuates the lumbar lordosis. This tilting increases the lumbosacral (L5-S1) angle above its normal 30° orientation (figure 8.28) and accentuates the shear loading on the intervertebral disks and surrounding structures.

Spondylolysis and Spondylolisthesis

Low-back pain arises from myriad causes, including structural abnormalities, chronic overuse, and trauma. Two specific conditions that especially afflict young and athletic populations are spondylolysis and spondylolisthesis. These conditions affect the bony structure of the vertebrae, especially at the L4-L5 and L5-S1 levels. Spondylolysis is defined as a defect in the area of the lamina between the superior and inferior articular facets known as the

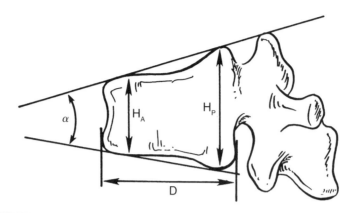

Figure 8.27   Vertebral wedging as measured by the angle α. The amount of wedging can also be measured by calculating the body height ratio (H_A/H_P).

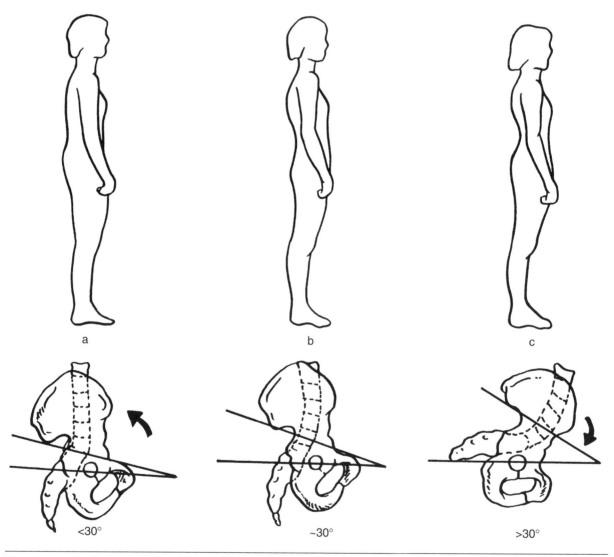

Figure 8.28   Effect of pelvic tilting on the lumbosacral (L5-S1) angle. (*b*) Normal standing creates a lumbosacral angle of approximately 30°. (*a*) Tilting the pelvis backward decreases the lumbosacral angle (< 30°) and flattens the lumbar spine. (*c*) Tilting the pelvis forward increases the lumbosacral angle (> 30°) and exaggerates the lumbar lordosis.

Reprinted from Lindh 1989.

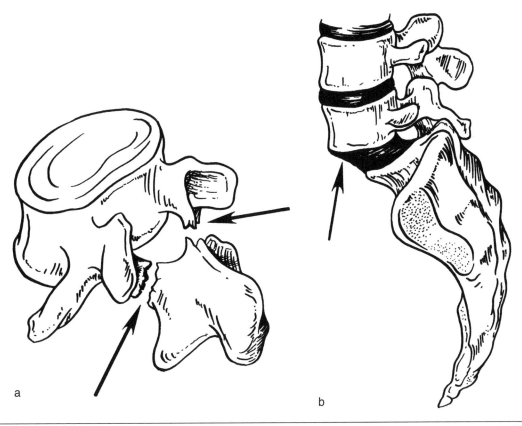

Figure 8.29   (*a*) Spondylolysis showing bilateral fracture of the pars interarticularis (arrows). (*b*) Spondylolisthesis exhibiting slippage (arrow) between the L5 and S1 vertebrae.

pars interarticularis (figure 8.29). Spondylolisthesis is translational motion, or slippage, between adjacent vertebral bodies. Most individuals with either condition remain asymptomatic.

Despite having been described in the literature for many years, spondylolysis and spondylolisthesis have remained a source of controversy. Recent advances in imaging techniques have permitted a better understanding of the pathogenesis of both conditions.

Classification of spondylolysis and spondylolisthesis according to their etiological and anatomical characteristics commonly identifies five types: dysplastic, isthmic, degenerative, traumatic, and pathological (Newman & Stone 1963; Wiltse, Newman, & MacNab 1976). The involved anatomic structures and pathogenesis for each type are presented in table 8.6. Of greatest concern to young athletes is the isthmic type, in which repeated loading of the pars region causes microfractures and eventual bone failure. Among the mechanisms responsible for these pars defect failures are repetitive spinal flexion, combined flexion and extension, forcible hyperextension, and lumbar spine rotation. Not sur-

prisingly, the populations most at risk are those whose training exposes them to repeated, high, compressive spinal loading, especially in combination with flexion-extension and rotational positions and movements. These include gymnasts, weight lifters, wrestlers, and divers. Spondylolysis is exacerbated by the stresses imposed on the vertebral laminae by the body's lumbar lordosis.

In spondylolisthesis, slippage occurs between adjacent vertebrae. The process involved in slippage differs between younger and older individuals (typically in women over 50 years old). In older populations, spondylolisthesis occurs most frequently at L4-L5, due in part to degenerative lesions associated with arthritis of the facet joints and to relative instability at this level compared to L5-S1. This instability may be due to a developmental predisposition to more sagitally oriented facet joints at the L4-L5 level (Grobler et al. 1993).

In young athletes the mechanism allowing spondylolisthesis differs from that observed in adults. In patients between 9 and 18 years old, Ikata and coworkers (1996) found end-plate lesions in all cases of vertebral slip between L5-S1 exceeding 5%. The

Table 8.6 Classification of Spondylolysis and Spondylolisthesis

Type	Name	Anatomic involvement	Etiology
I	Dysplastic	Neural arch dysplasia	Hereditary or congenital facet orientation anomalies, particularly L5-S1 facets and supporting structure
II	Isthmic	Pars interarticularis abnormality	Succession of microfractures; mechanical, hormonal, hereditary causes
III	Degenerative	Degenerative disk, facet, and ligamentous disease	Advanced pan-column degenerative changes
IV	Traumatic	Traumatic column instability with delayed translational changes	Trauma
V	Pathological	Pars and other components	Noncongenital or acquired (e.g., infection or neoplasm)

Adapted from Stillerman, Schneider, & Gruen 1993.

implicated mechanism was slippage between the osseous and cartilaginous end plates secondary to spondylolysis. The likelihood of progression (continuing slippage) depends on the type, stability, and degree of slippage, and slip angle (Bradford 1995; figure 8.30).

Lumbosacral Pathologies

Lumbosacral injuries can involve any of the many structures comprising the spinal column and in general involve three basic mechanisms: (1) spinal compression or weight bearing, (2) torsional loading, which results in various patterns of shearing in the transverse (horizontal) plane, and (3) tensile stresses resulting from excessive spinal motion (Watkins & Dillin 1994b). We present one class of lumbosacral injury (intervertebral disk pathologies) whose injury mechanisms are typical of other lumbosacral injuries.

Normal activities load the intervertebral disks in complex ways. The combined effects of spinal flexion-extension, lateral bending, and rotation exert considerable forces on the disks and their supporting structures. These forces are highest in the lumbar region, largely due to the compressive forces imposed by the weight of superior body segments.

Since disk morphology dictates mechanical response, it is important to understand some details of disk anatomy. The intervertebral disk is a viscoelastic structure consisting of two distinct structural elements, the *annulus fibrosus* and *nucleus pulposus*. The disk is separated from the vertebra by a thin layer of hyaline cartilage (*cartilaginous end plate*). The nucleus pulposus is a gelatinous mass consisting of fine fibers embedded in a mucoprotein gel, with water content ranging from 70% to 90%. Water and proteoglycan contents are highest in the young and decrease with age. The mechanical consequences of these losses include decreases in disk height, elasticity, energy storage ability, and load-carrying capacity. The lumbar nucleus pulposus occupies 30% to 50% of the total disk area in cross section and is located slightly posteriorly (rather than centrally) between adjacent vertebral bodies.

The annulus fibrosus is composed of fibrocartilage and consists of concentric bands of annular fibers that surround the nucleus pulposus and form the outer boundary of the disk. The collagen fibers of adjacent annular bands run in opposite directions (figure 8.31). This criss-crossed fiber orientation allows the annulus to accommodate multidirectional torsional and bending loads.

When subjected to compressive loading, the disk components respond differently. In an unloaded state, the nucleus pulposus exhibits an intrinsic pressure of $10 \, N \cdot cm^{-2}$ due to preloading provided by the longitudinal ligaments and the ligamenta flava. In a loaded state, the nucleus pulposus accepts 1.5 times the externally applied load, while the annulus experiences only 0.5 times the compressive load (figure 8.32). Due to the relative incompressibility of the nucleus pulposus, the load is transmitted (see Poisson's effect, chapter 3) as a tensile load to the fibers of the annulus fibrosus. These forces radiate circumferentially in what is described as a *hoop effect*.

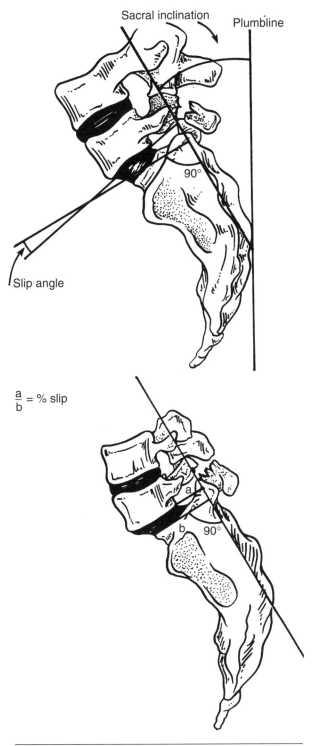

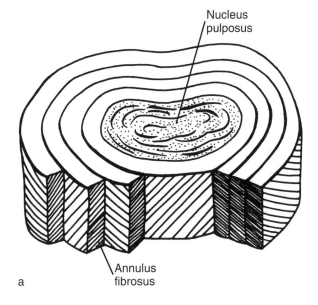

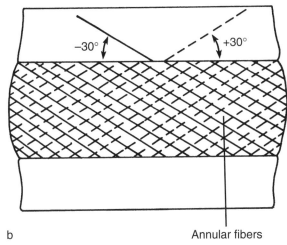

Figure 8.31 (*a*) Concentric rings of the annulus fibrosus surrounding the centrally located nucleus pulposus. (*b*) Alternating 30° angulation of annular fibers. This structural orientation enhances the ability of the annulus fibrosus to accommodate multidirectional loading.

Figure 8.30 Schematic of sacral inclination and slip angle (*top*) and percentage slip (*bottom*).
Adapted from Stinson 1993.

The resulting tensile stresses are four to five times greater than the externally applied compressive load (Nachemson 1975).

Many mechanisms have been suggested as being responsible for lumbar disk pathologies. In a classic work, Charnley (1955) presented a theoretical framework of potential pathoanatomic mechanisms responsible for intervertebral disk pathologies. These are summarized in table 8.7.

We will examine one of these factors (type IV, bulging disk) in detail here. In this mechanism the nucleus pulposus is displaced from its normal position within the annulus fibrosus. Rotational body movements produce shearing stress in the annular fibers and can lead to circumferential and radial tears. The resulting weakness in the annular layers reduces the ability of the annulus to contain the

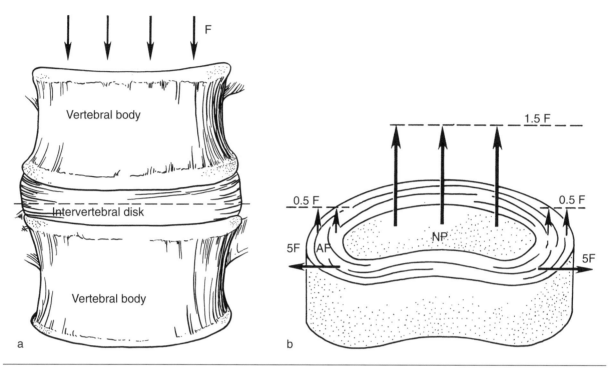

Figure 8.32 Uneven stress distribution across the lumbar intervertebral disk. A uniform compressive load (F) applied through the vertebral body (*a*) creates an axial stress of 1.5 F (per unit area) in the nucleus pulposus (NP) (*b*). The annulus fibrosus (AF), in contrast, generates an axial stress of only 0.5 F. The orthogonal stress in the annulus (perpendicular to the applied load) can reach levels up to five times the applied force (5F).

Reprinted from Nachemson 1975.

Table 8.7 Causal Factors in Intervertebral Disk Pathologies

Type	Name (description)
I	Acute back sprain (injury to annular fibers, other posterior ligaments, or musculotendinous structures)
II	Fluid ingestion (increased fluid uptake in the nucleus pulposus)
III	Posterolateral annulus disruption (annular disruption with consequent stimulation of sensory innervation by mechanical, chemical, or inflammatory irritants)
IV	Bulging disk (protrusion of the nucleus pulposus with impingement on neural structures)
V	Sequestered fragment (separated piece of tissue, or *sequestrum*, from the annulus fibrosus or nucleus pulposus that wanders within the joint space and causes irritation)
VI	Displaced sequestered fragment (displacement of sequestrum into the spinal canal or intervertebral foramen)
VII	Degenerating disk (progressive degeneration of the annulus fibrosus)

From *Clinical Biomechanics of the Spine* (2nd ed.) (p. 391-395) by A.A. White, III, & M.M. Panjabi, 1990, Philadelphia: J.B. Lippincott Company. Copyright 1990 by Lippincott-Raven. Adapted by permission.

nucleus pulposus. Compressive loads then squeeze the nucleus pulposus (disk prolapse) into the area of annular weakness. Sudden disk prolapse occurs acutely and typically is precipitated by a hyperflexion mechanism, often in conjunction with lateral bend-ing. This mechanism creates tensile stresses on the posterolateral aspect of the annulus fibrosus (figure 8.33), which, when combined with a compressive load, results in disk prolapse. Adams and Hutton (1982) suggested that sudden disk prolapse occurs

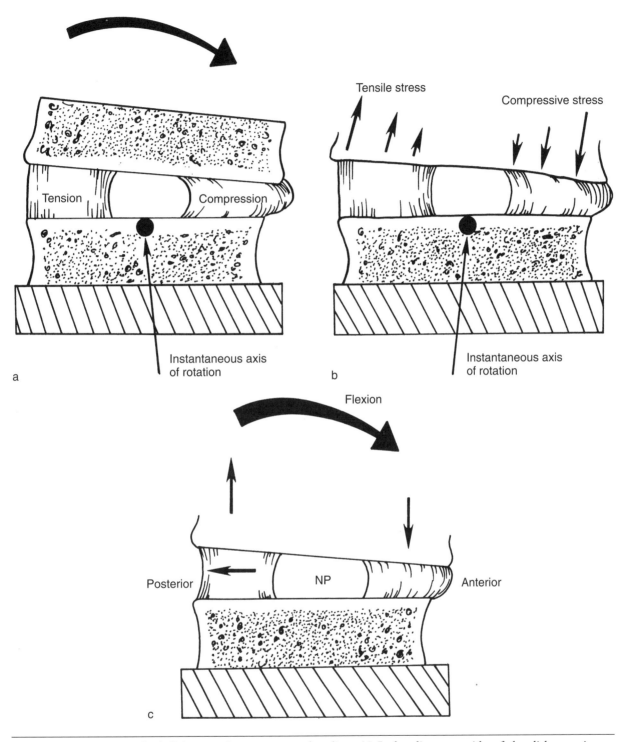

Figure 8.33 Intervertebral disk stress in response to bending. (*a*) In bending, one side of the disk experiences compression while the other side undergoes tension. (*b*) The compressive and tensile stresses are at a maximum at the outer borders of the disk and decrease toward the center of the disk. (*c*) Forward flexion of the spine tends to squeeze the nucleus pulposus (NP) posteriorly.

Parts (*a, b*) from *Clinical Biomechanics of the Spine* (2nd ed.) (Fig. 1-10, p. 15) by A.A. White & M.M. Panjabi, 1996, Philadelphia: J.B. Lippincott Company. Copyright 1990 by Lippincott-Raven. Adapted by permission.

most often in the lower lumbar region (L4-L5 or L5-S1) and is associated with disk degeneration.

The hyperflexion mechanism is not implicated in

most cases of gradual disk prolapse (i.e., where there is no identifiable precipitating event). These injuries have been associated with a weakened and

A Real Pain in the (Low) Back

By any measure, lower-back pain is the most costly musculoskeletal disorder in industrial societies. Up to 80% of the population will suffer from low-back pain in their lifetimes. For some people the pain is merely a temporary annoyance. For others, however, the pain associated with low-back pathologies can be completely debilitating.

The pain associated with low-back dysfunction arises from chemical or mechanical irritation of pain-sensitive nerve endings in structures of the lumbar spine. Chemical irritation is associated with the biochemical events of inflammatory diseases or subsequent to tissue damage. Mechanical irritation, in contrast, can result from stretching of connective tissues such as ligaments, periosteum, tendons, or the joint capsule. Compression of spinal nerves by a herniated intervertebral disk, damage to the disk itself, local muscle spasms, and zygapophyseal joint pathology can also result in low-back pain. Whatever its source, low-back pain either can be felt locally in the lumbar region or may be referred to the buttocks, lower extremities, or less commonly to the abdominal wall or groin.

The efficacy of various treatment strategies remains controversial, largely due to the fact that an estimated 85% of low-back pain cases remain unspecifically diagnosed. Conservative treatment (e.g., ice, rest, gentle activity), manipulative therapies, and therapeutic exercise interventions all have their proponents. Only rarely is surgical intervention indicated. The limited number of well-controlled, randomized studies addressing the issues of low-back pain treatment leave this area open to continuing debate and controversy.

degenerative annulus and other loading mechanisms (e.g., bending and twisting).

Whatever the causal mechanism, the bulging, or protruding, disk impinges on adjacent structures. Since many disk prolapse injuries occur in the posterolateral direction, the affected structure often is a nerve root. This results in mechanical, and possibly chemical and/or inflammatory, irritation of the nerve root with resultant pain in the back, buttocks, thigh, lower leg, and possibly even the foot. Lower-back pain, whether from disk pathology or other causes, will afflict about 80% of individuals at some time during their lives and is the most common occupationally related disability. Given the serious and pervasive nature of this musculoskeletal condition, knowledge of its causal mechanisms is essential in prescribing treatment programs and designing injury prevention strategies.

Concluding Comments

Of all the body's regions, the head, neck, and trunk have the greatest potential for catastrophic injury. As highlighted by the many examples in this chapter, the risks are real and considerable. Injuries to vital structures in these regions can readily compromise essential body functions and, in all too many cases, result in paralysis or death.

An understanding of injury mechanisms in all body regions can assist health professionals in effectively diagnosing and treating patients who suffer these unfortunate injuries and can facilitate the efforts of researchers and medical professionals to reduce the risk of injury and develop effective injury prevention programs. While our understanding of musculoskeletal injury has increased considerably in recent decades, much remains to be discovered. Among the challenges requiring further investigation are those related to the in vivo responses of biological tissues to mechanical loading, the relations between load volume (i.e., intensity, duration, frequency) and tissue response in real-world situations (e.g., ergonomic, sport), computer modeling of injury dynamics, and effective education programs across all strata of society. Our continuing efforts to understand the biomechanics of musculoskeletal injury are well worth the effort and resources expended. Injury prevention holds the key. After all, the best injury is the one that never happens.

Suggested Readings

Head, Neck, and Trunk

Becker, D.P., & Gudeman, S.K. (Eds.). (1989). *Textbook of Head Injury*. Philadelphia: Saunders.

Cooper, P.R. (Ed.). (1993). *Head Injury* (3rd ed.). Baltimore: Williams & Wilkins.

Hoerner, E.F. (Ed.). (1993). *Head and Neck Injuries in Sports*. Philadelphia: American Society for Testing and Materials.

Levine, R.S. (Ed.). (1994). *Head and Neck Injury*. Warrendale, PA: Society of Automotive Engineers.

Lonstein, J.E., Bradford, D.S., Winter, R.B., & Ogilvie, J.W. (Eds.). (1995). *Moe's Textbook of Scoliosis and Other Spinal Deformities* (3rd ed.). Philadelphia: Saunders.

Rizzo, M., & Tranel, D. (Eds.). (1996). *Head Injury and Postconcussive Syndrome*. New York: Churchill Livingstone.

Torg, J.S. (Ed.). (1991). *Athletic Injuries to the Head, Neck, and Face* (2nd ed.). St. Louis: Mosby-Year Book.

Vinken, P.J., Bruyn, G.W., & Klawans, H.L. (Eds.). (1990). *Head Injury*. New York: Elsevier.

General Sources

Browner, B.D., Jupiter, J.B., Levine, A.M., & Levine, P.G. (1992). *Skeletal Trauma*. Philadelphia: Saunders.

Feliciano, D.V., Moore, E.E., & Mattox, K.L. (Eds.). (1996). *Trauma* (3rd ed.). Stamford, CT: Appleton & Lange.

Fu, F.H., & Stone, D.A. (1994). *Sports Injuries: Mechanisms, Prevention, Treatment*. Baltimore: Williams & Wilkins.

Nicholas, J.A., & Hershman, E.B. (Eds.). (1995). *The Lower Extremity and Spine in Sports Medicine*. St. Louis: Mosby-Year Book.

Reference List

References for Chapter 1

Andersen, M.B., & Williams, J.M. (1988). A model of stress and athletic injury: Prediction and prevention. *Journal of Sport and Exercise Psychology, 10,* 294-306.

Committee on Trauma Research. (1985). *Injury in America: A Continuing Public Health Problem.* Washington, DC: National Academy Press.

Gielen, A.C. (1992). Health education and injury control: Integrating approaches. *Health Education Quarterly, 19(2),* 203-218.

Haddon, W., Jr., & Baker, S.P. (1981). Injury control. In: Clark, D., & MacMahon, B. (Eds.), *Preventive and Community Medicine.* New York: Little, Brown.

Heil, J. (1993). *Psychology of Sport Injury.* Champaign, IL: Human Kinetics.

Keele, K.D. (1983). *Leonardo da Vinci's Elements of the Science of Man.* New York: Academic Press.

LeVay, D. (1990). *The History of Orthopaedics.* Lancashire, England: Parthenon.

Max, W., Rice, D.P., & MacKenzie, E.J. (1990). The lifetime cost of injury. *Inquiry, 27,* 332-343.

Miller, A.P. (1979). Strains of the posterior calf musculature ("tennis leg"). *American Journal of Sports Medicine, 7(3),* 172-174.

National Center for Health Statistics. (1995). *Health United States 1994* (Department of Health and Human Services Publication No. PHS 95-1232). Washington, DC: U.S. Government Printing Office.

National Safety Council. (1994). *Accident Facts, 1994 edition.* Itasca, IL.

National Safety Council. (1996). *Accident Facts, 1996 edition.* Itasca, IL.

Rice, D.P., MacKenzie, E.J., and Associates (1989). *Cost of Injury in the United States: A Report to Congress.* Institute for Health and Aging, University of California, and Injury Prevention Center, Johns Hopkins University.

Runge, J.W. (1993). The cost of injury. *Emergency Medicine Clinics of North America, 11(1),* 241-253.

Sanders, M.S., & McCormick, E.J. (1993). *Human Factors in Engineering and Design* (7th ed.). New York: McGraw-Hill.

Sanders, M., & Shaw, B. (1988). *Research to Determine the Contribution of System Factors in the Occurrence of Underground Injury Accidents.* Pittsburgh: Bureau of Mines.

Steiner, D.L., Norman, G.R., & Blum, H.M. (1989). *PDQ Epidemiology.* Toronto: B.C. Decker.

Stussman, B.J. (1996). National Hospital Ambulatory Medical Care Survey: 1993 emergency department summary. *Advance Data, 271,* 1-15.

Suchman, E. (1961). On accident behavior. In: *Behavioural Approaches to Accident Research.* Washington, DC: Association for the Aid to Crippled Children.

Watson, G.S., Zador, P.L., & Wilks, A. (1980). The repeal of helmet use laws and increased motorcyclist mortality in the United States, 1975-1978. *American Journal of Public Health, 70(6),* 579-585.

References for Chapter 2

Åstrand, P.-O., & Rodahl, K. (1986). *Textbook of Work Physiology: Physiological Bases of Exercise* (3rd ed.). New York: McGraw-Hill.

Berchuck, M., Andriacchi, T.P., Bach, B.R., & Reider, B. (1990). Gait adaptations by patients who have a deficient anterior cruciate ligament. *Journal of Bone and Joint Surgery, 72A,* 871-877.

Bray, R., Frank, C.B., & Miniaci, A. (1991). Structure and function of diarthrodial joints. In: McGinty, J.B. (Ed.), *Operative Arthroscopy* (pp. 79-123). New York: Raven Press.

Caplan, A.I. (1988). Bone development. In: Wiley, J. (Ed.), *Cell and Molecular Biology of Vertebrate Hard Tissues* (CIBA Foundation Symposium 136) (p. 3). Chichester, UK. CIBA.

Carter, D.R., Fyhrie, D.P., & Whalen, R.T. (1987). Trabecular bone density and loading history: Regulation of connective tissue biology by mechanical energy. *Journal of Biomechanics, 20,* 785-794,

Cohen, B., Chorney, G.S., Phillips, D.P., Dick, H.M., Buckwalter, J.A., Ratcliffe, A., & Mow, V.C. (1992). The microstructural tensile properties and biochemical composition of the bovine distal femoral growth plate. *Journal of Orthopaedic Research, 10,* 263-275.

Eyre, D.R. (1980). Collagen: Molecular diversity in the body's protein scaffold. *Science, 207,* 1315-1322.

Fawcett, D.W. (1986). *Bloom and Fawcett: A Textbook of Histology* (11th ed.). Philadelphia: Saunders.

Garrett, W.E., Jr., & Best, T.M. (1994). Anatomy, physiology, and mechanics of skeletal muscle. In: Simon, S.R. (Ed.), *Orthopaedic Basic Science* (pp. 89-126). Park Ridge, IL: American Academy of Orthopaedic Surgeons.

Gross, P.M., Heistad, D.D., & Marcus, M.L. (1979). Neurohumeral regulation of blood flow to bones and marrow. *American Journal of Physiology, 237,* H440-H448.

Holtrop, M.E. (1992). Light and electron microscopic structure of bone-forming cells. *Bone, 1,* 1.

Johansson, H., Sjolander, P., & Sojka, P. (1991). Receptors in the knee joint ligaments and their role in the biomechanics of the joint. *CRC Critical Reviews in Biomedical Engineering, 18,* 341-368.

Martin, R.B., & Burr, D.B. (1989). *Structure, Function, and Adaptation of Compact Bone.* New York: Raven Press.

Miller, S.C., & Jee, W.S.S. (1992). Bone lining cells. *Bone, 4,* 1.

Mow, V.C., Ratcliffe, A., & Poole, A.R. (1992). Cartilage and diarthrodial joints as paradigms for hierarchical materials and structures. *Biomaterials, 13,* 67-97.

Muscher, E., Desaulles, P.A., & Schenk, R. (1965). Experimental studies on tensile strength of and morphology of the epiphyseal cartilage at puberty. *Annals of Pediatrics, 205,* 112.

Ogden, J.A. (1990a). Anatomy and physiology of skeletal development. In: Ogden, J.A. (Ed.), *Skeletal Injury in the Child* (2nd ed.) (p. 42). Philadelphia: Saunders.

Ogden, J.A. (1990b). Injury to the growth mechanisms. In: Ogden, J.A. (Ed.), *Skeletal Injury in the Child* (2nd ed.) (p. 97). Philadelphia: Saunders.

Ogden, J.A., & Grogan, D.P. (1987). Prenatal development and growth of the musculoskeletal system. In: Albright, J.A., & Brand, R.A. (Eds.), *The Scientific Basis of Orthopaedics* (2nd ed.) (pp. 47-89). Norwalk, CT: Appleton-Lange.

Ogden, J.A., Grogan, D.P., & Light, T.R. (1987). Postnatal development and growth of the musculoskeletal system. In: Albright, J.A., & Brand, R.A. (Eds.), *The Scientific Basis of Orthopaedics* (2nd ed.) (pp. 91-160). Norwalk, CT: Appleton-Lange.

Surve, I., Schwellnus, M.P., Noakes, T., & Lombard, C. (1994). A fivefold reduction in the incidence of recurrent ankle sprains in soccer players using the Sport-Stirrup orthosis. *American Journal of Sports Medicine, 22,* 601-606.

Tidball, J.G. (1983). The geometry of actin filament-membrane associations can modify adhesive strength of the myotendinous junction. *Cell Motility, 3,* 439-447.

Woo, S.L.-Y., An, K.-N., Arnoczky, S.P., Wayne, J.S., Fithian, D.C., & Myers, B.S. (1994). Anatomy, biology, and biomechanics of tendon, ligament, and meniscus. In: Simon, S.R. (Ed.), *Orthopaedic Basic Science* (pp. 45-87). Park Ridge, IL: American Academy of Orthopaedic Surgeons.

References for Chapter 3

Andreasson, G., Lindenberger, U., Renstrom, P., & Peterson, L. (1986). Torque developed at simulated sliding between sport shoes and an artificial turf. *American Journal of Sports Medicine 14(3),* 225-230.

Burstein, A.H., & Wright, T.M. (1994). *Fundamentals of Orthopaedic Biomechanics.* Baltimore: Williams & Wilkins.

Ekstrand, J., & Nigg, B.M. (1989). Surface-related injuries in soccer. *Sports Medicine, 8,* 56-62.

Hubbard, M. (1993). Computer simulation in sport and industry. *Journal of Biomechanics, 26* (Suppl. 1), 53-61.

Nash, W.A. (1994). *Strength of Materials* (3rd ed.). New York: McGraw-Hill.

Nigg, B.M., & Segesser, B. (1988). The influence of playing surfaces on the load on the locomotor system and on football and tennis injuries. *Sports Medicine, 5,* 375-385.

Nigg, B.M., & Yeadon, M.R. (1987). Biomechanical aspects of playing surfaces. *Journal of Sports Sciences, 5,* 117-145.

Robertson, L.S. (1992). *Injury Epidemiology.* New York: Oxford University Press.

Skovron, M.L., Levy, I.M., & Agel, J. (1990). Living with artificial grass: A knowledge update, Part 2: Epidemiology. *American Journal of Sports Medicine, 18(5),* 510-513.

Winter, D.A. (1990). *Biomechanics and Motor Control of Human Movement.* New York: Wiley.

References for Chapter 4

Amiel, D., Woo, S.L., Harwood, F.L., & Akeson, W.H. (1982). The effect of immobilization on collagen turnover in connective tissue. *Acta Orthopaedica Scandinavica, 53,* 325-332.

Åstrand, P.-O., & Rodahl, K. (1986). *Textbook of Work Physiology: Physiological Bases of Exercise* (3rd ed.). New York: McGraw-Hill.

Atteh, J.O., & Leeson, S. (1984). Effects of dietary saturated or unsaturated fatty acids and calcium level on performance and mineral metabolism of broiler chicks. *Poultry Science, 63,* 2252-2260.

Bailey, D.A., Faulkner, R.A., & McKay H.A. (1996). Growth, physical activity, and bone mineral acquisition. *Exercise and Sport Sciences Reviews, 24,* 233-266.

Bandy, W.D., & Dunleavy, K. (1996). Adaptability of skeletal muscle: Response to increased and decreased use. In: Zachazewski, J.E., Magee, D.J., & Quillen, W.S. (Eds.), *Athletic Injuries and Rehabilitation* (pp. 55-70). Philadelphia: Saunders.

Bilanin, J., Blanchard, M., & Russek-Cohen, E. (1989). Lower vertebral bone density in male long distance runners. *Medicine and Science in Sports and Exercise, 21,* 66-70.

Booth, F.W., & Gould, E.W. (1975). Effects of training and disuse on connective tissue. *Exercise and Sport Sciences Reviews, 3,* 83-112.

Brandt, K.D. (1992). The pathogenesis of osteoarthritis. *EULAR Bulletin, 3,* 75-81.

Bray, R., Frank, C.B., & Miniaci, A. (1991). Structure and function of diarthrodial joints. In: McGinty, J.B. (Ed.), *Operative Arthroscopy* (pp. 79-123). New York: Raven Press.

Buckwalter, J.A., Maynard, J.A., & Vailas, A.C. (1987). Skeletal fibrous tissues: Tendon, joint capsule, and ligament. In: Albright, J.A., & Brand, R.A. (Eds.), *The Scientific Basis of Orthopaedics* (2nd ed.) (pp. 387-405). Norwalk, CT: Appleton-Lange.

Burr, D.B., Milgrom, C., Fyhrie, D., Forwood, M., Nyska, M., Finestone, A., Saiag, E., & Simkin, A. (1995). Human in vivo strains during vigorous activity. *Transactions Orthopaedic Research Society, 20,* 204.

Butler, D.L., Grood, E.S., Noyes, F.R., & Zernicke, R.F. (1978). Biomechanics of ligaments and tendons. *Exercise and Sport Sciences Reviews, 6,* 125-181.

Christiansen, C. (1992). Prevention and treatment of osteoporosis: A review of current modalities. *Bone, 13,* S35-S43.

Cureton, K.J., Collins, M.A., Hill, D.W., McElhannon, F.M., Jr. (1990). Muscle hypertrophy in men and women. *Medicine and Science in Sports and Exercise, 20,* 338-344.

Currey, J.D. (1979). Mechanical properties of bone tissues with greatly differing functions. *Journal of Biomechanics, 12,* 313-319.

Currey, J.D. (1985). *The Mechanical Adaptations of Bones.* Princeton, NJ: Princeton University Press.

Currey, J.D. (1988a). The effect of porosity and mineral content on the Young's modulus of elasticity of compact bone. *Journal of Biomechanics, 21,* 131-139.

Currey, J.D. (1988b). Strain rate and mineral content in fracture models of bone. *Journal of Orthopaedic Research, 6,* 32-38.

Currey, J.D. (1990). Physical characteristics affecting the tensile failure properties of compact bone. *Journal of Biomechanics, 23,* 837-844.

Currey, J.D., & Alexander, R.M. (1985). The thickness of walls of tubular bones. *Journal of Zoology* (London), *206,* 453-468.

Curwin, S.L., Vailas, A.C., & Wood, J. (1988). Immature tendon adaptation to strenuous exercise. *Journal of Applied Physiology, 65,* 2297-2301.

Dalen, N., & Olsson, K.E. (1974). Bone mineral content and physical activity. *Acta Orthopaedica Scandinavica, 45,* 170-174.

Engelmark, V.E. (1961). Functionally induced changes in articular cartilage. In: Evans, F.G. (Ed.), *Biomechanical Studies of the Musculoskeletal System* (pp. 3-19). Springfield, IL: Charles C Thomas.

Ferretti, J.L., Tessaro, R.D., Delgado, C.J., Bozzini, C.E., Alippi, R.M., & Barcelo, A.C. (1988).

Biomechanical performance of diaphyseal shafts and bone tissue of femurs from protein-restricted rats. *Bone & Mineral, 4,* 329-339.

Forwood, M.R., & Burr, D. (1993). Physical activity and bone mass: Exercises in futility. *Bone & Mineral, 21,* 89-112.

Frank, C.B. (1996). Ligament injuries: Pathophysiology and healing. In: Zachazewski, J.E., Magee, D.J., & Quillen, W.S. (Eds.), *Athletic Injuries and Rehabilitation* (pp. 9-26). Philadelphia: Saunders.

Garn, S.M., & Kangas, J. (1981). Protein intake, bone mass, and bone loss. In: DeLuca, H.F., & Frost, H. (Eds.), *Osteoporosis: Recent Advances in Pathogenesis and Treatment* (pp. 257-263). Baltimore: University Park Press.

Garrett, W.E., Jr., & Best, T.M. (1994). Anatomy, physiology, and mechanics of skeletal muscle. In: Simon, S.R. (Ed.), *Orthopaedic Basic Science* (pp. 89-126). Park Ridge, IL: American Academy of Orthopaedic Surgeons.

Garrett, W.E., Jr., Nikolaou, P.K., Ribbeck, B.M., Glisson, R.R., & Seaber, A.V. (1988). The effect of muscle architecture on the biomechanical failure properties of skeletal muscle under passive extension. *American Journal of Sports Medicine, 16,* 7-12.

Garrett, W.E., Jr., Safran, M.R., Seaber, A.V., Glisson, R.R., & Ribbeck, B.M. (1987). Biomechanical comparison of stimulated and non stimulated skeletal muscle pulled to failure. *American Journal of Sports Medicine, 15,* 448-454.

Gregor, R.J., Komi, P.V., Browning, R.C., & Jarvinen, M. (1991). A comparison of the triceps surae and residual muscle moments at the ankle during cycling. *Journal of Biomechanics, 24 (5),* 287-297.

Heaney, P.R. (1988). Nutritional factors in bone health. In: Riggs, B., & Melton, L. (Eds.), *Osteoporosis: Etiology, Diagnosis, and Management.* New York: Raven Press.

Heaney, P.R., & Recker, R.R. (1982). Effects of nitrogen, phosphorus, and caffeine on calcium balance in women. *Journal of Laboratory and Clinical Medicine, 99,* 46-55.

Hetrick, G.A., & Wilmore, J.H. (1979). Androgen levels and muscle hypertrophy during an eight week weight training program for men/women. *Medicine and Science in Sports, 11,* 102.

Ikai, M., & Fukunaga, T. (1968). Calculation of muscle strength per unit cross-sectional area of human muscle by means of ultrasonic measurements. *Internationale Zeitschrift fur Angewandte Physiologie, 6,* 174-177.

Jones, H.H., Priest, J., Hayes, W.C., Tichenor, M.S., & Nagel, D.A. (1977). Humeral hypertrophy in response to exercise. *Journal of Bone and Joint Surgery, 59A,* 204-208.

Kahn, A.J., & Parfitt, A.M. (1992). Bone resorption in vivo. *Bone, 2,* 119.

Kaplan, F.S., Hayes, W.C., Keaveny, T.M., Boskey, A., Einhorn, T.A., & Iannotti, J.P. (1994). Form and function in bone. In: Simon, S.R. (Ed.), *Orthopaedic Basic Science* (pp. 185-218). Park Ridge, IL: American Academy of Orthopaedic Surgeons.

Kiiskinen, A. (1977). Physical training and connective tissue in young mice—physical properties of Achilles tendon and long bone growth. *Growth, 41,* 123-127.

Komi, P.V. (1992). *Strength and Power in Sport.* Oxford: Blackwell Scientific.

Krolner, B., Toft, B., Nielson, S.P., & Tondevold, E. (1983). Physical exercise as prophylaxis against involutional vertebral bone loss: A controlled trial. *Clinical Science, 64,* 541-546.

Lanyon, L.E. (1987). Functional strain in bone tissue as an objective and controlling stimulus for adaptive bone remodeling. *Journal of Biomechanics, 20,* 1083-1093.

Loitz, B.J., & Zernicke, R.F. (1992). Strenuous exercise-induced remodeling of mature bone: Relationships between in vivo strains and bone mechanics. *Journal of Experimental Biology, 170,* 1-18.

Loitz-Ramage, B.J., & Zernicke, R.F. (1996). Bone biology and mechanics. In: Zachazewski, J.E., Magee, D.J., & Quillen, W.S. (Eds.), *Athletic Injuries and Rehabilitation* (pp. 99-119). Philadelphia: Saunders.

MacDougall, J., Webber, C., Martin, J., Ormerod, S., Chesley, A., Younglai, E., Gordon, C., & Blimkie, C. (1992). Relationship among running mileage, bone density, and serum testosterone in male runners. *Journal of Applied Physiology, 73*, 1165-1170.

Mankin, H.J., Mow, V.C., Buckwalter, J.A., Iannotti, J.P., & Ratcliffe, A. (1994). Form and function of articular cartilage. In: Simon, S.R. (Ed.), *Orthopaedic Basic Science* (pp. 1-44). Park Ridge, IL: American Academy of Orthopaedic Surgeons.

Marcus, R., Cann, C., Madvig, P., Minkoff, J., Goddard, M., Bayer, M., Martin, M., Haskell, W., & Genant, H. (1985). Menstrual function and bone mass in elite women distance runners. Endocrine and metabolic features. *Annuals of Internal Medicine, 102*, 158-163.

Martin, R.B., & Burr, D.B. (1989). *Structure, Function, and Adaptation of Compact Bone*. New York: Raven Press.

Matsuda, J.J., Zernicke, R.F., Vailas, A.C., Pedrini, V.A., Pedrini-Mille, A., & Maynard, J.A. (1986). Morphological and mechanical adaptation of immature bone to strenuous exercise. *Journal of Applied Physiology: Respiratory, Environmental, and Exercise Physiology, 60*, 2028-2034.

McMaster, P.E. (1933). Tendon and muscle ruptures. *Journal of Bone and Joint Surgery, 15*, 705-722.

Michna, H. (1984). Morphometric analysis of loading-induced changes in collagen-fibril populations in young tendons. *Cell and Tissue Research, 236*, 465-470.

Mish, F.C. (Ed.). (1984). *Webster's Ninth New Collegiate Dictionary*. Springfield, MA: Merriam-Webster.

Mow, V.C., Ratcliffe, A., & Poole, A.R. (1992). Cartilage and diarthrodial joints as paradigms for hierarchical materials and structures. *Biomaterials, 13*, 67-97.

Noyes, F.R., Torvik, P.J., Hyde, W.B., & DeLucas, J.L. (1974). Biomechanics of ligament failure. *Journal of Bone and Joint Surgery, 56A*, 1406-1418.

Ormerod, S., MacDougall, J., & Webber, C. (1988). The effects of different forms of exercise on bone mineral content. *Canadian Journal of Sport Science, 13*, 74P.

Orwoll, E., Ware, M., Stribrska, L., Bikle, D., Sanchez, T., Andon, M., & H. Li. (1992). Effects of dietary protein deficiency on mineral metabolism and bone mineral density. *American Journal of Clinical Nutrition, 56*, 314-319.

Pirnay, F., Bodeux, M., Crielaard, J.B., & Franchimont, P. (1987). Bone mineral content and physical activity. *International Journal of Sports Medicine, 8*, 331-335.

Rambaut, P.C., & Goode, A.W. (1985). Skeletal changes during space flight. *Lancet, 2*, 1050-1052.

Robinson, T., Snow-Harter, C., Taafe, D., Gillis, D., Shaw, J., & Marcus, R. (1995). Gymnasts exhibit higher bone mass than runners despite prevalence of amenorrhea and oligomenorrhea. *Journal of Bone and Mineral Research, 19*, 26-35.

Rubin, C.T., & Lanyon, L.E. (1985). Regulation of bone mass by mechanical strain magnitude. *Calcified Tissue International, 37*, 411-417.

Säämänen, A.-M., Tammi, M., Kiviranta, I., Helminen, H., & Jurvelin, J. (1986). Moderate running increases but strenuous running prevents elevation of proteoglycan content in canine articular cartilage. *Scandinavian Journal of Rheumatology, 60* (Suppl.), 45.

Snow-Harter, C., & Marcus, R. (1991). Exercise, bone mineral density, and osteoporosis. *Exercise and Sport Sciences Reviews, 19*, 351-388.

Tammi, M., Paukkonen, K., Kiviranta, I., Jurvelin, J., Säämänen, A.-M., & Helminen, H.J. (1987). Joint loading–induced alterations in articular cartilage. In: Helminen, H.J., Kiviranta,

I., Tammi, M., Säämänen, A.-M., Paukkonen, K., & Jurvelin, J. (Eds.), *Joint Loading* (p. 82). Bristol: Wright.

Tidball, J.G. (1983). The geometry of actin filament-membrane associations can modify adhesive strength of the myotendinous junction. *Cell Motility, 3,* 439-447.

Tidball, J.G, & Chan, M. (1989). Adhesive strength of single muscle cells to basement membrane at myotendinous junction. *Journal of Applied Physiology, 67,* 1063-1069.

Tidball, J.G., Salem, G., & Zernicke, R.F. (1993). Site and mechanical conditions for failure of skeletal muscle in experimental strain injuries. *Journal of Applied Physiology, 74,* 1280-1286.

Tipton, C.M., Matthes, R.D., Maynard, J.A., & Carey, R.A. (1975). The influence of physical activity on tendons and ligaments. *Medicine and Science in Sports, 7,* 165-175.

Toss, G. (1992). Effect of calcium intake vs. other life-style factors on bone mass. *Journal of Internal Medicine, 231,* 181-186.

Tuukkanen, J., Wallmark, B., Jalovaara, P., Takala, T., Sjogren, S., & Vaananen, K. (1991). Changes induced in growing rat bone by immobilization and remobilization. *Bone, 12,* 113.

Vasan, N. (1983). Effects of physical stress on the synthesis and degradation of cartilage matrix. *Connective Tissue Research, 12,* 49-58.

Vogler, C., & Bove, K.E. (1985). Morphology of skeletal muscle in children. *Archives of Pathology and Laboratory Medicine, 109,* 238-242.

Walker, J.M. (1996). Cartilage of human joints and related structures. In: Zachazewski, J.E., Magee, D.J., & Quillen, W.S. (Eds.), *Athletic Injuries and Rehabilitation* (pp. 120-151). Philadelphia: Saunders.

Wells, C.L. (1991). *Women, Sport and Performance* (2nd ed.). Champaign, IL: Human Kinetics.

Williams, P.E., & Goldspink, G. (1981). Longitudinal growth of striated muscle. *Journal of Cell Science, 9,* 751-767.

Wilmore, J.H. (1979). The application of science to sport: Physiological profiles of male and female athletes. *Canadian Journal of Applied Sport Science, 4,* 103-115.

Woo, S.L.-Y., An, K.-N., Arnoczky, S.P., Wayne, J.S., Fithian, D.C., & Myers, B.S. (1994). Anatomy, biology, and biomechanics of tendon, ligament, and meniscus. In: Simon, S.R. (Ed.), *Orthopaedic Basic Science* (pp. 45-87). Park Ridge, IL: American Academy of Orthopaedic Surgeons.

Woo, S.L.-Y., Gomez, M.A., Woo, Y.K., & Akeson, W.H. (1982). Mechanical properties of tendons and ligaments: II. The relationships of immobilization and exercise on tissue remodeling. *Biorheology, 19,* 397-408.

Woo, S. L.-Y., Kuei, S., Amiel, D., Gomez, M., Hayes, W.C., White, F., & Akeson, W.H. (1981). The effect of prolonged physical training on the properties of long bone: A study of Wolff's Law. *Journal of Bone and Joint Surgery, 63A,* 780-787.

Woo, S.L.-Y., Matthews, J.V., Akeson, W.H., Amiel, D., & Convery, F.R. (1975). Connective tissue response to immobility. Correlative study of biochemical measurements of normal and immobilized rabbit knees. *Arthritis and Rheumatism, 18,* 257-264.

Woo, S.L.-Y., Ritter, M., Amiel, D., Sander, T.M., Gomez, M.A., Kuei, S.C., Garfin, S.R., & Akeson, W.H. (1980). The biomechanical and biochemical properties of swine tendon—long-term effects of exercise on the digital extensors. *Connective Tissue Research, 7,* 177-183.

Yamada, H. (1973). *Strength of Biological Materials.* Huntington, NY: Krieger.

Zamora, A.J., & Marini, J.F. (1988). Tendon and myo-tendinous junction in an overloaded skeletal muscle of the rat. *Anatomy and Embryology, 179,* 89-96.

Zernicke, R.F., Garhammer, J.J., & Jobe, F.W. (1977). Human patellar tendon rupture: A kinetic analysis. *Journal of Bone and Joint Surgery, 59A,* 179-183.

Zernicke, R.F., & Loitz, B.J. (1990). Myotendinous adaptation to conditioning. In: Leadbetter, W.B., Buckwalter, J.A., & Gordon, S.J. (Eds.), *Sports-Induced Inflammation: Clinical and Basic Concepts* (pp. 687-698). Park Ridge, IL: American Academy of Orthopaedic Surgeons.

Zernicke, R.F., McNitt-Gray, J., Otis, C., Loitz, B., Salem, G., & Finerman, G. (1994). Stress fracture risk assessment among elite collegiate women runners. *Journal of Biomechanics, 27,* 854.

Zioupos, P., & Currey, J.D. (1994). The extent of microcracking and the morphology of microcracks in damaged bone. *Journal of Materials Science, 29,* 978-986.

References for Chapter 5

Baker, S.P., O'Neill, B., Ginsburg, M.J., & Li, G. (1992). *The Injury Fact Book.* New York: Oxford University Press.

Committee on Trauma Research (1985). *Injury in America: A Continuing Public Health Problem.* Washington, DC: National Academy Press.

Coombs, R., Gristina, A., & Hungerford, D. (Eds.). (1990). *Joint Replacement: State of the Art.* St. Louis: Mosby-Year Book.

Crowninshield, R.D. (1990). Computer-assisted prosthetic design. In: Coombs, R., Gristina, A., & Hungerford, D. (Eds.), *Joint Replacement: State of the Art* (pp. 3-8). St. Louis: Mosby-Year Book.

Frank, C.B. (1996). Ligament injuries: Pathophysiology and healing. In: Zachazewski, J.E., Magee, D.J., & Quillen, W.S. (Eds.), *Athletic Injuries and Rehabilitation* (pp. 9-26). Philadelphia: Saunders.

Fulkerson, J.P., Edwards, C.C., & Chrisman, O.D. (1987). Articular cartilage. In: Albright, J.A., & Brand, R.A. (Eds.), *The Scientific Basis of Orthopaedics* (2nd ed.) (pp. 267-288). Norwalk, CT: Appleton-Lange.

Harris, W., & Mackie, R. (1972). A study of the relationships among fatigue, hours of service, and safety of operations of truck and bus drivers. (Rept. BMCS-RD-71-2). Washington, DC: Bureau of Motor Carrier Safety.

Haupt, H. (1991). Ergogenic aids. In: Reider, B. (Ed.), *Sports Medicine: The School-Age Athlete* (pp. 52-66). Philadelphia: Saunders.

Hipp, J.A., Cheal, E.J., & Hayes, W.C. (1992). Biomechanics of fractures. In: Browner, B.D., Jupiter, J.B., Levine, A.M., & Trafton, P.G. (Eds.), *Skeletal Trauma*, Vol. 1 (pp. 95-125). Philadelphia: Saunders.

Houston, C.S., & Swischuk, L.E. (1980). Varus and valgus—no wonder they are confused. *New England Journal of Medicine, 302*(8), 471-472.

Leadbetter, W.B. (1994). Soft tissue athletic injury. In: Fu, F.H., & Stone, D.A. (Eds.), *Sports Injuries: Mechanisms, Prevention, Treatment* (pp. 733-780). Baltimore: Williams & Wilkins.

National Institutes of Health. (1994). Total hip replacement. *NIH Consensus Statement, 12*(5), 1-31.

National Safety Council. (1996). *Accident Facts, 1996 edition.* Itasca, IL.

Ostrum, R.F., Chao, E.Y.S., Bassett, C.A.L., Brighton, C.T., Einhorn, T.A., Lucas, T.S., Aro, H.T., & Spector, M. (1994). Bone injury, regeneration, and repair. In: Simon, S.R. (Ed.), *Orthopaedic Basic Science* (pp. 277-323). Park Ridge, IL: American Academy of Orthopaedic Surgeons.

Praemer, A., Furner, S., & Rice, D.P. (1992). *Musculoskeletal Conditions in the United States.* Park Ridge, IL: American Academy of Orthopaedic Surgeons.

Salter, R.B. (1983). *Textbook of Disorders and Injuries of the Musculoskeletal System.* Baltimore: Williams & Wilkins.

Sanders, M., & Albright, J.A. (1987). Bone: Age-related changes and osteoporosis. In: Albright, J.A., & Brand, R.A. (Eds.), *The Scientific Basis of Orthopaedics* (2nd ed.). Norwalk, CT: Appleton-Lange.

Sanders, M.S., & McCormick, E.J. (1993). *Human Factors in Engineering and Design* (7th ed.). New York: McGraw-Hill.

Smith, L.L. (1991). Acute inflammation: The underlying mechanism in delayed onset muscle soreness? *Medicine and Science in Sports and Exercise, 23*(5), 542-551.

Sunderland, S. (1978). *Nerves and Nerve Injuries* (2nd ed.). Edinburgh: Churchill Livingstone.

Weissmann, G. (1988). Inflammation: Historical perspective. In: Gallin, J.I., Goldstein, I.M., & Snyderman, R. (Eds.), *Inflammation: Basic Principles and Clinical Correlates* (2nd ed.) (pp. 5-9). New York: Raven Press.

Woo, S.L.-Y., An, K.-N., Arnoczky, S.P., Wayne, J.S., Fithian, D.C., & Myers, B.S. (1994). Anatomy, biology, and biomechanics of tendon, ligament, and meniscus. In: Simon, S.R. (Ed.), *Orthopaedic Basic Science* (pp. 45-87). Park Ridge, IL: American Academy of Orthopaedic Surgeons.

References for Chapter 6

Ahmed, A.M., & Burke, D.L. (1983). In-vitro measurement of static pressure distribution in synovial joints: Part I. Tibial surface of the knee. *Journal of Biomechanical Engineering, 105*(3), 216-225.

Ahmed, A.M., Burke, D.L., & Yu, A. (1983). In-vitro measurement of static pressure distribution in synovial joints: Part II. Retropatellar surface. *Journal of Biomechanical Engineering, 105*(3), 226-236.

Andrews, J.R., Edwards, J.C., & Satterwhite, Y.E. (1994). Isolated posterior cruciate ligament injuries. *Clinics in Sports Medicine, 13*(3), 519-530.

Arendt, E., & Dick, R. (1995). Knee injury patterns among men and women in collegiate basketball and soccer. NCAA data and review of literature. *American Journal of Sports Medicine, 23*(6), 694-701.

Bouche, R.T., Sullivan, K., & Ichikawa, D.J. (1994). Athletic injuries. In: Oloff, L.M. (Ed.), *Musculoskeletal Disorders of the Lower Extremities* (pp. 234-259). Philadelphia: Saunders.

Brien, W.W., Kuschner, S.H., Brien, E.W., & Wiss, D.A. (1995). The management of gunshot wounds to the femur. *Orthopedic Clinics of North America, 26*(1), 133-138.

Burdett, R.G. (1982). Forces predicted at the ankle during running. *Medicine and Science in Sports and Exercise, 14*(4), 308-316.

Ciullo, J.V., & Shapiro, J.D. (1994). Track and field. In: Fu, F.H., & Stone, D.A. (Eds.), *Sports Injuries: Mechanisms, Prevention, Treatment* (pp. 649-677). Baltimore: Williams & Wilkins.

Crisco, J.J., Jokl, P., Heinen, G.T., Connell, M.D., & Panjabi, M.M. (1994). A muscle contusion injury model: Biomechanics, physiology, and histology. *American Journal of Sports Medicine, 22*(5), 702-710.

Croft, P., Cooper, C., Wickham, C., & Coggon, D. (1992). Osteoarthritis of the hip and occupational activity. *Scandinavian Journal of Work and Environmental Health, 18*, 59-63.

Cummings, S.R., Kelsey, J.L., Nevitt, M.C., & O'Dowd, K.J. (1985). Epidemiology of osteoporosis and osteoporotic fractures. *Epidemiologic Review, 7*, 178-208.

Dayton, P.D., & Bouche, R.T. (1994). Compartment syndromes. In: Oloff, L.M. (Ed.), *Musculoskeletal Disorders of the Lower Extremities* (pp. 726-736). Philadelphia: Saunders.

Felson, D.T., Anderson, J.J., Naimark, A., Walker, A.M., & Meenan, R.F. (1988). Obesity and knee osteoarthritis: The Framingham study. *Annals of Internal Medicine, 109*(1), 18-24.

Funsten, R.V., Kinser, P., Frankel, C.J. (1938). Dashboard dislocation of the hip: A report of 20 cases of traumatic dislocations. *Journal of Bone and Joint Surgery, 20A*, 124-132.

Garrett, W.E. (1995). Basic science of musculotendinous injuries. In: Nicholas, J.A., & Hershman, E.B. (Eds.), *The Lower Extremity and Spine in Sports Medicine* (pp. 39-51). St. Louis: Mosby-Year Book.

Garrett, W.E., Rich, F.R., Nikolaou, P.K., & Vogler, J.B. (1989). Computed tomography of hamstring muscle strains. *Medicine and Science in Sports and Exercise, 21(5)*, 506-514.

Garrett, W.E., Jr., Safran, M.R., Seaber, A.V., Glisson, R.R., & Ribbeck, B.M. (1987). Biomechanical comparison of stimulated and nonstimulated skeletal muscle pulled to failure. *American Journal of Sports Medicine, 15*, 448-454.

Gokcen, E.C., Burgess, A.R., Siegel, J.H., Mason-Gonzalez, S., Dischinger, P.C., & Ho, S.M. (1994). Pelvic fracture mechanism of injury in vehicular trauma patients. *Journal of Trauma, 36(6)*, 789-796.

Grood, E.S., Noyes, F.R., Butler, D.L., & Suntary, W.J. (1981). Ligamentous and capsular restraints preventing straight medial and lateral laxity in intact human cadaver knees. *Journal of Bone and Joint Surgery, 63A*, 1257-1269.

Gulli, B., & Templeman, D. (1994). Compartment syndrome of the lower extremity. *Orthopedic Clinics of North America, 25(4)*, 677-684.

Hait, G., Boswick, J.A., & Stone, J.J. (1970). Heterotopic bone formation secondary to trauma (myositis ossificans traumatica). *Journal of Trauma, 10*, 405-411.

Harris, W.H. (1986). Etiology of osteoarthritis of the hip. *Clinical Orthopaedics and Related Research, 213*, 20-33.

Hull, M.L., & Mote, C.D. (1980). Leg loading in snow skiing: Computer analyses. *Journal of Biomechanics, 13*, 481-491.

Hurschler, C., Vanderby, R., Jr., Martinez, D.A., Vailas, A.C., & Turnipseed, W.D. (1994). Mechanical and biochemical analyses of tibial compartment fascia in chronic compartment syndrome. *Annals of Biomedical Engineering, 22*, 272-279.

Inoue, M., McGurk-Burleson, E., Hollis J.M., & Woo, S.L.-Y. (1987). Treatment of the medial collateral ligament injury. *American Journal of Sports Medicine, 15(1)*, 15-21.

Ireland, M.L. (1994). Special concerns of the female athlete. In: Fu, F.H., & Stone, D.A. (Eds.), *Sports Injuries: Mechanisms, Prevention, Treatment* (pp. 153-187). Baltimore: William & Wilkins.

Jozsa, L., Balint, J.B., Kannus, P., Reffy, A., & Barzo, M. (1989). Distribution of blood groups in patients with tendon rupture. *Journal of Bone and Joint Surgery, 71B*, 272-274.

Kibler, W.B., & Chandler, T.J. (1994). Racquet sports. In: Fu, F.H., & Stone, D.A. (Eds.), *Sports Injuries: Mechanisms, Prevention, Treatment* (pp. 531-550). Baltimore: Williams & Wilkins.

Kibler, W.B., Goldberg, C., & Chandler, T.J. (1991). Functional biomechanical deficits in running athletes with plantar fasciitis. *American Journal of Sports Medicine, 19(1)*, 66-71.

Kujala, U.M., Jarvinen, M., Natri, A., Lehto, M., Nelimarkka, O., Hurme, M., Virta, L., & Finne, J. (1992). ABO blood groups and musculoskeletal injuries. *Injury, 23(2)*, 131-133.

Kvist, M. (1994). Achilles tendon injuries in athletes. *Sports Medicine, 18(3)*, 173-201.

Lawrence, R.C., Hochberg, M.C., Kelsey, J.L., McDuffie, F.C., Medsger, T.A., Jr., Felts, W.R., & Shulman, L.E. (1989). Estimates of the prevalence of selected arthritic and musculoskeletal diseases in the United States. *Journal of Rheumatology, 16(4)*, 427-441.

Levin, P.E., & Browner, B.D. (1991). Dislocations and fracture-dislocations of the hip. In: Steinberg, M.E. (Ed.), *The Hip and Its Disorders* (pp. 222-246). Philadelphia: Saunders.

Levy, A.S., Bromberg, J., & Jasper, D. (1994). Tibia fractures produced from the impact of a baseball bat. *Journal of Orthopaedic Trauma, 8(2)*, 154-158.

Mahan, K.T., & Carter, S.R. (1992). Multiple ruptures of the tendo Achillis. *Journal of Foot Surgery, 31(6)*, 548-559.

Moffatt, C.A., Mitter, E.L., & Martinez, R. (1990). Pelvic fractures crash vehicle indicators. *Accident Analysis and Prevention, 22(6)*, 561-569.

Noonan, T.J., & Garrett, W.E. (1992). Injuries at the myotendinous junction. *Clinics in Sports Medicine, 11(4)*, 783-806.

O'Donoghue, D.H. (1984). *Treatment of Injuries to Athletes* (4th ed.). Philadelphia: Saunders.

Piziali, R.L., Rastegar, J., Nagel, D.A., & Schurman, D.J. (1980). The contribution of the cruciate ligaments to the load-displacement characteristics of the human knee joint. *Journal of Biomechanical Engineering, 102(4)*, 277-283.

Praemer, A., Furner, S., & Rice, D.P. (1992). *Musculoskeletal Conditions in the United States*. Park Ridge, IL: American Academy of Orthopaedic Surgeons.

Robinovitch, S.N., McMahon, T.A., & Hayes, W.C. (1995). Force attenuation in trochanteric soft tissues during impact from a fall. *Journal of Orthopaedic Research, 13*, 956-962.

Rothwell, A.G. (1982). Quadriceps hematoma: A prospective clinical study. *Clinical Orthopaedics and Related Research, 171*, 97-103.

Scott, S.H., & Winter, D.A. (1990). Internal forces at chronic running injury sites. *Medicine and Science in Sports and Exercise, 22(3)*, 357-369.

Seedhom, B.B., & Wright, V. (1974). Functions of the menisci—a preliminary study. *Journal of Bone and Joint Surgery, 56B*, 381-382.

Seering, W.P., Piziali, R.L., Nagel, D.A., & Schurman, D.J. (1980). The function of the primary ligaments of the knee in varus-valgus and axial rotation. *Journal of Biomechanics, 13(9)*, 785-794.

Siegler, S., Block, J., & Schneck, C.D. (1988). The mechanical characteristics of the collateral ligaments of the human ankle joint. *Foot & Ankle, 8(5)*, 234-242.

Speer, K.P., Spritzer, C.E., Bassett, F.H., Feagin, J.A., & Garrett, W.E. (1992). Osseous injury associated with acute tears of the anterior cruciate ligament. *American Journal of Sports Medicine, 20(4)*, 382-389.

Speer, K.P., Warren, R.F., Wickiewicz, T.L., Horowitz, L., & Henderson, L. (1995). Observations on the injury mechanism of anterior cruciate ligament tears in skiers. *American Journal of Sports Medicine, 23(1)*, 77-81.

Spilker, R.L., Donzelli, P.S., & Mow, V.C. (1992). A transversely isotropic biphasic finite element model of the meniscus. *Journal of Biomechanics, 25(9)*, 1027-1045.

Stedman's Medical Dictionary (25th ed.). (1990). Baltimore: Williams & Wilkins.

Sterett, W.I., & Krissoff, W.B. (1994). Femur fractures in alpine skiing: Classification and mechanisms of injury in 85 cases. *Journal of Orthopaedic Trauma, 8(4)*, 310-314.

Swenson, T.M., & Harner, C.D. (1995). Knee ligament and meniscal injuries: Current concepts. *Orthopaedic Clinics of North America, 26(3)*, 529-546.

Upadhyay, S.S., Moulton, A., & Burwell, R.G. (1985). Biological factors predisposing to traumatic posterior dislocation of the hip. *Journal of Bone and Joint Surgery, 67B*, 232-236.

van den Kroonenberg, A.J., Hayes, W.C., & McMahon, T.A. (1995). Dynamic models for sideways falls from standing height. *Journal of Biomechanical Engineering, 117*, 309-318.

Vuori, J.-P., & Aro, H.T. (1993). Lisfranc joint injuries: Trauma mechanisms and associated injuries. *Journal of Trauma, 35(1)*, 40-45.

Walker, P., & Erkman, M. (1975). The role of the menisci in force transmission across the knee. *Clinical Orthopaedics, 109*, 184-192.

Winquist, R.A., & Hansen, S.T., Jr. (1980). Comminuted fractures of the femoral shaft treated by intramedullary nailing. *Orthopedic Clinics of North America, 11*, 633-648.

Winquist, R.A., Hansen, S.T., Jr., & Clawson, D.K. (1984). Closed intramedullary nailing of femoral fractures: A report of five hundred and twenty cases. *Journal of Bone and Joint Surgery, 66A,* 529-539.

Wiss, D.A., Brien, W.W., & Becker, V., Jr. (1991). Interlocking nailing for the treatment of femoral fractures due to gunshot wounds. *Journal of Bone and Joint Surgery, 73A,* 598-606.

Worrell, T.W. (1994). Factors associated with hamstring injuries: An approach to treatment and preventative measures. *Sports Medicine, 17(5),* 338-345.

Zernicke, R.F. (1981). Biomechanical evaluation of bilateral tibial spiral fractures during skiing—a case study. *Medicine and Science in Sports and Exercise, 13(4),* 243-245.

Zernicke, R.F., Garhammer, J., & Jobe, F.W. (1977). Human patellar-tendon rupture: A kinetic analysis. *Journal of Bone and Joint Surgery, 59A,* 179-183.

References for Chapter 7

Bado, J.L. (1967). The Monteggia lesion. *Clinical Orthopaedics and Related Research, 50,* 71-86.

Botte, M.J., & Gelberman, R.H. (1987). Fractures of the carpus, excluding the scaphoid. *Hand Clinics of North America, 3,* 149-161.

Branch, T., Partin, C., Chamberland, P., Emeterio, E., & Sabetelle, M. (1992). Spontaneous fractures of the humerus during pitching: A series of 12 cases. *American Journal of Sports Medicine, 20(4),* 468-470.

Burkhart, S.S. (1993). Arthroscopic debridement and decompression for selected rotator cuff tears. Clinical results, pathomechanics, and patient selection based on biomechanical parameters. *Orthopedic Clinics of North America, 24(1),* 111-123.

Burnham, R.S., May, L., Nelson, E., Steadward, R., & Reid, D.C. (1993). Shoulder pain in wheelchair athletes: The role of muscle imbalance. *American Journal of Sports Medicine, 21(2),* 238-242.

De Smet, L. (1994). Ulnar variance: Facts and fiction. Review article. *Acta Orthopaedica Belgica, 60,* 1-9.

DiFiori, J.P., Puffer, J.C., Mandelbaum, B.R., & Mar, S. (1996). Factors associated with wrist pain in the young gymnast. *American Journal of Sports Medicine, 24(1),* 9-14.

Fleisig, G.S., Andrews, J.R., Dillman, C.J., & Escamilla, R.F. (1995). Kinetics of baseball pitching with implications about injury mechanisms. *American Journal of Sports Medicine, 23(2),* 233-239.

Fu, F.H., Harner, C.D., & Klein, A.H. (1991). Shoulder impingement syndrome: A critical review. *Clinical Orthopaedics and Related Research, 269,* 162-173.

Galeazzi, R. (1934). Uber ein besonderes syndrom bei verltzunger im bereich der unterarmknochen. *Archiv Fur Orthopadische und Unfall-Chirurgie., 35,* 557-562.

Giangarra, C.E., Conroy, B., Jobe, F.W., Pink, M., & Perry, J. (1993). Electromyographic and cinematographic analysis of elbow function in tennis players using single- and double-handed backhand strokes. *American Journal of Sports Medicine, 21(3),* 394-399.

Harryman, D.T., II, Sidles, J.A., Clark, J.M., McQuade, K.J., Gibb, T.D., & Matsen, F.A., III. (1990). Translation of the humeral head on the glenoid with passive glenohumeral motion. *Journal of Bone and Joint Surgery, 72A(9),* 1334-1343.

Horvath, F., & Kery, L. (1984). Degenerative deformations of the acromioclavicular joint in elderly. *Archives of Gerontology and Geriatrics, 3(3),* 259-265.

Hotchkiss, R.N. (1996). Fractures and dislocations of the elbow. In: Rockwood, C.A., Green, D.P., Bucholz, R.W., & Heckman, J.D. (Eds.), *Rockwood and Green's Fractures in Adults* (pp. 929-1024). Philadelphia: Lippincott-Raven.

Jobe, F.W., & Pink, M. (1993). Classification and treatment of shoulder dysfunction in the overhead athlete. *Journal of Orthopaedic and Sports Physical Therapy, 18(2)*, 427-432.

Jupiter, J.B., & Fernandez, D.L. (1996). *Fractures of the Distal Radius.* New York: Springer-Verlag.

Jupiter, J.B., Leibovic, S.J., Ribbans, W., & Wilk, R.M. (1991). Posterior Monteggia lesion. *Journal of Orthopaedic Trauma, 5(4)*, 395-402.

Kannus, P., & Jozsa, L. (1991). Histopathologic changes preceding spontaneous rupture of a tendon. *Journal of Bone and Joint Surgery, 73A*, 1517-1525.

Kibler, W.B. (1995). Pathophysiology of overload injuries around the elbow. *Clinics in Sports Medicine, 14(2)*, 447-457.

Koh, T.J., Grabiner, M.D., & Weiker, G.G. (1992). Technique and ground reaction forces in the back handspring. *American Journal of Sports Medicine, 20*, 61-66.

Kristensen, S.S., Thomassen, E., & Christensen, F. (1986). Ulnar variance determination. *Journal of Hand Surgery, 11B(2)*, 255-257.

Lippitt, S., & Matsen, F. (1993). Mechanisms of glenohumeral joint stability. *Clinical Orthopaedics and Related Research, 291*, 20-28.

Markolf, K.L., Shapiro, M.S., Mandelbaum, B.R., & Teurlings, L. (1990). Wrist loading patterns during pommel horse exercises. *Journal of Biomechanics, 23(10)*, 1001-1011.

Meeuwisse, W.H. (1994). Assessing causation in sport injury: A multifactorial model. *Clinical Journal of Sports Medicine, 4*, 166-170.

Morris, M., Jobe, F.W., Perry, J., Pink, M., & Healy, B.S. (1989). Electromyographic analysis of elbow function in tennis players. *American Journal of Sports Medicine, 17*, 241-247.

Nakamura, R., Tanaka, Y., Imaeda, T., & Miura, T. (1991). The influence of age and sex on ulnar variance. *Journal of Hand Surgery, 16B(1)*, 84-88.

National Safety Council. (1996). *Accident Facts, 1996 edition.* Itasca, IL.

Praemer, A., Furner, S., & Rice, D.P. (1992). *Musculoskeletal Conditions in the United States.* Park Ridge, IL: American Academy of Orthopaedic Surgeons.

Priest, J.D., Braden, J., & Gerberich, S.G. (1980). The elbow and tennis. *The Physician and Sportsmedicine, 8*, 80-85.

Ptasznik, R., & Hennessy, O. (1995). Abnormalities of the biceps tendon of the shoulder: Sonographic findings. *American Journal of Roentgenology, 164*, 409-414.

Rockwood, C.A., Jr., Williams, G.R., & Young, D.C. (1996). Injuries to the acromioclavicular joint. In: Rockwood, C.A., Green, D.P., Bucholz, R.W., & Heckman, J.D. (Eds.), *Rockwood and Green's Fractures in Adults* (pp. 1341-1413). Philadelphia: Lippincott-Raven.

Safran, M.R. (1995). Elbow injuries in athletes: A review. *Clinical Orthopaedics and Related Research, 310*, 257-277.

Silverstein, B.A., Fine, L.J., & Armstrong, T.J. (1987). Occupational factors and carpal tunnel syndrome. *American Journal of Industrial Medicine, 11(3)*, 343-358.

Snijders, C.J., Volkers, A.C.W., Mechelse, K., & Vleeming, A. (1987). Provocation of epicondylalgia lateralis (tennis elbow) by power grip or pinching. *Medicine and Science in Sports and Exercise, 19(5)*, 518-523.

Speer, K.P. (1995). Anatomy and pathomechanics of shoulder instability. *Clinics in Sports Medicine, 14(4)*, 751-760.

Weber, E.R., & Chao, E.Y. (1978). An experimental approach to the mechanism of scaphoid waist fractures. *Journal of Hand Surgery, 3*, 142-148.

Werner, S.L., Fleisig, G.S., Dillman, C.J., & Andrews, J. (1993). Biomechanics of the elbow during baseball pitching. *Journal of Orthopaedic and Sports Physical Therapy, 17(6)*, 274-278.

Williams, G.R., Nguyen, V.D., & Rockwood, C.A., Jr. (1989). Classification and radiographic analysis of acromioclavicular dislocations. *Applied Radiology*, (Feb.), 29-34.

Wilson, F.D., Andrews, J.R., Blackburn, T.A., & McCluskey, G. (1983). Valgus extension overload in the pitching elbow. *American Journal of Sports Medicine*, *11(2)*, 83-88.

References for Chapter 8

Adams, M.A., & Hutton, W.C. (1982). Prolapsed intervertebral disc. A hyperflexion injury. *Spine*, *7(3)*, 184-191.

Adams, R.D., & Victor, M. (1993). *Principles of Neurology*. New York: McGraw-Hill.

Barnsley, L., Lord, S., & Bogduk, N. (1994). Whiplash injury. *Pain*, *58*, 283-307.

Bradford, D.S. (1995). Kyphosis in the elderly. In: Lonstein, J.E., Bradford, D.S., Winter, R.B., & Ogilvie, J.W. (Eds.), *Moe's Textbook of Scoliosis and Other Spinal Deformities* (pp. 639-641). Philadelphia: Saunders.

Charnley, J. (1955). Acute lumbago and sciatica. *British Medical Journal*, *4904(1)*, 344-346.

Courville, C.B. (1942). Coup-contrecoup mechanism of craniocerebral injuries: Some observations. *Archives of Surgery*, *45*, 19-43.

Culham, E.G., Jimenez, H.A., & King, C.E. (1994). Thoracic kyphosis, rib mobility, and lung volumes in normal women and women with osteoporosis. *Spine*, *19(11)*, 1250-1255.

Cutler, W.B., Friedmann, E., & Genovese-Stone, E. (1993). Prevalence of kyphosis in a healthy sample of pre- and postmenopausal women. *American Journal of Physical Medicine and Rehabilitation*, *72(4)*, 219-225.

Damasio, A.R. (1994). *Descartes' Error: Emotion, Reason, and the Human Brain*. New York: Grosset/Putnam.

Dawson, S.L., Hirsch, C.W., Lucas, F.V., & Sebek, B.A. (1980). The contrecoup phenomenon: Reappraisal of a classic problem. *Human Pathology*, *11*, 155-166.

Denis, F. (1983). The three column spine and its significance in the classification of acute thoracolumbar spinal injuries. *Spine*, *8(8)*, 817-831.

Denny-Brown, D., & Russell, W.R. (1941). Experimental cerebral concussion. *Brain*, *64*, 93-164.

Grobler, L.J., Robertson, P.A., Novotny, J.E., & Pope, M.H. (1993). Assessment of the role played by lumbar facet joint morphology. *Spine*, *18(1)*, 80-91.

Hampson, D. (1995). Facial injury: A review of biomechanical studies and test procedures for facial injury assessment. *Journal of Biomechanics*, *28(1)*, 1-7.

Hart, C., & Williams, E. (1994). Epidemiology of spinal cord injuries: A reflection of changes in South African society. *Paraplegia*, *32(11)*, 709-714.

Haug, R.H., Adams, J.M., Conforti, P.J., & Likavec, M.J. (1994). Cranial fractures associated with facial fractures: A review of mechanism, type, and severity of injury. *Journal of Oral and Maxillofacial Surgery*, *52*, 729-733.

Holbourn, A.H.S. (1943). Mechanics of head injuries. *Lancet*, *2*, 438-441.

Holdsworth, F.W. (1963). Fractures, dislocations, and fracture-dislocations of the spine. *Journal of Bone and Joint Surgery*, *45B*, 6-20.

Holdsworth, F.W. (1970). Fractures, dislocations, and fracture-dislocations of the spine. *Journal of Bone and Joint Surgery*, *52A*, 1534-1541.

Ikata, T., Miyake, R., Katoh, S., Morita, T., & Murase, M. (1996). Pathogenesis of sports-related spondylolisthesis in adolescents. *American Journal of Sports Medicine*, *24(1)*, 94-98.

Kim, P.E., & Zee, C.S. (1995). The radiologic evaluation of craniocerebral missile injuries. *Neurosurgery Clinics of North America*, *6(4)*, 669-687.

Lim, L.H., Lam, L.K., Moore, M.H., Trott, J.A., & David, D.J. (1993). Associated injuries in facial fractures: Review of 839 patients. *British Journal of Plastic Surgery, 46(8)*, 635-638.

Miller, J.D. (1993). Traumatic brain swelling and edema. In: Cooper, P.R. (Ed.), *Head Injury* (3rd ed.) (pp. 331-354). Baltimore: Williams & Wilkins.

Myers, B.S., McElhaney, J.H., & Nightingale, R. (1994). Cervical spine injury mechanisms. In: Levine, R.S. (Ed.), *Head and Neck Injury* (pp. 107-156). Warrendale, PA: Society of Automotive Engineers.

Nachemson, A. (1975). Towards a better understanding of low-back pain: A review of the mechanics of the lumbar disc. *Rheumatology and Rehabilitation, 14(3)*, 129-143.

Newman, P.H., & Stone, K.H. (1963). The etiology of spondylolisthesis with special investigation. *Journal of Bone and Joint Surgery, 45B*, 39-59.

Ommaya, A.K., & Gennarelli, T.A. (1974). Cerebral concussion and traumatic unconsciousness: Correlations and experimental and clinical observations on blunt head injuries. *Brain, 97*, 633-654.

Ommaya, A.K., Grubb, R.L., Jr., & Naumann, R.A. (1971). Coup and contre-coup injury: Observations on the mechanics of visible brain injuries in the rhesus monkey. *Journal of Neurosurgery, 35*, 503-516.

Padman, R. (1995). Scoliosis and spine deformities. *Delaware Medical Journal, 67(10)*, 528-533.

Panjabi, M.M., Oxland, T.R., Lin, R.-M., & McGowen, T.W. (1994). Thoracolumbar burst fracture: A biomechanical investigation of its multidirectional flexibility. *Spine, 19(5)*, 578-585.

Praemer, A., Furner, S., & Rice, D.P. (1992). *Musculoskeletal Conditions in the United States.* Park Ridge, IL: American Academy of Orthopaedic Surgeons.

Puche, R.C., Morosano, M., Masoni, A., Jimeno, N.P., Bertoluzzo, S.M., Podadera, J.C., Podadera, M.A., Bocanera, R., & Tozzini, R. (1995). The natural history of kyphosis in postmenopausal women. *Bone, 17(3)*, 239-246.

Roaf, R. (1960). A study of the mechanism of spinal injuries. *Journal of Bone and Joint Surgery, 42B*, 810-823.

Shirado, O., Kaneda, K., Tadano, S., Ishikawa, H., McAfee, P.C., & Warden, K.E. (1992). Influence of disc degeneration on mechanism of thoracolumbar burst fractures. *Spine, 17(3)*, 286-292.

Sturzenegger, M., DiStefano, G., Radanov, B.P., & Schnidrig, A. (1994). Presenting symptoms and signs after whiplash injury: The influence of accident mechanisms. *Neurology, 44*, 688-693.

Tran, N.T., Watson, N.A., Tencer, A.F., Ching, R.P., & Anderson, P.A. (1995). Mechanism of the burst fracture in the thoracolumbar spine: The effect of loading rate. *Spine, 20(18)*, 1984-1988.

Valsamis, M.P. (1994). Pathology of trauma. *Neurosurgery Clinics of North America, 5(1)*, 175-183.

Ward, W.T. (1994). Boxing. In: Fu, F.H., & Stone, D.A. (Eds.), *Sports Injuries: Mechanisms, Prevention, Treatment* (pp. 235-259). Baltimore: Williams & Wilkins.

Watkins, R.G., & Dillin, W.M. (1994a). Cervical spine and spinal cord injuries. In: Fu, F.H., & Stone, D.A. (Eds.), *Sports Injuries: Mechanisms, Prevention, Treatment* (pp. 853-876). Baltimore: Williams & Wilkins.

Watkins, R.G., & Dillin, W.M. (1994b). Lumbar spine injuries. In: Fu, F.H., & Stone, D.A. (Eds.), *Sports Injuries: Mechanisms, Prevention, Treatment* (pp. 877-893). Baltimore: Williams & Wilkins.

Wiltse, L.L., Newman, P.H., & MacNab, I. (1976). Classification of spondylolysis and spondylolisthesis. *Clinical Orthopaedics and Related Research, 117*, 23-29.

Index

About the Authors

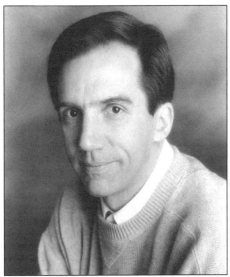

William C. Whiting

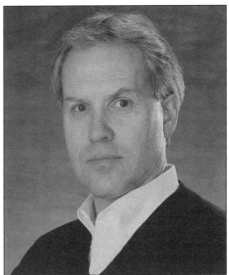

Ronald F. Zernicke

William C. Whiting is director of the Biomechanics Laboratory and assistant professor of kinesiology at California State University, Northridge. Dr. Whiting earned his PhD in kinesiology at UCLA. He has taught courses in biomechanics for more than 10 years, and has published 25 articles and 20 research abstracts.

Dr. Whiting currently serves on the editorial board of the *Journal of Strength and Conditioning Research*, and he has served as a reviewer for a number of other scholarly journals. Dr. Whiting is a Fellow of the American College of Sports Medicine and a member of the American Society of Biomechanics; the International Society of Biomechanics; the National Strength and Conditioning Association; and the American Alliance for Health, Physical Education, Recreation, and Dance.

Dr. Whiting has coached basketball and volleyball at the interscholastic and intercollegiate levels for 20 years and received a basketball Coach of the Year award in 1992 from the Southern California Community Newspapers. Dr. Whiting enjoys reading, camping, and hiking. He lives in Glendale, California.

Ronald F. Zernicke has taught courses in biomechanics and injury mechanisms at the university level for more than 25 years. He is the Wood Professor for Joint Injury Research at the University of Calgary, where he holds appointments in the departments of surgery (division of orthopaedics), mechanical engineering, civil engineering, and kinesiology. He also chairs the Joint Injury and Arthritis Research Group.

Dr. Zernicke has published more than 120 research papers, 145 research abstracts, and one other book. He has served on the editorial boards of the *Journal of Motor Behavior*, the *Exercise and Sport Sciences Reviews*, the *Journal of Biomechanics*, and the *Clinical Journal of Sport Medicine*. He is a Fellow of the American College of Sports Medicine, a charter member and former president of the International Society of Biomechanics, and a member and former president of the American Society of Biomechanics. Dr. Zernicke is also a member of the Canadian Society of Biomechanics, the Orthopaedic Research Society, and the Society for Neuroscience.

Dr. Zernicke lives in Calgary, Alberta, with his wife, Kathleen, and twins, Kristin and Eric. In his leisure time he enjoys reading, hiking, and cross-country skiing.